Language and Literacy Development

English Learners with Communication Disorders, from Theory to Application

SECOND EDITION

T0290904

Language and Literacy Development

English Learners with Communication Disorders, from Theory to Application

SECOND EDITION

Linda I. Rosa-Lugo, EdD, CCC-SLP
Florin M. Mihai, PhD
Joyce W. Nutta, PhD

PLURAL
PUBLISHING
INC.

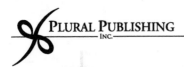

5521 Ruffin Road
San Diego, CA 92123

e-mail: information@pluralpublishing.com
Website: https://www.pluralpublishing.com

Typeset in 11/13 Garamond Book by Flanagan's Publishing Services, Inc.
Printed in the United States of America by Integrated Books International

Library of Congress Cataloging-in-Publication Data:
Names: Rosa-Lugo, Linda I., author. | Mihai, Florin, author. | Nutta, Joyce W., author.
Title: Language and literacy development : English learners with communication disorders, from theory to application / Linda I. Rosa-Lugo, Florin M. Mihai, Joyce W. Nutta.
Description: Second edition. | San Diego, CA : Plural Publishing, Inc., [2020] | Includes bibliographical references and index.
Identifiers: LCCN 2019047348 | ISBN 9781635501537 (paperback) | ISBN 9781635501551 (ebook)
Subjects: MESH: Communication Disorders | Language Development
Classification: LCC RC423 | NLM WL 340.2 | DDC 616.85/5—dc23
LC record available at https://lccn.loc.gov/2019047348

Contents

Contents

Foreword

When I wrote the Foreword for the first edition of this book, I began with the recognition that the cultivation of a literate citizenry was a significant challenge facing our nation. Unfortunately, in 2020 it remains so. Perhaps even more today the well-being of our democracy depends on it. The idea that the work of educational institutions on meeting this challenge is complicated by the needs of English learners (ELs), as well as students with communication disorders, remains relevant and, in fact, is more germane, as EL populations increase in schools. Although many states no longer use the Common Core State Standards, all states continue to emphasize preparation of children and adolescents to meet the high expectations of postsecondary education and the workforce. Therefore, when addressing the literacy needs of children and adolescents with communication disorders who are also learning English as another language, educators continue to face the enormous challenges of intense curricular demands. Hence, educators from a variety of disciplines and with different job responsibilities seeking to help these youth become literate need support and resources for this work. They will be pleased with the additional content of this second edition.

Although it is true that considerable attention has been paid in the literature to the education of ELs and to the problems of students with communication disorders, rarely has the work of both disciplines been integrated sufficiently to create a comprehensive context for addressing their literacy needs. The 2012 edition was the first book to do so. This second edition ups the ante by providing additional practical information. There is a lot to know in meeting the needs of students with communication disorders who are also learning English as another language. Integrating all relevant information to take appropriate action in assessing, intervening, and monitoring progress is not an easy task for practitioners. Exhorting them to approach assessment, intervention, and progress monitoring in particular ways has to be grounded in sound theoretical constructs and evidence-based practice, which this edition continues to provide. However, the additional material addressing application of sound principles will be even more attractive to those on the front lines. The AIM Framework and case studies presented in this edition provide specific guidance. Although a major audience for this book is the speech-language pathologist (SLP) working in schools, I am convinced that the content will be a great asset to a variety of professionals in schools, as well as to researchers formulating inquiries about effective practices.

In writing about the first edition, I argued that the complexity of facilitating literacy proficiency in ELs with communication disorders calls for approaches involving meaningful collaboration among all professionals working with these students, but that special partnerships among ESOL professionals and SLPs are essential to this work. Even greater attention is being paid to collaboration in educational literature and research, than was the case eight years ago. However, practitioners need concrete collaboration practices. The content of this edition provides even more guidance in this arena.

What I continue to value about this book is that the medium is the message; that is, Drs. Rosa-Lugo, Mihai, and Nutta have continued meaningful collaboration themselves to bring together these professional worlds in order to guide professionals in meeting the complex needs of English learners with communication disorders. In fact, I would argue that they have stepped up their game and once again provide a model of the kind of substantive interdisciplinary work that is sorely needed to solve the complex problems educators face in helping youth prepare for a productive future.

—Barbara J. Ehren, Ed.D., CCC-SLP,
    ASHA Fellow and Honoree,
    Board Certified Specialist in Child Language
Former Professor and Director of the Doctoral Program
School of Communication Sciences and Disorders
University of Central Florida

Foreword

I am delighted to write a Foreword for the second edition of *Language and Literacy Development: English Learners with Communication Disorders, from Theory to Application*, a timely and important book that fully and clearly explains how to effectively address the language acquisition and literacy development needs of English learners with communication disorders.

We all know that increasing numbers of students in U.S. classrooms are English learners, a trend that presents unique challenges as well as opportunities for English for speakers of other languages (ESOL) teachers, literacy specialists, and speech-language pathologists. How should schools effectively respond to the cultural, linguistic, and literacy needs of English learners, particularly those with communication disorders? The answer to this question is a central aim of this book.

Three unique features set the second edition of this book apart from other books that address English learner education. First, a glance through the pages of this book will show that it is an unusual type of publication. The vision for effectively addressing the needs of English learners with communication disorders is conceived and led by a formidable cross-disciplinary team of professionals representing the fields of speech-language pathology, ESOL education, and literacy development. The basic premise behind this cross-disciplinary approach is that the education of English learners crosses multiple areas of expertise and that teamwork and collaboration are paramount to addressing the needs of these students.

Second, the second edition of *Language and Literacy Development: English Learners with Communication Disorders, from Theory to Application* outlines a carefully studied approach to reaching and teaching English learners with communication disorders. The authors have compiled essential cross-disciplinary insights from research, policy, and best practices that teams of educators within schools need to know to effectively reach and teach English learners with communication disorders. They carefully outline how teachers can address more precisely the specific needs and varied backgrounds of English learners. This includes knowing English learners in terms of levels of English proficiency, age at initial exposure to learning English, literacy levels in first language, nature of students' first language and its unique features, prior education in or outside the United States, and cultural and experiential background. Knowing students in terms of these characteristics enables teachers to be more intentional about designing, implementing, and evaluating instructional interventions that work for these students.

Finally, when all is said and done, the most important feature of this book is its practicality. It is grounded in credible research about speech-language pathology, language acquisition, literacy development, identification, assessment, and intervention, but it is ultimately an action-oriented guide to help teachers and speech-language pathologists work collaboratively to effectively support English learners with communication disorders. The authors have given us the opportunity to apply essential knowledge as well as strategies known to stimulate growth in the interconnected processes of developing oral proficiency in a second language, learning to read and write in that language, and using that language to learn.

During the past several years, I have had the enormous privilege of working with the authors on three projects involving the education of English learners, and I witnessed firsthand several of the approaches and action-oriented practices discussed in this book. This is a must-read for anyone who wants to improve teaching and learning for English learners with or without communication disorders.

—Kouider Mokhtari, PhD
   Anderson-Vukelja-Wright Endowed Chair
      of Literacy Education
   The University of Texas at Tyler

Organization of the Text

After publishing our first book, *Language and Literacy Development: An Interdisciplinary Focus on English Learners with Communication Disorders*, which gives a comprehensive overview of the theory and practice of serving English learners (ELs) with communication disorders, readers asked us for a second book that would provide the nuts and bolts of *how* to meet ELs' needs. We were excited to update this book, *Language and Literacy Development: English Learners with Communication Disorders, from Theory to Application*, because although we are university-based faculty, we spend a great deal of time in schools, working side-by-side with school-based professionals to serve real students with real needs, and we wanted to share all the best practices we've seen that have had a positive impact on ELs' education.

In this book, we discuss language and literacy development for ELs with communication disorders and bring you the most useful, current information on best practices—how to conduct assessment, intervention, and progress monitoring for ELs with communication disorders. Continuing the perspective of our previous book, we emphasize the importance of interprofessional collaboration. Particularly, we focus on speech-language pathologist (SLP) and English for speakers of other languages (ESOL) professionals.

After reading this book, you will be informed about the most important theory, policies, and practices for meeting the educational needs of ELs with communication disorders. More importantly, you will be able to apply the knowledge you gained through understanding and analyzing the actual mechanics and practicalities of assessment, intervention, and progress monitoring for ELs with communication disorders from a variety of backgrounds.

Chapter 1 provides the backdrop for the merging of two particular disciplines, speech-language pathology and English as a second language to address the needs of English learners in general and English learners with communication disorders.

Chapter 2, The Context of Working with English Learners with Communication Disorders, provides an overview of ELs in pre-K–12 schools and current demographics of EL students and their families. This chapter defines and analyzes key terms associated with ELs and English learners with communication disorders (ELCDs) and discusses their varying characteristics. The educational contexts generally associated with ELs and ELCD students and the legislative initiatives that have influenced their education in the United States are also presented in relationship to the increasing impact of common standards, school accountability measures, and college and career readiness initiatives. We close Chapter 2 by considering some of the challenges faced by SLPs and ESOL professionals in working with ELs and ELCDs.

Chapter 3, English Learners—Perspectives from Two Disciplines, considers the role and responsibilities of SLPs and ESOL professionals in working with ELs and ELCDs. In particular, we provide an overview of the specialized competencies necessary for SLPs and ESOL professionals to work with ELs and ELCD students and examine the commonalities and differences between the two fields in theoretical as well as practical domains. Recommended competencies and preferred practices found in the ASHA Practice Portal and TESOL website are used to guide our discussions on the standards set for each of the professions. Specifically, we acknowledge the challenges they face in determining whether EL student language behavior reflects normal second language development patterns or if there is evidence of a language disorder.

Chapter 4, First and Second Language Acquisition: Theoretical and Practical Considerations, provides the readers with basic information on first and second language acquisition. Armed with an understanding and knowledge of the developmental trajectory of language in EL children and adolescents offers the reader the opportunity to engage in purposeful collaboration to distinguish between typically developing EL students and those with a communication disorder.

Chapter 5, Literacy Development in a Second Language, offers a definition of literacy and provides the reader with a general overview of literacy development in English learners. Although L1 and L2 reading share basic elements, they also differ in several important ways. To better understand L2 reading similarities and differences in L2, emphasis is placed on L2 reading, writing, and schema and how these operations contribute to literacy development of ELs and ELs with communication disorders.

Chapter 6, Assessing Language Proficiency Levels for Identification and Disability Determination, provides the framework that guides this chapter, the AIM (assessment, intervention, and monitoring) framework. We consider assessment from the perspective of identification practices for ELs in general, to the educational identification of a speech-language impairment and the procedures used to determine the need for special education services, related services and placement for ELs with communication disorders. Specifically, a goal of this chapter is to provide information about procedures and instruments used in the assessment and identification of ELs' different language proficiency levels. In particular, we discuss the importance of assessing language proficiency and how the assessment of language proficiency impacts the identification, placement, and exit of ELs from special programs.

Chapter 7, Intervention and Monitoring—Approaches and Practical Strategies to Facilitate and Monitor Language and Literacy Development in English Learners, focuses on the other two components of our AIM (assessment/intervention/monitoring) framework, intervention and monitoring. It offers practices, strategies, and techniques used to facilitate language and literacy instruction for ELs and consider their application with ELCDs.

The final chapter, Chapter 8, Directions for an Effective Collaborative Practice Between SLPs and ESOL Professionals—The Power of Two+, reiterates an important premise throughout this book, that all professionals—speech-language pathologists, general education teachers, special education and literacy specialists, administrators, and English as a second language (ESL) and bilingual educators—share responsibility for the assessment, intervention, and monitoring (AIM) of ELs and ELCDs. We stress the importance of a collaborative "shared decision-making" framework for working with ELs and ELs with communication disorders. We anticipate that after reading this book, your perspective will be expanded regarding ELs and ELCDs and how SLP and ESOL professionals can support their success at school with the collaboration of other professionals.

This revised edition includes ancillary resources on a PluralPlus companion website at https://www.pluralpublishing .com/publication/lld2e. Specifically, we provide three examples of students with different English proficiency levels based on EL students we have worked with in the public school setting. Subsequently, we include useful references and tools that can be used by the reader to guide their work in promoting language.

List of Important Terms

AAE—African American English

ACE—Award for Continuing Education

AIM—Assessment, Intervention, Monitoring

AMAO—Annual Measurable Achievement Objective

ASHA—American Speech-Language-Hearing Association

ASL—American Sign Language

BEA—Bilingual Education Act

BICS—Basic Interpersonal Communication Skills

BID—briefing, interaction, and debriefing

CAA—Council on Academic Accreditation in Audiology and Speech Language Pathology

CAEP—Council for the Accreditation of Educator Preparation

CAL—Center for Applied Linguistics

CALP—Cognitive Academic Language Proficiency

CCC—Certificate of Clinical Competence

CCSS—Common Core State Standards

CEB—Continuing Education Board

CF—Clinical Fellowship

CFCC—Council for Clinical Certification

CIERA—Center for the Improvement of Early Reading Achievement

CLD—Culturally and Linguistically Diverse

CSD—Communication Sciences and Disorders

CST—Child Study Team

CUP—Common Underlying Proficiency

DA—Dynamic Assessment

DHH—Deaf and Hard of Hearing

EAL—English as an Additional Language

EBP—Evidence-Based Practice

EL—English Learner

ELs—English learners

ELCD—English learners with communication disorders

ELD—English Language Development

ELL—English Language Learner

ELP—English Language Proficiency

ENL—English as a New Language

ESEA—Elementary and Secondary Act

ESL—English as a Second Language

ESOL—English for Speakers of Other Languages

ESSA—Every Student Succeeds Act

FAPE—Free and Appropriate Public Education

FES—Fluent English Speaker

FLEP—Formerly Limited English Proficient

HLS—Home Language Survey

IDEA—Individuals with Disabilities Education Act

IEP—Individual Education Plan

IFSP—Individual Family Service Plan

IPP—Interprofessional Collaborative Practice

L1—First language

L2—Second Language

LAD—Language Acquisition Device

LEA—Language Experience Approach

LEP—Limited English Proficient

LES—Limited English Speaker (or Limited English speaking)

LI—Language Impairment

LEA—Language Experience Approach

LRE—Least Restrictive Environment

MAE—Mainstream American English

MLR—Mean Length of Response

MLU—Mean Length of Utterance

MTSS—multitiered system of support

NCLB—No Child Left Behind Act

NELP—National Early Reading Panel

NES—Native English Speaker

NES—Non-English Speaker

NRP—National Reading Panel

OELA—Office of English Language Acquisition

OMA—Office of Multicultural Affairs

RtI—Response to Intervention

SIFE—Students with Inconsistent/Interrupted Formal Education

SLA—Second Language Acquisition

SLI—Specific Language Impairment

SLP—Speech-Language Pathologist

SUP—Separate Underlying Proficiency

TESOL—Teachers of English to Speakers of Other Languages

TTR—Type-Token Ratio

T-Units—Terminal Units

WIDA—World-Class Instructional Design and Assessment

ZPD—Zone of Proximal Development

Acknowledgments

Much has happened in our respective disciplines since the publication of the first edition of our book, *Language and Literacy Development: An Interdisciplinary Focus on English Learners with Communication Disorders*. English learners (ELs) continue to represent a growing part of the U.S. student body, the most prevalent disability categories continue to be specific learning disability (SLD) and speech or language impairment, and more students with special needs are integrated into general-education classrooms requiring professionals who have both the knowledge and the skills to work collaboratively to improve language and literacy educational outcomes. Thus, this second edition has as its primary mission to provide an update for professionals charged with this responsibility and who are committed to making a difference in their work with bilingual children and their families.

Many people have contributed to this book. We are grateful to all who have guided our work and supported its completion. We are sincerely appreciative to Plural Publishing for their guidance and patience as we worked tirelessly to "get it right."

We greatly appreciate the collegiality and generosity of Drs. Barbara Ehren and Kouider Mokhtari, who composed complementary Forewords that set a high bar for the scholarship presented. Their expertise in first and second language literacy development is sterling, and we are humbled to have our work summarized and foreshadowed by their eloquent essays.

From the first steps in updating, expanding, and redesigning the first edition to the finishing touches on the galley proofs of the second, we are thankful to all the University of Central Florida (UCF), School of Communication Sciences and Disorders Graduate Assistants (Joanne Medina, Laura Flores, Paula Uribe, Juliana Hirn, Donna Reynolds, and Erika Daly) for their efficient, meticulous work in proofreading and suggestions. We thank the students in the UCF Master's Program in Communication Sciences and Disorders who asked questions and provided feedback about what they wanted included in the second edition.

Many thanks are owed to our colleagues who talked through ideas and read early drafts with us, giving valuable insights generously and encouragingly. Again, a special thank you to Omar D. Martinez for the book cover design and the parents of the children on the cover for allowing them to be photographed as they worked in classrooms.

The first author is indebted to the University of Central Florida for support of a one-year sabbatical leave to work on this second edition and to the Central Florida school districts who allowed me into classrooms to observe and work with their speech-language pathologists (SLPs), ESOL professionals, and EL students. Specifically, we thank the USDOE, OSEP office for funding the grants awarded to Dr. Rosa-Lugo that prepare SLPs to provide services to English Learners with communication disorders (Project SLP_ELL), listening and spoken language in children with hearing loss who come from linguistically diverse homes (Project SLP_LSL), and special educators and SLPs to collaboratively gain the knowledge and competencies to assess and address the language, literacy, and academic needs of diverse students with high intensity needs (Project SPEECH).

A special thank you to the Office of English Language Acquisition (OELA) for funding two National Professional Development federal grants "Micro-credentialing of English Learner Teaching Skills (MELTS)" and "Dual Language Support through Technology Enhanced Programs and Strategies (DL STEPS), awarded to Drs. Nutta and Mihai. These grant projects have been instrumental in developing our assessment, intervention, and monitoring (AIM) model focused on English learners and English learners with communication disorders. We particularly thank the teachers and teacher candidates who participated in the grants and shared their experiences and those of their English learners, most prominently our colleague Leslie Mendez and the graduate certificate candidates in the Dual Language STEPS program.

Equally supportive have been the students in our UCF SLP/ESOL Endorsement program, who brought us their anecdotes, cases, and insights.

These opportunities and grant initiatives continue to allow the three authors to develop and share high impact practices and engage in collaborative scholarly work. Simply put, we continue to work with "real student and their families," engage in life-long learning, and share this with our respective colleagues and students.

Finally, our families and friends have been silent partners in this long-term endeavor, and we thank them for enduring time without us as we toiled away at researching, writing, and polishing this new edition.

Linda I. Rosa-Lugo
Florin M. Mihai
Joyce W. Nutta

1
English Learners— The Merging of Two Disciplines

Introduction

English learners (ELs) is a broad term that is often used to refer to students with limited English proficiency. These students are diverse, vary in native language backgrounds, and face distinct educational experiences, given that states and schools differ in how they identify, teach, and reclassify EL students (Bialik, Scheller, & Walker, 2018; Estrada & Wang, 2018; Garcia & Kleifgen, 2018). Despite the variation, ELs continue to represent the fastest growing segment of the school-age population in the United States. According to the most recent data from the U.S. Department of Education (2018), there were approximately 5 million EL students in U.S. public schools, with an average of 14.0% of total public school enrollment in cities, 9.1% in suburban areas, 6.5% in towns, and 3.6% in rural areas. This figure has more than doubled in the last few decades, and it is predicted that by 2030, 40% of all K–12 students will be considered EL students (McFarland et al., 2018).

Almost 45% of U.S. teachers have at least one student designated as an EL in their classrooms (Hopstock & Stephenson, 2003; Master, Loeb, Whitney, & Wyckoff, 2016). These students represent various backgrounds and experiences. They are either newly arrived immigrants or refugees (learning the language and getting acquainted with U.S. culture), U.S. born in households where English is not the primary language of communication, or sojourners (people from other countries who are working or studying in the United States for a finite period of time) (Capps, Fix, Murray, Ost, Passel, & Herwantoro, 2005; de Jong & Harper, 2005, 2011). Most EL students are not new to the country but were born in the United States. In fact, more than 75% of EL students in Grades K–5 are second- or third-generation Americans. Within the designation of "English learners" in K–12, these students represent over 400 language backgrounds; however, Spanish speakers are the fastest growing EL population in the United States, followed by Asians and Pacific Islanders (McFarland et al., 2018).

In the United States, ELs are educated in a variety of instructional environments in the school setting. These can include (1) all-English instruction with some support related to their limited English proficiency, (2) all-English instruction with no support related to their limited English proficiency, or (3) programs that make some use of their home language. If ELs have special needs, such as a communication disorder, then a number of well-delivered research-based instruction, intervention, and delivery models are considered and implemented to address their communication disorder (e.g., pull-out speech-language therapy in a small group or one-on-one; classroom based; see Chapter 6 for more information on program options) (ASHA, 2010a; Cirrin et al., 2010; Kangas, 2014; Moore & Montgomery, 2018). Despite the array of instructional environments, intervention designs, and delivery methods for ELs, there are critical questions educators should ask themselves. First, is the amount, quality, and design of the support and instruction ELs receive appropriate? Additionally, do the instructional practices and service delivery models that are being used in the public school setting address the L2 educational needs of ELs, and student achievement, specifically for ELs with communication disorders (Brandel & Loeb, 2011; Goldenberg, 2008; Kangas, 2014).

In the absence of careful planning and implementation of effective instructional practices, ELs are at risk of becoming academic underachievers with limited vocational and economic opportunities. The level of academic achievement among ELs, measured as a subgroup, is lower than that of proficient

English-speaking learners. This is not surprising given that they are learning a new language. Language learning is a complex, dynamic process that forms the foundation for academic skills. In fact, students classified as English learners are often deemed to have lower academic abilities and may be placed in lower ability groups than native English-speaking peers (President's Advisory Commission on Educational Excellence for Hispanic Americans, 2003). These students often do not meet state norms for reading in English according to education agency reports from 41 states (Kindler, 2002). Although ELs eventually acquire adequate conversational language and informal writing skills in English, they often lack the academic language that is essential for high levels of achievement in the content areas (Coleman & Goldenberg, 2012; Goldenberg & Coleman, 2010).

Beginning with basic communication skills, ELs face an uphill battle to acquire the sophisticated verbal skills needed for college entry or career success. Moreover, there is a wide range of educational policies and practices that either help or hinder this process. The challenge for school professionals is to determine how best to work together to provide appropriate and effective instruction for students who are ELs (Casteel & Ballantyne, 2010) and specifically ELs with a communication disorder (Rosa-Lugo, Mihai, & Nutta, 2017). The emphasis on shared responsibility for all students demands a foundation of shared knowledge from which school professionals can work (Mann, 2018).

To build this foundation, this book focuses on the knowledge, skills, and competencies of two specific school professionals: speech-language pathologists (SLPs) and English for speakers of other languages (ESOL) professionals who work with ELs in the public school setting. Although we concentrate on the role of these two professionals in the public school setting and how their disciplines interact in working with ELs in language and literacy, we also emphasize the importance of collaboration among all professionals. Possible ways in which they may collaborate to work with school-age children who are developing English proficiency and literacy and who exhibit communication disorders are also explored. The roles and responsibilities of each professional as defined by their respective national organizations (e.g., ASHA [American Speech-Language-Hearing Association]

and TESOL [Teachers of English to Speakers of Other Languages])
and the collaboration that is required of the SLP and the ESOL
in the identification, assessment, and intervention of ELs are
discussed as we consider the use of evidence-based approaches
and practical strategies that can be used to facilitate language
and literacy in ELs by the SLP and ESOL professionals.

Are SLP and ESOL Professionals Prepared to Work with ELs?

A *Changing Society*

ELs present a specific challenge to school professionals due
to the linguistic diversity and proficiency they possess in their
first and second languages (Collier, 2000; Klingner et al., 2005;
Roseberry-McKibbin, 2000). These students are required to grap-
ple with the dual demands of learning to speak English and
achieve academically. Yet they often do not enter school with
similar English language skills and academic preparedness as
their English-speaking counterparts. ELs lag significantly behind
their fluent English-speaking peers in language and literacy and
are at risk for underachievement and subsequently dropping out
of high school (August, 2003; Callahan, 2013; Haskins & Rouse,
2005). To obtain an understanding of the challenges faced by ELs
and the role of each professional (e.g., speech-language pathologist and English as a second language professional) in working
with these children and specifically ELs with communication
disorders, the following question is posed: *How well are SLPs
and ESOL professionals prepared to work with ELs?*

EL-Focused Professional Preparation

In the absence of qualified ESL or bilingual education teachers,
teaching English language skills and academic content to EL students has become the responsibility of *all* school staff. Research
has shown that there has been limited availability of school
professionals with adequate preparation in effective practices

to work with ELs (Barron & Menken, 2002; Calderón, 2007) and more specifically to work with ELs with communication disorders (Edgar & Rosa-Lugo, 2007; Kimble, 2013; Roninson, 2003; Rosa-Lugo, Mihai, & Nutta, 2017; Rosa-Lugo, Rivera, & McKeown, 1998). Providing quality instruction to ELs requires professionals who are skilled in a variety of curricular and instructional strategies (Valdés, Kibler, & Walqui, 2014). Research on teacher training and preparedness suggests that educators who do not hold bilingual or ESL certification are not well prepared to meet the needs of these children (Ballantyne, Sanderman, & Levy, 2008; Karabenick & Clemens Noda, 2004; Menken & Atunez, 2001; Reeves, 2006; U.S. Department of Education [NCES], 1997, 1999, 2001; Zehler et al., 2003). Consequently, it is essential that school-based SLPs and ESOL engage in professional development as well as self-inquiry that will lead to implementation of culturally responsive instructional practices.

School professionals do not necessarily come from the same cultural and linguistic backgrounds as their students. Because of this, it is essential that professionals make conscious and sustained efforts to learn about their students and to commit to becoming a culturally competent professional. There is growing evidence that professionals are not as well prepared as they should be for the changing demographics reflected in the classrooms across the United States. Despite the abundance of research and availability of professional development focusing on working with ELs, professionals note that they have not received adequate information on addressing the needs of ELs and feel inadequate and ill prepared to meet the needs of these students (Flynn & Hill, 2005; Lewis et al., 1999).

Professional staff development has been one method that has been used to develop culturally competent professionals. Mainstream teachers in urban areas with large numbers of ELs report that they have participated in professional development focusing on the needs of ELs. However, they note that training has not been enough to prepare them to foster English-language acquisition while also teaching the content knowledge and skills these students need to achieve academically (Cosentino de Cohen, Deterding, & Clewell, 2005).

Lynch and Hanson (1998) suggest that effective staff development requires attention to participants' cultural self-awareness, attitudes/expectations, beliefs, knowledge, and skills as well as a foundation of shared knowledge from which professionals can work together. Twenty states currently require that new teachers have some EL preparation: however, states' requirements vary considerably, with some peripherally mentioning ELs in their standards for preservice teachers and others (Arizona, California, Florida, Pennsylvania, and New York) requiring specific course-work or separate certification to address the educational needs of ELs (Ballantyne, Sanderman, & Levy, 2008; Education Commission of the States, 2014; Samson & Collins, 2012). In a survey of postsecondary institutions offering EL teacher preparation, Menken and Atunez (2001) in conjunction with the American Association of Colleges for Teacher Education (Brisk, Barnhardt, Herrera, & Rochon, 2002) found that less than one-sixth of all postsecondary institutes required EL-oriented content in their preparation of mainstream teachers. Unfortunately, most states continue to lack explicit requirements for teacher preparation relevant to ELs.

At the state and district levels, staff development opportunities for practicing teachers are similarly underrepresented. A 2001 National Center for Education Statistics (NCES) study of staff development reported that EL education was the least likely topic of focus (U.S. Department of Education, 2001). Although 80% of those surveyed had participated in staff development that related to their state or district curriculum, only 26% had staff development relating to ELs. Zehler et al. (2003) found that of teachers who had at least three ELs in their classroom, 62% had reported attending training related to ELs within the past 5 years with the median amount of training being only 4 hours.

Surveys of attitudes and feelings of preparedness indicate that teachers are uneasy with their lack of knowledge in this area. In the 2001 NCES survey, only 27% of teachers felt that they were "very well prepared" to meet the needs of ELs, whereas 12% reported that they were "not at all prepared" (U.S. Department of Education, NCES, 2001). In a separate survey of over 1,200 teachers, 57% indicated that they needed more information to work effectively with ELs (U.S. Department of Education, 1999, p. 10). In research conducted with 279 teachers in a school district with a minimal number of ELs, Reeves (2006) found that 81.7% believed that they did not have adequate training to work effectively with ELs, and 53% wanted more preparation. Given the steady increase in the EL population, it is safe to assume that a growing number of teachers continue to see the need for—and feel the lack of—professional development (Johannessen, Guzman, Thorsos, & Dickinson, 2016).

Schools in suburban and rural communities have historically enrolled very few students for whom English is a second or new language. Although low numbers of ELs have been characteristic of most schools situated in suburban and rural schools, a recent study of EL students suggests that the biggest increase (in EL students) is occurring in these school systems (Gill, Posamentier, & Hill, 2016). This shift calls for a dramatic need for quality interventions for EL students. Professional staff is likely to be unprepared for the changing realities of having children of limited English proficiency in the classroom. Like the need expressed by teachers in urban areas, teachers in suburban and rural schools report a need for competence in EL methodology, multiculturalism, EL curriculum development, EL assessment, and second language acquisition theory (Berube, 2000, 2002; Field, 2008; Gill, Posamentier, & Hill, 2016).

Smaller-scale attitudinal surveys of teachers have often focused on teacher attitudes toward and knowledge about ELs as a proxy for preparedness, reasoning that if teachers do not have accurate information about the cultural, linguistic, and learning characteristics of ELs, then they are not well prepared to teach them. Teachers of ELs often hold beliefs of this population that have either been disproven or are seriously contested. For example, Reeves (2006) found that 71.1% of teachers surveyed believed that ELs should be able to learn English within 2 years. In a survey of 729 teachers in a school district in which almost one third of students were ELs, Karabenick and Clemens Noda (2004) found that a majority (52%) believed that speaking one's first language at home inhibited English language development. Nearly one third (32%) thought that if students are not able to produce fluent English, they are also unable to comprehend it. The authors also reported that many mainstream teachers do not "distinguish between oral communication proficiencies and cognitive academic language capabilities" (p. 63). Several researchers, including those above (see also Bartolomé, 2002; Lee & Oxelson, 2006; Phuntsog, 2001), have found that culturally sensitive and comprehensive training of educators leads to a shift in attitudes toward ELs.

The need to prepare SLPs to work with ELs and to demonstrate cultural competence has also been addressed in the literature (ASHA, 1985, 2011b, 2011c, 2017a; Battle, 2002; Kayser, 1996, 2008). Several researchers have examined the preparedness of SLPs to work with ELs (Artiles & Klingner, 2006; Campbell, Brennan, & Steckol, 1992; McConnell-Stephen, Weiler, Sandman, & Dell'aira, 1994; Nixon, McCardle, & Leos, 2007; Rosa-Lugo & Fradd, 2000; Roseberry-McKibbin, Brice, & O'Hanlon, 2005; Roseberry-McKibben & Eicholtz, 1994). Studies note that a significant percentage of SLPs are not proficient enough in a language other than English to provide services to ELs, do not feel competent or confident in conducting nonbiased assessment or using alternate assessments, and do not feel prepared to provide evidence-based culturally and linguistically appropriate treatment (Caesar & Kohler, 2007; Chabon & Lee-Wilkerson, 2007; Guiberson & Atkins, 2012; Kohnert et al., 2003; Kritikos, 2003; Roseberry-McKibbin, 2018). On the other hand, ESOL professionals are adequately prepared to work with ELs but often do not have the preservice or in-service preparation to work with ELs with communication disorders (Turkan & Schramm-Possinger, 2014).

To summarize, there is a pressing need for further professional preparation for teachers and SLPs at all stages in their careers. In studying the preparedness of educators and SLPs to work with ELs, several recommendations have been offered. Preservice and/or in-service initiatives such as inclusion of coursework and clinical practice with individuals from diverse backgrounds is one such recommendation, as is an increased emphasis on research on communication disorders in diverse populations (Coleman, 2000; Horton-Ikard, Munoz, Thomas-Tate, & KellerBell, 2009; Stockman, Boult, & Robinson, 2004). Other researchers have recommended modifications of traditional assessment practices and the use of culturally appropriate intervention strategies and evidence-based practices in working with ELs (Farrugia-Bernard, 2018; Roseberry-McKibben, 2013, 2018).

A recommendation most offered for SLP and other key professionals is that they should develop "cultural competence" or become "culturally competent" to work with ELs (Anderson,

1992; ASHA, 1985; Campbell, Brenna, & Steckol, 1992; Crowley, Guest & Sudler, 2015). To better understand this recommendation and the competencies and skills set needed by SLPs and ESOL professionals to work with ELs, it is important to understand what is meant by "cultural competence."

Development of Culturally Competent Professionals

What Is a Culturally Competent Professional?

Cultural competence, as defined by Lynch and Hanson (1998), is described "as having respect for difference, eagerness to learn, and a willingness to accept that there are many ways of viewing the world" (p. 356). ASHA (2019a) describes cultural competence as "understanding and appropriately responding to the unique combination of cultural variables" that can occur in all professional/client interactions across identification, assessment, and intervention. ASHA (2019a) specifically points out that culture and cultural diversity incorporate a variety of factors, such as "age, disability, ethnicity, gender identity (encompasses gender expression), national origin (encompasses related aspects e.g., ancestry, culture, language, dialect, citizenship, and immigration status), race, religion, sex, sexual orientation, and veteran status. Linguistic diversity can also accompany cultural diversity."

Although the term "cultural competence" has been used interchangeably with other terms (i.e., cultural humility, sensitivity, and/or cross-cultural competence), they all refer to ways of thinking and behaving that enable members of one cultural, ethnic, or linguistic group to work effectively with members of another. Cross, Bazron, Dennis, and Isaacs (1989) describe a path toward cultural competence that illustrates that cultural competence is a process with varied rules and facts to be learned. They describe several stages within the continuum of cultural competence, such as cultural destructiveness, cultural incapacity, cultural blindness, cultural precompetence, cultural competency, and cultural proficiency. In general, cultural competence includes (1) an awareness of one's own cultural limitations; (2) openness, appreciation, and respect for cultural differences; (3) a view of intercultural interactions as learning opportunities; (4) the ability to use cultural resources in interventions; and (5) an acknowledgment of the integrity and value of all cultures (Green, 1982, p. 356).

Attaining cultural competence is an ongoing process and requires systematic study of individuals, including the impact that their cultural and linguistic background has had on academic achievement and/or clinical service (Battle, 2002; Farrugia-Bernard, 2018). Numerous books, chapters, and journal articles have been used to raise critical issues and offer solutions when working with ELs. For example, authors have written about (a) the general characteristics of racial, ethnic, and cultural groups (Kayser, 2008; Lynch & Hanson, 1998; Roseberry-McKibben, 2018; Taylor, 1986); (b) the nature of linguistic differences among certain culturally and linguistically diverse groups and the implications for SLPs and other professionals (Battle, 2002; Centeno, Anderson, & Obler, 2007; Coleman, 2000; Goldstein, 2004; Goldstein & Washington, 2001; Kohnert, 2008; Rivers, Rosa-Lugo, & Hedrick, 2004; Seymour, Bland-Stewart, & Green, 1998); and (c) the impact cultural characteristics have on the language and literacy development of ELs (Brisk & Harrington, 2007; Calderon, 2007; Curtin, 2009; Diaz-Rico & Weed, 2006; Farrell, 2009; Freeman, Freeman, & Ramirez, 2008; Klingner, Hoover, & Baca, 2008; Peregoy & Boyle, 2005; Quiocho & Ulanoff, 2009; Roseberry-McKibben, 2018).

National organizations such as the American Speech-Language-Hearing Association (ASHA) and Teachers of English to Speakers of Other Languages (TESOL) have outlined the professional standards and the knowledge, skills, and competencies expected of professionals who work with ELs and ELs with communication disorders (see ASHA Practice Portal, https://www.asha.org/practice-portal/ and the TESOL website, https://www.tesol.org/advance-the-field/advocacy-resources/position-statements). Specifically, ASHA's Code of Ethics (ASHA, 2017a) includes specific statements of minimally acceptable as well as unacceptable professional conduct for speech-language pathologists and audiologists in a variety of areas. The Code of Ethics addresses the need for professionals to provide culturally and linguistically competent services with individuals with communication disorders across the life span and settings.

These resources serve as starting points for learning about different cultural groups, their linguistic characteristics, and the role of families and the community in the development of language and literacy in ELs, specifically those with communication disorders. Although these resources provide valuable information, simply reading them will not lead one to become a culturally competent professional. They can, however, serve to facilitate discussion, generate questions, and propel us to reexamine our cultural competence.

Although it is impossible for an individual to be knowledgeable about all the cultural and linguistic characteristics of ELs, it is recommended that professionals strive for increased cultural sensitivity toward people whose cultural, linguistic, and social backgrounds are different from their own (Verdon, Wong, & McLeod, 2016). Strategies such as obtaining information about a family's culture and language, working with people from the cultural community who can guide service providers in culturally appropriate interactions with clients and their families, examining similarities and differences in students and their families, and evaluating our own values and assumptions have proven helpful in developing cultural competency (Crowley, Guest, & Sudler, 2015; Roseberry-McKibben, 2018). The practice of viewing individuals from a narrow lens can be dangerous. When people are viewed as "representative" of a specific cultural and/ or linguistic group without considering the great heterogeneity that exists within cultural groups, this can lead to subjective and erroneous stereotypes and/or generalizations (Riquelme, 2013). Simply put, a "culturally competent professional" recognizes that each person in any cultural group is first an individual and is willing to explore and question their biases and perceptions when working with individuals who are different from their own cultural and linguistic background (Preis, 2013).

Key Terms and Concepts

EL Terminology

As in other professions, working with students for whom English is not the primary language requires mastering a unique jargon. A culturally competent professional must be familiar with key terminology related to working with ELs. Often, the term "EL" specifically refers to students who are learning English and already have a native language, but other labels have been used to describe these students. For example, within the public schools in the United States, common terms include "language-minority," "English as a Second Language (ESL)" students, "limited English proficient," "second-language learners," "culturally and linguistically diverse (CLD)," and/or "bilingual." The terms "language-minority," "limited English speaking," and "limited English proficient (LEP)" have been official designations under federal law. The term "LES" or "LEP" was used in the first authorization of the Bilingual Education Act (Title VII of ESEA, prior to No Child Left Behind) in 1968 (Bardack, 2010). However, the expression English language learner (ELL) has replaced these terms to avoid the implication that nonnative English-speaking students are deficient (National Council of Teachers of English, 2008). However, each of these labels is problematic because there is inconsistent uniformity in defining and describing ELs. To ensure some continuity, a consistent definition of what constitutes an EL is necessary (Short & Fitzsimmons, 2006).

Description of English Learners

Several terms are often used to *describe* ELs. For example, terms such as "culture," "race," and "ethnicity" have been causing miscommunications or misunderstandings. **Culture** is the shared beliefs, traditions, and values of a group of people; learned patterns of thoughts and behavior (Payne, 1986); and the framework that guides and bounds life practices (Hanson, 1992). Culture is associated with or influenced by factors such as age, gender, religion, education, child-rearing practices, geographic region, and socioeconomic status (SES). Presently, culture has taken on various shades of meaning in the social science literature, and several definitions have been proposed (see Frisby, 1992; Garcia, 1982; Goldman & McDermott, 1987). Scholars note that the term "culture" has sometimes been erroneously used synonymously with race—however, the terms are not the same. Two people may be of the same race and yet identify with two very different cultural groups.

Race has traditionally been defined as a classification that distinguishes one group of people from another based on physical characteristics (e.g., skin color, facial features) (Kammey, Ritzer, & Yetman, 1990). Physical characteristics are one means of differentiating people; however, the criteria used to distinguish one racial group from another vary from one society to another (Kammey et al., 1990). It appears that categorizing people by race has been discredited and is not useful in addressing the linguistic needs of ELs with communication disorders (Kendall, 1997).

Ethnicity is another term that has often been confused with culture and race. Ethnicity is the social definition of groups of people based on cultural similarities. Ethnicity includes race and factors such as customs, nationality, language, and heritage (Coleman & McCabe, 2000). Sociologists suggest that ethnic groups share five main characteristics: (1) unique cultural traits (e.g., language, clothing, holidays); (2) a sense of community; (3) a feeling of ethnocentrism or a belief that one's own culture and way of life are superior to all others; (4) ascribed membership—a status conferred at birth; and (5) territoriality, defined as a tendency to occupy a distinct geographic area (such as Chinatown) by choice or for self-protection (Kammey et al., 1990).

Several other terms have been included in the *description* of ELs. Wei (2006) outlined approximately 35 terms that have been used to describe ELs. For example, terms have been used to describe (a) their language proficiency (non-English speaking [NES]; limited English speaking [LES]; fluent English speaker [FES]; emergent bilingual); (b) their stage of language proficiency (preproduction, emergent production; bridging); (c) the conditions under which bilingualism occurs (simultaneous; sequential); (d) the types of bilingualism (semilingual, additive bilingualism, subtractive bilingualism, dual language); (e) the instructional environments (sheltered English; dual-language instruction); (f) the way they organize, classify, and assimilate information in a language (learning style, field dependent, field independent); and (g) how they have transitioned into the mainstream culture (acculturation, assimilation). As Goldstein (2004) points out, scholars (see Abedi, 2003; Baker, 2001; de Houwer, 1990; García & Kleifgen, 2018; Hakuta, 1986; Linquanti & Cook, 2013; Romaine, 1995; Valdes & Figueroa, 1994) have defined and described ELs in a variety of ways. These descriptions highlight the complexity of issues associated with this student population from the perspective of SLPs and ESOLs.

Recommended Competencies for SLPs and ESOL Professionals

What Competencies Are Critical in Working with ELs?

ASHA has recognized the need for practitioners and professionals who work with ELs to develop specific competencies and a skill set to help ELs achieve high academic standards since 1985. In 2004, the knowledge and skills needed by SLPs and audiologists to provide culturally and linguistically appropriate identification, assessment, and intervention services were outlined and described by ASHA (2004a). The knowledge and skills to acquire professional cultural competency focused on three fundamental knowledge domains: knowledge of self, knowledge of others, and knowledge of the theoretical and empirical literature on dual-language development, use, and disorders (Kohnert et al., 2003; Rosa-Lugo & Champion, 2007). Specifically, ASHA (2004a) suggested knowledge and skills that SLPs should develop in order to work with ELs. SLPs should:

A. Engage in self-scrutiny.
B. Demonstrate an understanding of cultural characteristics and the impact that these characteristics have on students' performance in the classroom learning environment.
C. Be able to distinguish between normal characteristics of second language acquisition, a communication difference, and/or a communication disorder using appropriate assessment measures.
D. Provide appropriate, culturally responsive, and evidence-based practices (Battle, 2002; Kayser, 1995;

Kohnert et al., 2003; Roseberry-McKibben, 2018; Roth, 2015).

Over the years, additional policy, professional documents, and scholarly publications have informed all aspects of work with students for whom English is not the primary language to include evidence-based assessment and treatment practices (ASHA, 2013; Ortiz & Robertson, 2018; Paradis, 2016; Rosa-Lugo, Mihai, & Nutta, 2017; Roseberry-McKibben, 2018).

Similarly, the knowledge and skills needed by ESOL professionals to effectively work with ELs were outlined in several position papers by Teachers of English to Speakers of Other Languages (TESOL, 2003a, 2003b, 2005a, 2005b, 2007a, 2008, 2010a). Specifically, the position papers stressed the need for ESOL professionals to (a) engage in lifelong learning, (b) understand the academic and linguistic needs of ELs with special needs, and (c) access and apply research-based approaches from a variety of disciplines to improve the achievement and academic success of ELs.

To equip SLPs and ESOL professionals with explicit, research-based pedagogical knowledge and skills that they can use in the classroom, professional development related to diversity must go beyond cultural humility, sensitivity, and appreciation (Garcia & Guerra, 2004). Both professionals must be provided with opportunities to obtain knowledge and develop expertise in the basic constructs of language proficiency, bilingualism, and second language development; the role of the first language and culture in learning; the demands found in the general education curriculum for ELs placed in mainstream English-only classrooms (Clair & Adger, 1999); the academic and linguistic demands of ELs with special needs (Antunez, 2002b); and evidence-based approaches and strategies (Valdés, Kibler, & Walqui, 2014). Thus, the primary goals of SLP and ESOL professionals are to address the language development, instructional, and literacy needs of ELs (ASHA, 2001a; TESOL, 2003a, 2003b, 2008, 2010a) and to use evidence-based approaches to facilitate the academic success of school-age ELs (Rosa-Lugo, Mihai, & Nutta, 2017). These shared goals present opportunities to discuss the implementation of evidence-based approaches and strategies that can be used by SLPs and ESOL professionals to work with ELs with communication disorders. This is addressed further in Chapter 7.

Evidence-Based Practice

What Is the Significance of Evidence-Based Approaches and Strategies in Working with ELs?

The current climate of accountability, particularly in our nation's schools, emphasizes personal and institutional responsibility for actions and decisions concerning our nation's schoolchildren. This climate stems, in part, from the spiraling costs of special education services. The No Child Left Behind Act (NCLB) of 2001 (NCLB, 2002) placed a strong emphasis on accountability and emphasized the need for school-based professionals to deliver instruction and interventions that have demonstrated efficiency (the time taken to reach a desired outcome) and effectiveness (the likelihood that the desired outcome will be achieved). The NCLB Act also required that all school districts use instructional strategies that are rooted in scientifically based research.

New education initiatives such as the Common Core State Standards (CCSS; Council for Clinical Certification in Audiology and Speech-Language Pathology of the Council of Chief State School Officers, 2010), released in 2010 (for mathematics, English language arts and literacy in history/social studies, science, and technical subjects), set high benchmarks for what K–12 students need to know to compete in a global, knowledge-based economy (Hanushek, Peterson, & Woessmann, 2012). The standards, adopted by 45 states, require students to demonstrate high levels of competency in language and literacy skills. Specifically, ELs are required to demonstrate complex literacy and content skills that are highly dependent upon language ability. The Every Student Succeeds Act (ESSA) (2015), a federal K–12 legislation, replaced the No Child Left Behind Act (NCLB) of 2001 and requires states to (a) include the acquisition of English language proficiency by ELs as one factor in their accountability framework; (b) demonstrate accountability regarding recently arrived ELs; (c) set uniform EL identification and exit criteria, as well as a timeline for ELs to reach English language proficiency; and (d) disaggregate ELs with a disability from ELs in particular.

School-based SLPs and professionals in many other disciplines embody the 21st century's emphasis on reform based on accountability and research. Together, these concepts contextualize discussions of evidence-based practice (EBP) as it applies to meeting the needs of school-age ELs, specifically those with communication disorders.

The term "evidence-based practice" (EBP) refers to an approach in which current, high-quality research evidence is integrated with practitioner expertise and client preferences and values in the process of making clinical decisions (ASHA, 2005b). Research refers to a spirited inquiry and systematic investigation that contributes to the knowledge base of a field. For example, research-based knowledge provides a principled basis for understanding language teaching and learning and making decisions about policies, plans, and actions. Research has the potential to help English language teaching professionals improve the processes, outcomes, and conditions for language teaching, learning, and assessment. It also can help the profession address urgent social and political issues around the world, improve the materials used for second language teaching in schools, and clarify debates and debunk myths regarding second language acquisition. A strong commitment to research as a means of improving professional knowledge is vital to the field of teaching of English to speakers of other languages (TESOL, 2005b) and the discipline of speech-language pathology.

The goal of evidence-based practice is to integrate clinical expertise and best current evidence (ASHA, 2005b). In response to the evidence-based practice movement, ASHA created a framework for ranking levels of evidence that is specific to the field of communication disorders and sciences (*ASHA Leader*, 2007; Justice & Fey, 2004). For example, currently, evidence-based systematic reviews have been completed for specific areas of intervention or service delivery models (see Cirrin et al., 2010; Gorman, 2007; Mullen 2007; Thomason, Gorman, & Summers, 2007). Similarly, summaries of studies that have been peer-reviewed and published in professional journals have provided school-based SLPs with evidence-based support for the use of specific interventions (Gillam & Gillam, 2006; Powell, 2018; Schraeder, 2008). General clinical strategies and techniques are available for use by SLPs across a variety of intervention programs regardless of the student's disability type (Schraeder, 2008). ASHA has published policy statements related to the designation of competencies associated with the various needs (disorders or conditions) of persons being served. Each policy statement, derived from the ASHA Code of Ethics (ASHA, 2010a), details the scope of practice, the necessary education and training, precautions, and knowledge and skills needed in service delivery.

Application of EBP by the SLP involves more than simply making clinical decisions based on literature reviews. To date, a systematic review of what works with ELs with communication disorders, and specifically across disability type, is not readily available. However, with the establishment of ASHA's (2019b) National Center for Evidenced-Based Practice in Communication Disorders (N-CEP), it is anticipated that systematic reviews, and recommendations extracted from the professional literature of peer-reviewed and published studies specific to working with ELs (Guiberson & Ferris, 2019; Justice & Fey, 2004; Restrepo & Towle-Harmon, 2008) will be useful in making clinical decisions.

Specifically, it is recommended that school-based SLPs should:

1. Be culturally competent (ASHA, 2004a, 2005c, 2010c, 2019; Battle, 2002; Roseberry-McKibben, 2018; Schraeder, 2008).
2. Reflect on their cultural competence (ASHA, 2019a; McCarthy, 2003).
3. Collaborate with other school professionals to work with ELs (Anaby et al., 2019; Bauer, Iyer, Boon, & Fore, 2010; Blosser, 2006; Hegde & Davis, 1995; Rosa-Lugo & Fradd, 2000; Rosa-Lugo, Mihai, & Nutta, 2017).

Given the continued focus on accountability and current gaps that exist in the research on what works with ELs, and specifically ELs with communication disorders (ELCDs), it is important for readers to obtain a better understanding of ELs in general and then ELCDs specifically.

The next chapter provides an overview of ELs in preK–12 schools and current demographics of EL students and their families. Key terms and characteristics of ELs and ELCDs are discussed. Several significant legislation initiatives that have influenced the education of ELs and ELCDs in the United States are examined in relationship to the increasing impact of common standards, school accountability measures, and college and career readiness initiatives.

2

The Context of Working with English Learners with Communication Disorders

Introduction

Speech-language pathologists (SLPs) are often challenged with differentiating the performance of bilingual children with language impairment (LI) from those who may display a language difference. This is often exacerbated due to the variability observed in bilingual children in the United States who are in the process of acquiring English. The heterogeneous levels of experiences and use of each language require that SLPs be well informed about the differences often seen in the performance of ELs on language and literacy tasks.

In order to build the context for understanding English learners with communication disorders (ELCDs), this chapter provides a brief demographic overview of ELs and ELCD students in preK–12 schools and key terms associated with ELs and ELCDs. The expected variability and educational context associated with ELs in general and ELCDs specifically are described. The legislative initiatives that have influenced their education in the United States in very important ways are presented in relationship to the increasing impact of common standards, school accountability measures, and college and career readiness initiatives. We close this chapter by considering some of the challenges faced by SLPs and ESOL professionals in working with ELs and ELCDs.

Building the Context for Understanding ELs

Demographics

Children who are classified as ELs are the fastest growing segment of the school population in the United States. Over the past decade, ELs have increased by more than 15 million students (Flynn & Hill, 2005; Matthews & Ewen, 2006). Today, ELs represent more than 10% of the U.S. public school population in prekindergarten through the 12th grade (Bunch, Kibler, & Pimentel, 2013; McFarland et al., 2018; National Clearinghouse for English Language Acquisition, 2011; U.S. Department of Education, 2018b). This very significant percentage of public school students who are learning English is heterogeneous. Therefore, a list of characteristics that apply to all ELs in the United States is complex. Clearly, the EL student population is fluid and quite difficult to predict in terms of growth and diversity (Frey, 2015). One reason for this variation in identification are the different data sets that are used to capture the size and diversity of the EL population. For example, results of questions on the U.S. Census estimates that the number of ELs in the United States is approximately 2.6 million, whereas the U.S. Department of Education data sets suggest approximately 4.9 million (U.S. Census Bureau, 2015b; U.S. Department of Education, 2016b).

Children of immigrants have been the fastest growing and most diverse segments of the child population in the United States (Capps, 2015; Capps et al., 2005). They have played a significant role in the changing landscape of the U.S. population of school-age children and youth, Nonetheless, tougher law enforcement of illegal immigration and declining economic opportunities have resulted in challenges determining the total number of ELs enrolled at all stages in the educational pipeline (Flores, Park, Viano, & Coca, 2017). One impact associated with demographic trends has been in the distribution of languages spoken in the United States. The percentage of the U.S. population speaking only English has declined, while the percentage speaking a language other than English has increased (Gonzalez-Barrera & Lopez, 2013; Rumbaut & Massey, 2013). Although EL students speak over 350 native languages, almost 80% identify Spanish as their native language (Hopstock & Stephenson, 2003; Uro & Barrio, 2013; U.S. Census Bureau, 2015b).

Although the immigration surge might be slowing temporarily, the fact that so many immigrants have chosen to settle in states that were not traditional immigration magnets is an emerging feature of the geographic distribution of ELs. Historically, ELs migrated to large urban areas, but a recent migration shift in the United States has been to small towns and rural destinations (Uro & Barrio, 2013). It is important to note that there are notable variations within and among immigrant groups that can result in significant changes in school populations.

Thus, it is essential for decision makers at the state level to monitor the demographic statistics carefully in order to ensure that there are sufficient resources allocated to meet the needs of the changing student population.

English Learners: In Search of Common Terminology

There are various terms and definitions associated with ELs. However, these terms lack uniformity in defining and describing ELs. To facilitate the building of common EL terms, definitions associated with ELs at the federal and state level are presented.

The terms "EL" and "LEP" (limited English proficient) have been used quite extensively in the educational literature to describe students who are not yet proficient in English and who require instructional support in order to fully access academic content in their classes. The term most commonly used in the literature is EL, although federal legislation continues to use the term LEP (e.g., No Child Left Behind Act [NCLB], 2001). Students referred to as LEP are often seen as a subset of ELs who have not yet attained English language proficiency (as measured by the particular assessment procedures of their state). For example, in Florida, the term "LEP" was changed from limited English proficiency to language-enriched pupils in an attempt to deemphasize the language deficit of EL and emphasize language accomplishment (*Florida Department of Education, the League of United Latin American Citizens et al. v. Florida Board of Education,* 2019). However, to date, Florida has followed a national trend to use the term "EL" instead of "LEP." Despite the labels used by educators to describe nonnative English speakers, such as ELLs (English language learners), ESL (English as a second language), ESOL (English for speakers of other languages), and/or culturally and linguistically diverse (CLD) students, these group of students continue to need support in acquiring and using language in the classroom, particularly with complex academic language that leads to successful high school graduation and higher education opportunities (Francis, Rivera, Lesaux, Kieffer, & Rivera, 2006).

Due to the variety of terms used to describe this specific group of students, researchers have argued that it would be advantageous to have standardized EL definitions and terms that could be used nationally. For example, Short and Fitzsimmons (2007) argue that a common definition of an EL is necessary to have clear and consistent national standards that will define this student population and allow valid and reliable cross-state comparisons vis-à-vis EL academic achievement and English language proficiency. ELs are described and defined both at the federal and state levels, with some differences between the two. Definitions associated with ELs at the federal and state levels are reviewed here in order to facilitate the building of a common definition of ELs.

Federal

At the federal level, ELs are described as national origin minority students who are limited English proficient (LEP). Public Law 107-110, also known as the No Child Left Behind Act (NCLB) (2001) and reauthorized as Every Student Succeeds Act (ESSA) (2015), defines an LEP student in its Title IX, Part A, Sec. 9101, (25) as "an individual:

1. who is aged 3 through 21;
2. who is enrolled or preparing to enroll in an elementary school or secondary school;
3. (i) who was not born in the United States or whose native language is a language other than English;
   (ii) (I) who is a Native American or Alaska Native, or a native resident of the outlying areas; and
       (II) who comes from an environment where a language other than English has had a significant impact on the individual's level of English language proficiency; or
   (iii) who is migratory, whose native language is a language other than English, and who comes from an environment where a language other than English is dominant; and
4. whose difficulties in speaking, reading, writing, or understanding the English language may be sufficient to deny the individual
   (i) the ability to meet the State's proficient level of achievement on State assessments;
   (ii) the ability to successfully achieve in classrooms where the language of instructions is English; or
   (iii) the opportunity to participate fully in society."

There are several laws affecting the education of ELs, but two of them stand out: The Bilingual Education Act (BEA, 1968) and the No Child Left Behind Act (NCLB, 2001). The Bilingual Education Act (BEA), also known as Title VII of the Elementary and Secondary Education Act, was passed by the U.S. Congress in 1968. It was the first time the needs of low-income students whose dominant language was not English were recognized at the federal level. The act was reauthorized several times, with each reauthorization bringing forth important changes. The 1974 and 1978 reauthorizations specifically focused on the inclusion of ELs to be served. The 1984 reauthorization included not only the EL students but also their families by providing funding for family English literacy programs. Additionally, it funded the development of two-way bilingual programs. These two-way bilingual programs focused on the development of dual-language proficiency. In this bilingual model, students receive instruction in English and another language in classrooms that are usually composed of half native speakers of English and half native speakers of another language. The 1994 and final reauthorization of the BEA strongly endorsed the idea that ELs should not just be transitioned to full-language proficiency in English but should have dual-language proficiency (Stewner-Manzanares, 1988). However, the push for evidence-based practices, standards, and accountability set the stage for policies governing K–12 education for EL students.

In 1994, Congress passed the Goals 2000: Educate America Act of 1994, which established state standards. This shift toward systemic changes and standards (Cohen, 1995; Cross, 2015) resulted in the Improving America's Schools Act of 1994. This legislation addressed the accountability of states and school districts to prescribe the content of instruction for states and districts, since the federal government does not have the authority to prescribe the content of instruction for state standards.

The second important piece of legislation, NCLB (NCLB, 2001), passed by the U.S. Congress in 2001, was a reauthorization of the Elementary and Secondary Education Act (ESEA). A key focus of this act was to hold schools, local districts, and states accountable for the performance of ELs. Specifically, two goals of NCLB were critical for EL students' attainment of standards. The first goal required that by the year 2014, all children, ELs included, reach grade-level proficiency in English language arts and mathematics. The second goal required that all EL students become proficient in English and reach high academic standards, at a minimum attaining proficiency or better in reading/language arts and mathematics. Titles I and III of the law contained most of the important provisions affecting ELs.

Under Title I (Improving the Academic Achievement of the Disadvantaged) of the NCLB Act (NCLB, 2001), schools faced a federal mandate to properly meet the educational needs of ELs. Research-based language instruction curricula were required to determine the academic progress of ELs (Flynn & Hill, 2005). Title I wanted "to ensure that all children have a fair, equal, and significant opportunity to obtain a high-quality education and reach, at a minimum, proficiency on challenging state academic achievement standards and state academic assessments"

(NCLB, 2001). To achieve this purpose, the following steps were recommended:

◆ Align curriculum, teaching, and assessment to state standards.
◆ Meet the educational needs of low-achieving children from the following categories: low-income, ELs, migratory, special education, Indian, and so on.
◆ Strive to close the achievement gap between minority and nonminority children, with a focus on low-income students.
◆ Hold schools accountable for not improving the academic achievement of their students.
◆ Focus on improving teaching, learning, and assessment by using statewide assessment instruments aligned to state achievement and content standards.
◆ Promote effective scientifically based instructional strategies and challenging academic content.
◆ Provide ample opportunities to teachers and administrators for professional development.
◆ Encourage parental participation in the education of their children.

Beginning in third grade, Title I requires schools to improve the performance of ELs in reading and math as measured by state assessments. Although the outcomes of instruction are measured in third-grade improvement, activities begin long before then. These improvement activities are in response to the reauthorization of the Individuals with Disabilities Education Act (IDEA) of 2004 that requires early intervening services and response to intervention approaches (RtI) to support struggling learners. If schools constantly fail to improve the performance of their students, they are subject to various types of interventions, ranging from allowing parents to send their children to other schools or to offer additional services (e.g., from after-school programs to more extreme measures such as restructuring or closing).

Title III, Language Instruction for Limited English Proficient and Immigrant Students, had three parts: Part A, English Language Acquisition, Language Enhancement, and Academic Achievement Act; Part B, Improving Language Instructional Programs for Academic Achievement Act; and Part C, General Provisions (NCLB, 2001).

Part A, English Language Acquisition, Language Enhancement, and Academic Achievement Act, had several goals. First, it aimed to make sure that ELs develop high levels of academic achievement in English and content areas, as measured by state standards. It also focused on developing, establishing, implementing, and sustaining language instructional programs and programs of English language development for ELs.

Part B, Improving Language Instructional Programs for Academic Achievement Act, intended to "help ensure that limited English proficient children master English and meet the same rigorous academic standards for academic achievement as all children are expected to meet, including meeting challenging State academic content and student academic achievement standards" (NCLB, 2001). This purpose was to be fulfilled by developing and promoting accountability systems for educational programs serving ELs, developing language skills and multicultural understanding, and focusing on the development of English proficiency of ELs and, to the extent possible, the native language proficiency of ELs.

Part C, General Provisions, contained a listing of definitions used in Parts A and B, outlined procedures for parental notification, and established a national clearinghouse to disseminate information about ELs.

Finally, the 2015 reauthorization of the ESEA enactment, Every Student Succeeds Act (ESSA, 2015), changed the term "English learner" as a replacement for the term "limited English proficient" used in Section 9101 of the ESEA, as amended by the No Child Left Behind Act (NCLB) (2001).

State

At the state level, there is no consistent definition of the EL student population. States and school districts use a wide range of standards and language proficiency tests to determine eligibility for programs for ELs. This often results in a wide variation in the definition of who is considered to be limited English proficient and who is qualified to receive appropriate services. Thus, the definition varies from state to state. For example, some states such as Alaska, Louisiana, and Oregon use the federal definition illustrated above, while others use their own definition. For example, the New York State Education Department (see http://www.nysed.gov) defines ELs as students who speak a language other than English by reason of foreign birth or ancestry and either understand and speak little English or score below a specific threshold on a proficiency exam. Starting in 2015 to 2016, the following categories were added to reflect the heterogeneity within its EL population:

◆ Newcomer English language learners—students who have been identified as English language learners (ELLs) and received English as a new language instruction and/or bilingual instruction for a total of zero to 3 continuously enrolled school years in the United States.

◆ Students with inconsistent/interrupted formal education (SIFE)—ELLs who have attended schools in the United States for fewer than 12 months and who, upon initial enrollment, are 2 or more years below grade level in literacy in their home language and/or 2 or more years below grade level in math due to inconsistent or interrupted schooling prior to arrival in the United States.

◆ Developing English language learners—students who have been identified as ELLs and received English as a new language instruction and/or bilingual instruction for a total of 4 to 6 continuously enrolled school years in the United States.

◆ Long-term English language learners—students identified as ELLs and received English as a new language and/or bilingual instruction for 7 or more continuously enrolled school years in the United States (also referred to as "emergent bilinguals").

◆ Former English language learners—students identified as ELLs and subsequently exited from ELL status.

The fact that there is no common definition used at both the federal and state levels is also reflected in the various terms used to identify English learners. For example, Arizona and California use the term "English learner" (EL), derived from English language learner or ELL. Arkansas and Colorado use the term "ELL," while Iowa and Kansa use "limited English proficient" or LEP. Another term used in the literature that is inclusive and culturally sensitive is "culturally and linguistically diverse" (CLD) student. According to Herrera, Murry, and Morales Cabral (2007) and Rosa-Lugo, Mihai, and Nutta (2012), this term effectively describes students who require differentiated instruction and assessment because of their diversity of language and culture. The Office of English Language Acquisition (OELA) has used the term "EL" since 2011 (Nutta, Mokhtari, & Strebel, 2012) and it is the term we use in this book.

Legislation Affecting ELs

We have discussed specific laws and guidelines in order to contextualize the terms and definitions associated with ELs. Now we briefly review landmark court rulings that have played a major role for EL students, their families, and communities (Wright, 2015). Particularly, we focus on two Supreme Court cases and one federal court case that have had a significant impact on the education of ELs: *Lau v. Nichols, Plyer v. Doe,* and *Castañeda v. Pickard* (Table 2–1).

In a ruling that addressed equal opportunities for ELs, *Lau v. Nichols* (1974) examined whether or not same education was fair education for ELs. Plaintiffs representing 1,800 students of Chinese descent sued the San Francisco school district for not providing access to education by not implementing language accommodations for ELs. The Supreme Court ruled in favor of the plaintiffs and stated that the San Francisco school district did not comply with Title VI of the Civil Rights Act (1964). According to the Supreme Court, the school district in question denied non-English-speaking students of Chinese origin a meaningful opportunity to participate in the public school system. Providing students with equal access to desks, books, teachers, and curricula did not mean an equal educational opportunity if the students had limited English skills. The decision of the Supreme Court in the 1974 *Lau v. Nichols* case had significant and immediate effects in the United States. It directly led to the

Table 2–1. ELs and the Courts

Case	Description	Ruling
Lau v. Nichols (1974)	Supreme Court case started as a class action suit filed on behalf of Chinese-speaking children attending San Francisco schools	Identical education (same materials, teachers, curriculum, etc.) does not add up to equal education under Title VI of the 1964 Civil Rights Act.
Plyer v. Doe (1982)	Supreme Court Case considering revisions of Texas laws withholding state funds for educating children who had not been legally admitted to the United States and authorizing local school districts to deny enrollment to such students.	US public schools are prohibited to deny free public education to undocumented immigrant children.
Castañeda v. Pickard (1981)	A federal court case against ethnicity-based discriminatory practices that took place in the school district in Raymondville, Texas.	Creation of the Castañeda Test (theory, practice, results) to determine the quality of programs for EL students.

establishment of standards for identifying ELs, for assessing their language proficiency, and for meeting their instructional needs. Additionally, even though the decision did not require any specific solution to address the limited English proficiency of ELs, it favored the establishment of bilingual programs in states like Texas or California as a way of avoiding violations of Title VI of the Civil Rights Act (1964).

The second Supreme Court case, *Plyer v. Doe* (1982), ruled on a Texas statute that denied access to education to children of illegal immigrants. The Texas statute was a 1975 revision of education laws that allowed the withholding of state funds for educating children who had not been legally admitted to the United States. Additionally, the revision authorized school districts to deny enrollment to students who could not produce documentation of their legal status in the United States. The Supreme Court struck down the statute and ensured that all immigrant school-age children, whether here illegally or legally, who live in the United States have the right to attend public schools. Therefore, public schools in the United States are not allowed to deny admission to schools to any student based on immigration status, require students or parents to produce evidence of their immigration status, or require Social Security numbers of students.

The third case, *Castañeda v. Pickard* (1981), was a federal court case against the school district in Raymondville, Texas. The plaintiff claimed his Mexican American children were discriminated by the school district because of their ethnicity. Reversing an initial ruling in the federal district court, the U.S. Court of Appeals for the Fifth District agreed with the plaintiff and created a set of specific criteria for quality programming and for determining whether or not a school district is following the Equal Educational Opportunity Act. This compliance test has been known as the Castañeda Test and requires the satisfaction of three criteria for ensuring quality programming for ELs. The first criterion is theory: The school programs must be based on sound educational theory or legitimate experimental strategy. The second criterion is practice: The school programs must be implemented with adequate instructional practices, resources, and staff. The last criterion is results: The school program must demonstrate its effectiveness through evaluation, not only in the teaching of English but also in the broad access to the content areas of the curriculum (Alexander & Alexander, 2018).

In the three decades since these (and other) rulings were issued, states and localities have passed numerous measures and adopted unofficial policies that sought to deny immigrant children a public education. For example, in 2011, the state of Alabama enacted a law requiring school administrators to determine the immigration status of newly enrolling students. However, a federal appellate court blocked its implementation (U.S. Department of Education & U.S. Department of Justice, 2011). Despite efforts to provide equitable educational opportunities to EL students, in general, court decisions have made it quite clear that schools must address the needs of EL students.

Building the Context for Understanding English Learners with a Communication Disorder (ELCDs)

So far, this chapter has examined several important characteristics of ELs to understand this growing student population. To understand the category of ELs who are enrolled in special education programs, particularly ELCDs, it is important to describe and analyze key terms associated with ELCDs, provide a brief demographic overview of ELCD students in preK–12 schools, and explain legislative initiatives that have influenced the education of ELs with a communication disorder (ASHA, n.d.-a, n.d.-b, 2016a).

Terminology

The term "communication disorders" encompasses speech and language disorders across the life span. A communication disorder may range in severity from mild to profound, may be developmental or acquired, and/or may demonstrate one or any combination of communication disorders. A communication disorder may result in a primary disability or it may be secondary to other disabilities (ASHA, 1993).

A speech disorder is an impairment of the articulation of fluency, speech sounds, and/or voice, whereas a language disorder is the impaired comprehension and/or use of spoken, written, and/or other symbol systems. The disorder may involve the form, content, and/or function of language in communication (Law, Boyle, Harris, Harkness, & Nye, 2000). This term, "communication sciences and disorders," has come into consistent use only since the 1980s. The term "speech pathology" has been used and recognized for much longer (Guilford, 2003; Moeller, 1976). Early pioneers in speech-language pathology came from a variety of disciplines (e.g., education, psychology, linguistics), and the blending of knowledge through research and clinical application in diagnosis and treatment of communication disorders resulted in enhancing the practice of speech-language pathology (Duchan, 2002).

Communication disorders are among the most common disabilities in the United States. In 2015 to 2016, the number of students ages 3 to 21 receiving special education services was

6.7 million, or 13% of all public school students. Among students receiving special education services, 34% had specific learning disabilities. According to the 40th Annual Report to Congress on the Implementation of Individuals with Disabilities Education Act of 2018, "speech or language impairment" was the most prevalent disability category in schools, accounting for 42.6% of all preschoolers served in 2016 (U.S. Department of Education, 2018b). For students ages 6 through 21 who were served under IDEA, "speech or language impairment" (16.8%) was the second largest category of students served in a federally supported program for the disabled after "specific learning disabilities" (38.6%) (U.S. Department of Education, 2018c). Interestingly, in a 2018 report entitled *The Condition of Education* issued by the National Center for Education Statistics, it was reported that approximately 20% of children and youth receiving services under IDEA had speech or language impairments (McFarland et al., 2018). Thus, communication disorders continue to be one of the most prevalent disability types, remaining constant around 3%, with variations of less than 1 percentage point.

School-age children who are diagnosed with a special need are often served in special education settings or receive special education services. These settings are dictated by the mandates set forth by the NCLB Act (2001). Legislation notes that services for children with special needs must be offered in the least restrictive environment (LRE). According to the federal definition, special education is specially designed instruction that is provided to children with disabilities to meet their unique needs at no cost to the parents (NCLB, 2001). This includes instruction conducted in the classroom, in the home, in hospitals and institutions, and in other settings, as well as instruction in physical education. Special education may include a related service, if the service is considered special education rather than a related service under state standards (i.e., speech-language pathology services). The content, methodology, or delivery of instruction is often adapted to meet the needs of the child with special needs and to address the unique needs of the child that result from the child's disability. This ensures that the child has access to the general curriculum, so that the child can meet educational standards. In general, special education refers to a range of educational and social services provided by various educational entities to individuals with disabilities between the ages of 3 and 21 years of age.

The 1975 Education for All Handicapped Children Act (EAHCA) and the Individuals with Disabilities Education Act (IDEA) of 1997, which came into being when the EAHCA was renamed IDEA in 1997, are two important pieces of legislation governing the identification, assessment, and instruction of students with special needs in general and ELs with special needs. They contain key terminology used to describe children with special needs. These laws do not specifically address ELs with special needs; however, they provide an exclusionary statement that cautions professionals against misidentification of ELs. Multidisciplinary teams must provide assurances that students' problems are not the result of limited English proficiency, cultural or environmental disadvantage, or lack of educational opportunity or experiences. The exclusionary clause is one of the most important safeguards for ELs being considered for special education placement.

ELs with Communication Disorders (ELCDs)

English learners with communication disorders belong to the broader category of English learners and students with special needs. English learners (ELs) with special needs include students who are learning English and have disabilities for which they receive services or supports through an Individualized Education Program (IEP) or 504 accommodations plans. ELs with IEPs include those students (a) whose native language is other than English or whose English language proficiency has been affected by another language or languages as a result of bilingualism/ multilingualism, regardless of whether they were born in the United States or abroad; (b) whose difficulties in speaking, listening, reading, or writing in the English language may be sufficient to deny them the ability to successfully achieve in classrooms where the language of instruction and assessment is English; and (c) whose disabilities represent one or more disability categories listed in Table 2–2 (Snyder, de Brey, & Dillow, 2016).

Table 2–2. List and Percentage of Disabilities

Disability	Description	Percentage
Autism	Having a developmental disability significantly affecting verbal and nonverbal communication and social interaction, generally evident before age 3 that adversely affects a child's educational performance. Other characteristics often associated with autism are engagement in repetitive activities and stereotyped movements, resistance to environmental change or change in daily routines, and unusual responses to sensory experiences.	8.3
Deaf-blindness	Having concomitant hearing and visual impairments causing such severe communication, developmental, and educational problems that the child cannot be accommodated in programs exclusively designed for the deaf or for the blind.	0.2
Developmental delay	Having developmental delays in one or more of the following areas: physical development, cognitive development, communication development, social or emotional development, or adaptive development.	6.3
Emotional disturbance	Having a condition exhibiting one or more of the following characteristics, displayed over a long period of time and to a marked degree: • An inability to learn that cannot be explained by intellectual, sensory, or health factors • An inability to build or maintain satisfactory interpersonal relationships with peers or teachers • Inappropriate types of behavior or feelings under normal circumstances • A general pervasive mood of unhappiness or depression	5.5

Table 2–2. continued

Disability	Description	Percentage
Emotional disturbance *continued*	• A tendency to develop physical symptoms or fears associated with personal or school problems	5.5
Hearing impairment	Having a hearing impairment, whether permanent or fluctuating, that is not included under the definition of deafness.	1.2
Intellectual disability	Having significantly subaverage general intellectual functioning existing concurrently with deficits in adaptive behavior and manifested during the developmental period.	6.6
Multiple disabilities	Having a combination of impairments (with the exception of deaf-blindness) causing such severe educational problems that the child cannot be accommodated in a special education program designed only for one of the impairments.	2.0
Orthopedic impairment	Having a severe orthopedic impairment (amputation, absence of a limb, cerebral palsy, poliomyelitis, bone tuberculosis, etc.).	0.9
Other health impairment	Having limited strength, vitality, or alertness due to chronic or acute health problems (heart condition, rheumatic fever, asthma, hemophilia, leukemia, etc.).	12.6
Specific learning disability	Having a disorder in one or more of the basic psychological processes involved in understanding or in using language, spoken or written, that may manifest itself in an imperfect ability to listen, think, speak, read, write, spell, or do mathematical calculations. The term includes such conditions as perceptual disabilities, brain injury,	35.0

continues

Table 2–2. *continued*

Disability	Description	Percentage
Specific learning disability *continued*	minimal brain dysfunction, dyslexia, and developmental aphasia. It does not include children who have learning problems that are primarily the result of visual, hearing, or motor disabilities; mental retardation; or environmental, cultural, or economic disadvantage.	35.0
Speech or language impairment	Having a communication disorder such as stuttering, impaired articulation, language impairment, or voice impairment.	20.6
Traumatic brain injury	Having an acquired injury to the brain caused by an external physical force, resulting in total or partial functional disability or psychosocial impairment, or both. The term applies to open or closed head injuries resulting in impairments in one or more areas, such as cognition; language; memory; attention; reasoning; abstract thinking; judgment; problem-solving; sensory, perceptual, and motor abilities; psychosocial behavior; physical functions; information processing; and speech.	0.4
Visual impairment	Having impairment in vision (including blindness) that, even with correction, adversely affects a child's educational performance. The term includes both partial sight and blindness.	0.4

In terms of identification of ELs with special needs, the Individuals with Disabilities Education Improvement Act (IDEA) (2004) states that neither "lack of appropriate instruction in reading or math" nor "limited English proficiency" can result in eligibility of any disability category (34 C.F.R. Section 614(b)(5)(C)). In addition, to prevent against misdiagnosis or overrepresentation of EL population, the assessments and other evaluation materials used to assess a child must be selected and administered so as not to be discriminatory on a racial or cultural basis (34 C.F.R. Section 614(b)(3)(A)(i)). Moreover, these materials must be administered in a professional manner by competent personnel and must use the language and form most likely to yield accurate information on what the child knows and can do academically, developmentally, and functionally, unless it is not feasible to so provide or administer (34 C.F. R. Section 614(b)(3)(A)(ii–v)).

Demographics

We have stated that in general, ELs with communication disorders are members of both English learners and students with special needs. These two groups of U.S. students face difficulties in achieving academic success in K–12 schools and beyond (e.g., college enrollment, degree completion, and employment) and are often found eligible for special education, support services, and ESL or bilingual education services. Identifying and providing access to appropriate educational opportunities for students who identified as both ELs and students with communication disorders are complex undertakings, further complicated by limited knowledge about the diverse demographics of members of this group (Trainor, Murray, & Kim, 2014). To better understand this population, it is important to look at the demographics pertaining to English learner students in preK–12 schools in general and English learners with special needs in particular.

In 2016, the number of English learners in the K–12 school system in the United States was around 4.8 million students or approximately 10% of the entire school population. This number was higher than in 2003 to 2004 (4.2 million students or 8.8%) and 2012 to 2013 (4.4 million students or 9.2%) school years (Kena et al., 2016). Most ELs in K–12 are found at the elementary level, as illustrated in Table 2–3.

Table 2–3. *English Learners Enrolled in Public Schools by Grade*

Grade Level	Percentage of ELs
Kindergarten	13.5
Grade 1	13.5
Grade 2	12.8
Grade 3	11.3
Grade 4	8.9
Grade 5	7.3
Grade 6	6.0
Grade 7	5.4
Grade 8	4.9
Grade 9	5.3
Grade 10	4.1
Grade 11	3.4
Grade 12	3.3
Ungraded	0.2

Currently, ELs are concentrated in 10 states (Kena et al., 2015), which represent more than 70% of the total number of ELs in the United States. Table 2–4 lists the 10 states with the highest number of ELs.

According to the 2018 Condition of Education (U.S. Department of Education, 2018a), of the number of ELs in K–12, Hispanic EL students constituted over three quarters (77.7%) of the EL students enrolled in the public school. Asian EL students constituted the next largest group (10.5%) of EL students, with White EL students (6.1% of EL students) and Black EL students (3.7% of EL students) following. In each of the other racial/ethnic groups for which data were collected (Pacific Islanders,

Table 2–4. *States with the Highest Number of ELs*

State	Total Number of Students	Number of ELs	Percentage of ELs
California	6,235,520	1,392,263	22.3
Texas	5,232,065	949,074	18.1
Florida	2,496,165	260,746	10.4
New York	2,649,039	217,804	8.2
Illinois	2,046,857	211,619	10.3
Georgia	1,883,387	142,334	7.6
Colorado	889,006	126,840	14.3
Washington	1,162,019	119,844	10.3
North Carolina	1,567,424	99,513	6.3
Virginia	1,273,000	97,268	7.6

American Indians/Alaska Natives, and individuals of two or more races), fewer than 40,000 students were identified as ELs.

In school year 2015 to 2016, approximately 713,000 EL students were identified as students with disabilities (U.S. Department of Education, 2018a). These students represented 14.7% of the total EL population enrolled in U.S. public elementary and secondary schools as students served under the Individuals with Disabilities Education Act (IDEA) or 504 accommodations plans (Snyder et al., 2016). Interestingly, a higher percentage of students ages 3 to 21 received special education services under IDEA for specific learning disabilities than for any other type of disability (Snyder & Dillow, 2015; U.S. Department of Education, 2018b) with speech or language impairments accounting for the next population of students receiving services.

Thus, approximately 10% of the K–12 student population is identified as EL students and receives language assistance at school. Approximately 9% of students who receive special education are identified as ELs as well (National Center on Educational Outcomes, 2011). They have one or more disability categories recognized in federal policy, with the distribution of percentages shown in Table 2–5.

As previously stated, at the federal level, the percentage of ELs with IEPs is at about 9% of all students with disabilities and below the average of general education non-EL students. However, at the state level, as seen in Table 2–6, there is quite a bit of variation when we look at the proportion of the ELs with special needs from the total number of ELs in the 10 states with the most EL concentration (Snyder et al., 2016).

Students who are ELs and have a disability are underrepresented in special education programs (Morgan et al., 2015), although there are cases of overrepresentation and great variety across states, depending on the EL population within school districts. There is evidence in some states and districts that ELs are overrepresented, particularly in the mild disability categories

Table 2–5. *Disability Categories Recognized in Federal Policy*

Disability	Percentage of ELs with Disabilities
Autism	7
Deaf-blind	6
Developmental delay	9
Emotional disturbance	3
Hearing impairment and deafness	12
Intellectual disability	9
Multiple disabilities	5
Other health impairment	5
Orthopedic impairment	12
Specific learning disability	12
Speech-language impairment	12
Traumatic brain injury	6
Visual impairment and blindness	9

Table 2–6. *Percentage of ELs with Special Needs*

State	Percentage of ELs with Special Needs
California	15.4
Texas	7.4
Florida	12.0
New York	20.8
Illinois	9.7
Georgia	8.8
Colorado	5.6
Washington	12.6
North Carolina	15.5
Virginia	17.9

(Ortiz & Artiles, 2010). EL overrepresentation in special education programs typically occurs in school districts with small EL populations, as almost 16% of EL students receive special education in these districts. On the other hand, EL underrepresentation usually happens in school districts with EL populations of 100 or more as about 9% of EL students receive special education services in these districts (Keller-Allen, 2006).

Grade levels also seem to be directly interconnected with the EL disproportionality in special education. Using a nationally representative sample of kindergarten, first-grade, and third-grade students, Samson and Lesaux (2009) investigated proportional representation, identification rates, and predictors of ELs in special education. They found ELs were underrepresented in special education in kindergarten and first grade but were overrepresented in third grade across all disability categories. This dramatic increase in representation may be an indicator that existing assessments and measures to identify ELs with disabilities properly are not valid and reliable. Sullivan (2011) identified several reasons for disproportionality of ELs in special education. First, teachers may be hesitant to refer students who are learning English for disability identification given the fact that there are similarities between linguistic difference and disorder. Second, there may be insufficient access to EL services in school districts and poorly understood educational needs. Then, as also noted by Samson and Lesaux (2009), there may be few if any nondiscriminatory, reliable, and valid assessment tools and practices specific to the EL population.

In particular, ELs continue to be both overidentified and underidentified with language disorders (Sullivan & Bal, 2013). One reason for misidentification can partially be attributed to the false notion that there is a strict dichotomy between language difference and disorder. Because funding for special education and English language learning support comes from different sources, in some school districts, children are routinely channeled to different programs to avoid "double dipping" or providing special education and English language services. This is unfortunate because children with disabilities who are ELs are entitled to appropriate educational services, including English language services and special education services (Lhamon & Gupta, 2015). Federal legislation has been instrumental in addressing and improving educational outcomes for all students with special needs.

Legislation Affecting ELs with Special Needs

Federal Legislation

There have been several efforts to ensure that special education students in general and ELs with special needs in particular have equitable access to education and receive appropriate assessment and services tailored to their needs. One crucial piece of legislation has been pivotal in addressing the needs of children with special needs: the 1975 Education for All Handicapped Children Act (EAHCA), now known as the Individuals with Disabilities Education Act (IDEA). The 1975 law was a basic bill of rights for children with disabilities; these children had to demonstrate at least one disability to qualify for special services. This legislation was developed with the purpose of providing access to educational services to students.

The 1975 law had several important provisions (EAHCA, 1975). The first provision was *Zero Reject*. This provision implied that all children, regardless of disability and severity, were provided access to free and appropriate public education (FAPE). The second provision of the law was *Nondiscriminatory Assessment*, which stipulated that students must be diagnosed using nondiscriminatory standardized evaluation to be administered in the student's native language by properly trained administrators. It is important to note that the law clearly prohibited any test to be administered in any language other than the primary language spoken by the student.

Procedural Due Process and *Parental Participation* were two more important components of the Education for All Handicapped Children Act; they guaranteed parents' participation in educational decisions affecting their children, as well as parents' protection if they disagreed with school decisions. Parents were responsible for giving permission for testing and evaluation of their children for special services, participated in deciding whether or not their child should receive special education services, and advocated for their child (Birnbaum, 2008).

Another component of the law was the *Least Restrictive Environment (LRE)*, which stated that the best placement for a child with special needs was in the regular classroom. Only when the nature or the severity of the disability prevented the student from being educated in a regular classroom should the student be placed in a more restricted setting or in an environment outside the public school classroom.

Perhaps the most important part of the EAHCA was the call for an *Individualized Education Program (IEP)*, a legal document expressly written for a student requiring special services. When students were eligible for special education services, the school was required to convene an IEP team and develop an appropriate educational plan for the child. The IEP team included the student's parents or guardians, a special education teacher, at least one general education teacher, a school or district representative with knowledge regarding the availability of school resources, a professional qualified to interpret the instructional implications of the child's evaluation results (e.g., the school psychologist), and a translator for parents with limited English proficiency. The 2004 reauthorization of IDEA required the IEP to be written to meet the needs of the student and to include the following:

- ◆ The student's current level of academic and functional performance
- ◆ A statement of annual goals, including academic and functional goals
- ◆ Procedures for evaluation of goals
- ◆ A list of special education services, related services, and supplementary aids to be provided to the student, as well as program modifications or supports provided to school personnel on behalf of the child
- ◆ The dates for the beginning of services; the frequency, duration, and location for the provision of services; and the extent to which the student is able to participate in the general curriculum
- ◆ List of accommodations to be provided during assessments that measure the student's academic and functional performance

The reauthorization of IDEA in 2004 reflected a number of amendments added between the original authorization of the Education for All Handicapped Children Act in 1975 and the current legislation. A 1986 reauthorization expanded the original legislation to cover children between ages 3 and 5, and a 1990 reauthorization encouraged the use of "person-first" language when describing disabilities. Additionally, through its 1990 amendments, for the first time IDEA specifically addressed the needs of students who are ELs and disabled.

Studies have documented apparent discrepancies in the levels of referral and placement of limited English-proficient children in special education. The Department of Education has found that services provided to limited English-proficient students often do not respond primarily to the pupils' academic needs. These trends pose special challenges for special education in the referral, assessment, and services for our nation's students from non-English language backgrounds (IDEA, 1997).

In 1991, IDEA was again reauthorized and now required the development of an *Individualized Family Service Plan (IFSP)* for children and their families between birth and age 3. This plan required information about the child's status, family information, outcomes, early intervention services, dates and duration of services, and service coordinator. The IDEA changes of 1996 served to address and protect the educational rights of students who were disabled, but challenges continued in meeting the needs of school-age ELs, especially children with communication disorders (Murdick, Gartin, & Crabtree, 2014). Subsequent reauthorizations of IDEA (IDEA, 2004) augmented and amplified requirements for students with special needs with a focus on participation and achievement in the general education curriculum, nondiscriminatory assessment that focused on disability determination rather than lack of instruction in reading or math or limited English proficiency, and appropriate identification and support services to EL and underrepresented students to achieve their potential.

Standards-Driven Assessment and Instruction: The Influence on ELs

The fact that there is a lack of valid and reliable assessment tools specific for ELs and ELCDs is of high importance in an educational context dominated by standards. In the past two decades, we have seen a constant orientation of educational initiatives and legislation toward accountability through standardized testing as well as instructional standards. The first example is represented by the No Child Left Behind Act (2001). This act put in place measures that exposed achievement gaps among traditionally underserved students and their peers with a focus on accountability. NCLB had rigorous and ambitious goals, the most important being that all public school students had to achieve grade-level proficiency in English language arts and mathematics by 2014. As a result, all states had to create testing instruments to measure the progress of all students, including ELs and ELCDs.

Because all ELs were required to learn the same content and pass the same exams as non-EL students, classroom instruction for ELs became more focused on both English language proficiency improvement and academic content learning. Before NCLB, language programs for ELs focused mainly on language proficiency, whereas general education teachers concentrated on academic goals. Because of NCLB, language program teachers started to incorporate academic content more and content-area teachers started to actively promote language proficiency development in their classrooms.

NCLB expired in 2007 and was reauthorized in 2015. Before its reauthorization, states received waivers of the 2014 proficiency deadline if they implemented several education reforms. These reforms required states to adopt common core standards for college and career readiness, improve the lowest 15% of their lowest performing schools, and create guidelines for the evaluation of teacher performance.

The Common Core State Standards (CCSS), adopted by many states, described the knowledge and skills that public school education should provide to students so that they would graduate college- and career-ready. Specifically, the CCSS advocated shared responsibility for what students were expected to learn and detailed appropriate benchmarks for all students in language and literacy across disciplines, educators, and modalities (i.e., listening, speaking, reading, and writing; Murza, Malani, & Hahs-Vaugh, 2014).

States' adoption of the CCSS has had a tremendous influence on all aspects of teaching and assessment. The CCSS have also influenced EL education. For example, WIDA (World-Class Instructional Design and Assessment), a multistate consortium focused on academic language development and academic achievement for EL students, has designed and implemented EL K–12 proficiency standards and assessments. The WIDA English Language Development (ELD) standards that promote social and instructional language as well as academic language proficiency in four content areas—language arts, mathematics, science, and social studies—have been updated to align with the CCSS. Many states have been also revising their English language proficiency standards to align them with the CCSS, creating new language proficiency assessments and providing professional development for teachers. For example, TESOL International Association, the organization devoted to advancing the expertise of professionals who teach English to speakers of other languages in multilingual contexts worldwide, has also been developing supplementary information for its language proficiency standards to show the connection between them and the CCSS.

Every Students Succeeds Act (ESSA, 2015) is the most recent education initiative replacing the previous Elementary and Secondary Education Act (ESEA) reauthorization, also known as the No Child Left Behind Act of 2001. This piece of legislation has significant implications for ELs in assessment and accountability, educational standards, teacher quality, and program innovation. ESSA has incorporated the goals of CCSS and requires that all public school students be taught to high academic standards that will prepare them to succeed in college and careers. To measure K–12 students' progress toward those high standards, ESSA has continued the requirement of annual statewide assessments so that important information is provided to educators, families, students, and communities. The law has also sustained and expanded investments in increasing access to high-quality preschool. Moreover, it has kept the expectation that there will be accountability and action in lowest performing schools where students are not making progress and graduation rates are low.

In terms of accountability and assessment, ESSA has influenced ELs in several ways. First, it has given states two options for delaying ELs' inclusion in accountability systems while they are learning English. The first option allows states to exclude ELs from taking the reading/English language arts test and from counting results of either or both the math and English language arts tests for 1 year. The second option allows states to report ELs' test results in reading/English language arts and math but exclude their results from the accountability system for the first year, include a measure of student growth on both tests for the second year, and include both tests in the accountability system for the third year of enrollment. Additionally, ELs who have attained English proficiency and are no longer part of the EL category can be included in the EL group for accountability purposes for 4 years.

Second, ELs' language proficiency and academic achievement are more included as parts of the accountability and assessment system of schools and districts. The transition of these two parts from Title III (grants to states to support the education of

English learner and immigrant students) to Title I (provision to all children with opportunity to receive a fair, equitable, and high-quality education and to close achievement gaps), while maintaining and increasing Title III funding, emphasizes the importance the law places on all ELs' academic and language needs (Pompa & Villegas, 2017).

All SLPs and educators need to be prepared to address the academic and language needs of ELCDs not only in the classroom but also when they design and implement assessment techniques, instruments, and intervention plans. ESSA has become a law that permits a great deal of flexibility and prospect for pedagogical improvement to meet the challenges ELCDs and their SLPs and teachers face in schools today.

Court Rulings

Case law concerning the linguistic and educational needs of EL students has also had a major impact on federal and state policy for EL students, their families, and their communities. Although the court rulings of *Lau v. Nichols, Plyer v. Doe*, and *Castañeda v. Pickard* did not specifically address ELs with disabilities, the rulings made it more likely that students who were ELs would not be referred to special education because of a lack of educational opportunity or appropriate instruction. An important case that specifically dealt with the identification and placement of ELs in special education programs was *Diana v. State Board of Education* (1970). Plaintiffs, on behalf of Mexican American children in Monterey County, California, complained that the school system was wrongly identifying Spanish-speaking students as mentally challenged based on IQ tests administered in English. The judge ordered that an IQ test for Mexican American children be developed and all Mexican American children who had been placed in special education be reassessed in their first language and in English, or by using nonverbal IQ tests.

Fernandez (1992) identified two other important court cases that involved ELs with special needs (Table 2–7). The first one was *Jose P. v. Ambach* (1983), which was a class action suit on behalf of students who claimed they were denied access to adequate education because of the school's failure to evaluate and place

Table 2–7. *ELs with Special Needs and the Courts*

Case	Description	Ruling
Diana v. State Board of Education (1970)	A California District Court case in which the plaintiffs, on behalf of Mexican American children, complained that IQ tests in English were unfair.	The judge ordered IQ tests to be developed in students' native language, plus students who were misplaced were reassessed.
Jose P. v. Ambach (1979)	Federal District Court class action suit where plaintiffs claimed they were denied access to educational programs due to the inability of schools to evaluate and place them in special programs.	The schools were required to use bilingual resources to identify SpEd ELs, provide bilingual nondiscriminatory evaluations, provide bilingual alternatives at each stage of special education placement process, protect the rights of parents and students, and hire community workers to help with the involvement of parents in the assessment process and development of their IEPs.
Y. S. v. School District of Philadelphia (1986)	A federal class action suit where plaintiffs claimed educational decisions were incorrect because they were based on tests developed for English speakers.	The settlement included drastic changes in evaluation, curriculum, planning, and counseling of ELs and SpEd ELs.

them in special programs. The judge ordered several measures to provide language-appropriate services. The school board was required to complete a survey of all students with disabilities, recording by language the number of those who were ELs. The judge also required the school board to put together a description of each program for students with disabilities, including bilingual programs for ELs. An outreach office was created with the purpose of distributing information in English and other languages about special education programs. Procedures were to be developed for the provision of competent interpreters for EL parents, for evaluations of EL students, and for identifying appropriate bilingual tests.

The second case, *Y. S. v. School District of Philadelphia* (1986), was a federal class action suit. Y., a Cambodian refugee, was one of the students named in the case; Y. was enrolled in ESOL courses but received no other bilingual services. Three years after enrolling in school, Y. was placed in a class for students who were mentally challenged. Plaintiffs claimed that the decision to classify Y. was incorrect, because the decision was made based on a test developed for English-speaking students. The settlement reached between plaintiffs and school district officials required the district to implement several changes. First, the placement of all EL Asian students in general and special education was reviewed. Then, a remedial plan to address the needs of such students was developed. It included evaluation and counseling in their native language, a revised curriculum for the district's ESOL program, and a special education component of the remedial plan. The district agreed to hire and train bilingual staff and to improve communication with the students. It also agreed that all oral and written communication to parents would be provided in the parents' native language.

English Learners with Communication Disorders: Trends and Challenges

Determining the population of children and adults with speech and language disorders has been problematic because there are several populations that may have communication disorders secondary to another disability (i.e., autism, learning disability) (U.S. Department of Education, 2005). Specifically, when ELs struggle academically, professionals must consider a myriad of variables to determine if a child's learning problems can be attributed to a disorder that is affecting his or her ability to acquire language skills or if the student is progressing through the stages of learning a second language.

Distinguishing between a language difference and the presence of a language disorder is often a demanding task and requires specific knowledge and competencies to accurately distinguish a communication difference from a disorder. Researchers have described possible indicators of a communication disorder in ELs, such as (a) difficulty learning language at a normal rate, even with support and assistance in both languages; (b) gaps in vocabulary and decreased mean lengths of utterances; (c) difficulties communicating with peers as well as in the home; (d) difficulty across literacy events; (e) lack of organization in the use of language to convey thoughts; and (f) poor academic achievement despite having adequate academic proficiency in English. Researchers concur that typical language abilities serve as the focal point for determining a language disorder (Blake & McLeod, 2019; Fitton et al., 2016; Harry & Klingner, 2006; Kayser, 2002; Paradis, Genesee, & Crago, 2011; Roseberry-McKibbin, 2007, 2008). The literature consistently suggests that if a student has a language disorder, he or she will usually demonstrate problems not only in English but in English and the primary language, or the acquisition of any language (Goldstein, 2004; Klingner & Eppolito, 2014; Kohnert, 2008; Martinez-Alvarez, 2019; Roseberry-McKibben, 2018).

Summary

In order to understand the larger population to which ELs with communication disorders belong, this chapter examined several important characteristics of ELs. It looked at definitions and key terms, as well as federal legislation and legal action centered on ELs. Then, in order to build the context for understanding ELs with communication disorders further, the same parameters were applied. At the end of the analysis of ELs and ELs with communication disorders in the school-age population, one idea has become very clear: The notion that English learners are a monolithic group is unmistakably false.

What, then, are the important factors that SLPs and ESOL professionals must consider when working with ELs with communication disorders?

Federal legislation is clear in its stipulations that students must be assessed using measures that are "culturally and linguistically appropriate." SLPs play a critical role in identifying whether children with limited English proficiency have an underlying communication disorder. This monumental responsibility requires that the SLPs know normal language acquisition, recognize the signs of progressing second language acquisition, and consider the indicators of a communication disorder to better understand ELs with communication disorders (ASHA, 2004a). This means that the SLP must use procedures, materials, and protocols that will reduce the likelihood that an EL student will be misdiagnosed as having a communication disorder resulting from limited English exposure.

The ESOL professional must use appropriate measures to identify students appropriately as an EL student. Both professionals must pool their expertise and resources to appropriately and accurately identify and assess EL students. To accomplish this, they must share a knowledge base and work collaboratively to identify EL students, as well as to determine whether there is a language disorder or a language difference.

Given the importance of ensuring that ELs and ELs with communication disorders are appropriately identified and provided with appropriate education, it is critical to understand the professional preparation and characteristics of two professionals, the SLP and ESOL providers, that serve EL and ELCD students—in particular, the competencies of each, their respective roles and responsibilities, and how they influence educational decisions and student language and learning outcomes. The following chapter provides an overview of both disciplines and discusses EL students from the perspective of each of the disciplines.

3

English Learners—
Perspective from
Two Disciplines

Introduction

The discipline of communication sciences and disorders (CSD) includes the study of the human communication process, the science of human communication, breakdowns in the processes of human communication (referred to as communication differences or disorders), and the efficacy of the applied disciplinary practices (Guilford, Graham, & Scheuerle, 2007). Three primary professions are represented under the umbrella term "communication sciences and disorders." These include speech, language, and hearing sciences; audiology; and speech-language pathology. Other disciplines, such as deafness and deaf education, are often included as related areas of practice because many of these professionals develop and apply educational and rehabilitative techniques for individuals with severe and profound hearing impairments (Gillam & Marquardt, 2015; Guilford, 2003).

What Is the Profession of
Communication Sciences and Disorders?

The term "speech-language pathology" has primarily been used to describe the role of professionals primarily concerned with individuals who could not communicate. Early efforts in establishing the professional discipline of speech-language pathology came from psychology, education, medical science, and linguistics. Currently, this professional field focuses on the prevention, etiology, diagnosis, prognosis, and treatment of communication delays, disorders, or differences across the scope of practice (ASHA, 2007). The term "communication sciences and disorders" has consistently been used since the 1980s. It is offered as a program of study in approximately 300 U.S. graduate programs in the discipline; however, not all of these programs offer both speech-language pathology and audiology degrees.

Speech-language pathology is a dynamic and continuously developing profession. The goal of the profession of speech-language pathology and its members is the provision of the highest quality treatment and other services consistent with the fundamental right of those served to participate in decisions that affect their lives (ASHA, 2016a; Lubinski & Fratteli, 2001). Over the past 25 years, the client populations, work settings, and assessment and treatment methods have changed dramatically. Passage of educational legislation (i.e., Individuals with Disabilities Education Act [IDEA] and No Child Left Behind [NCLB]) focusing on the rights of school-age children have had a strong impact on the profession. Additionally, legislation focusing on individuals with disabilities and their communicative needs has resulted in the establishment of comprehensive diagnostic and treatment procedures for individuals across the life span.

An important characteristic of the practice of speech-language pathology is that, to the extent possible, clinical decisions are based on the best available evidence (Douglas & Burshnic, 2019). ASHA has defined evidence-based practice in speech-language pathology as an approach in which current, high-quality research evidence is integrated with practitioner expertise and the individual's preferences and values into the process of clinical decision making (ASHA, 2004a, 2005a). A high-quality basic, applied, and efficacy research base in communication sciences and disorders and related fields of study is essential to providing evidence-based clinical practice and quality clinical services (Campbell & Douglas, 2017).

Currently, SLPs provide services in settings that are deemed appropriate, including but not limited to health care, educational, community, vocational, home settings, and private practices (ASHA, n.d.-a, 2016b). As of 2018, more than half of SLPs (54.2%) are employed in educational settings, including 51.4% in schools and 2.7% in colleges and universities. An additional 39.3% are employed in health care settings, including 17.1% in nonresidential health care facilities, 12.5% in hospitals, and 9.7% in residential health care facilities. More than one fifth (21.1%) are employed full- or part-time in private practice (ASHA, 2019b).

Professional Association—American Speech-Language-Hearing Association (ASHA)

The American Speech-Language-Hearing Association (ASHA) is the professional, credentialing, and scientific organization for SLPs, audiologists, and speech/language/hearing scientists in the United States and internationally. Founded in 1925, it currently provides an array of membership services and has numerous scholarly journals and publications, special-interest divisions, and educational activities that support lifelong learning to its current 191,675 members (ASHA, 2019c). The purpose, nature, and scope of ASHA can be found in its bylaws (ASHA, 2017a) and governance structure (see ASHA governance chart at https://www.asha.org/uploadedFiles/ASHA-Governance-Structure.pdf).

The competencies needed by SLPs and audiologists are essential if patients and clients are to receive appropriate and quality care. Competencies are based on the professional body of knowledge and application of this knowledge to the assessment and treatment of individuals with communication disorders (Ehren, Lefkowitz, & Roth, 1997). SLPs must have the requisite knowledge, specialized skills, and techniques to work with a diverse population across the life span and settings. Graham and Guilford (2000) offer a model of clinical expertise that outlines five factors and associated indicators often cited as critical to the development of expertise within the profession. These five factors include interpersonal skills, professional skills, problem-solving skills, technical skills, and knowledge and experience. Although expertise in speech-language pathology is a broad concept, Graham (1998) notes that the factors and associated indicators represented in their model provide an overview of the competencies necessary for all SLPs in the development of expertise in the profession of speech-language pathology.

One important role served by ASHA is the assurance that newly certified SLPs entering independent professional practice have the relevant clinical activities, professional skills, and knowledge areas to provide optimum services to individuals with communication disorders. Specifically, the Council on Academic Accreditation in Audiology and Speech-Language Pathology (CAA) of the American Speech-Language-Hearing Association is the accrediting agency for audiology and speech-language pathology education programs. In general, they formulate standards for the accreditation of graduate education programs that provide entry-level professional preparation in audiology and/ or speech-language pathology (CAA, 2017). The Council for Clinical Certification in Audiology and Speech-Language Pathology (CFCC), a semiautonomous credentialing body of ASHA, is charged with defining the standards for clinical certification, applying those standards in granting certification to individuals, withdrawing certification in cases where certification was granted on the basis of inaccurate information, and administering the certification maintenance program (CFCC, 2013).

Graduates of an accredited program in speech-language pathology require academic and clinical education that reflects current knowledge, skills, technology, and scope of practice. The ASHA 2014 Standards required students to demonstrate that they had acquired a specific set of knowledge and skills standards through participation in their graduate program. Every academic program accredited by the CAA required graduates to demonstrate that they possessed a core set of knowledge and skills necessary to qualify for state and national credentials for independent professional practice. Thus, for ASHA Standards IV (the knowledge portion) and V (the skills portion), the emphasis focused on the acquisition of knowledge and skills, not on completion of specific course work. The Skills portion relating to clinical competencies across nine specific areas, often referred to as "the Big Nine" are outlined in Table 3–1.

In 2016, revisions were made to the 2014 ASHA standards. Specifically, the revisions expanded the definition of supervised clinical experiences, allowed students to obtain up to 20% (i.e.,

Table 3–1. *ASHA Standards for Speech-Language Pathology, Standard IV-C (2014)*

Std. IV-C: The applicant must have demonstrated knowledge of communication and swallowing disorders and differences, including the appropriate etiologies, characteristics, anatomical/physiological, acoustic, psychological, developmental, and linguistic and cultural correlates in the following areas:

"Big Nine" Clinical Areas	
Clinical Area	Descriptor
Articulation	Articulation and phonology
Fluency	Fluency, stuttering
Voice	Voice and resonance, including respiration and phonation
Language	Receptive and expressive language (phonology, morphology, syntax, semantics, and pragmatics) in speaking, listening, reading, writing, and manual modalities
Hearing	Hearing, including the impact on speech and language
Swallowing	Swallowing (oral, pharyngeal, esophageal, and related functions, including oral function for feeding; orofacial myofunction)
Cognitive aspects	Cognitive aspects of communication (attention, memory, sequencing, problem solving, executive functioning)
Social aspects	Social aspects of communication (including challenging behavior, ineffective social skills, lack of communication opportunities)
Communicative modalities	Communication modalities (including oral, manual, augmentative, and alternative communication techniques and assistive technologies)

Source: Council for Clinical Certification in Audiology and Speech-Language Pathology of the American Speech-Language-Hearing Association. (n.d.). 2016 Revisions to the 2014 Standards for the Certificate of Clinical Competence in Speech-Language Pathology. Retrieved from http://www.asha.org/Certification/2014-Speech-Language-Pathology-Certification-Standards/. All rights reserved. Adapted with permission.

59

75 hours) of direct contact hours using alternative clinical experiences (e.g., standardized patients, virtual patients, digitized mannequins, immersive reality, task trainers, computer-based interactive), and established clinical fellowship (CF) report due dates. In 2017, ASHA partnered with the Council for Clinical Certification (CFCC) and the Council on Academic Accreditation in Audiology and Speech-Language Pathology (CAA) to conduct a practice and curriculum analysis. The goal of this study was to determine if the current academic and clinical standards for speech-language pathology and the ASHA certification process accurately reflected the current state-of-the-art in speech-language pathology. The analysis was used to inform the CAA and CFCC on the academic and clinical standards for the profession of speech-language pathology and the content and weighting of the national Praxis® examination (ASHA, 2017a). The outcome of this analysis resulted in changes to the 2016 ASHA standards. The revisions to the standards and implementation procedures for the CCC in speech-language pathology are now in effect (January 1, 2020), and are referred to as the 2020 ASHA standards (CFCC, 2018).

A summary of the 2020 changes to the speech-language pathology standards includes:

- Changes in requirements to serve as Clinical supervisors and Clinical Fellowship mentors.
- Course requirements that require knowledge in basic physics or chemistry.
- Changes in knowledge and skills within the current nine core content areas (e.g., speech sound production, fluency disorders, literacy, and feeding) (Table 3–2).
- Incorporating interprofessional education and interprofessional practice into their clinical practicum and clinical fellowship experience.
- Earning one of their 30 required certification maintenance hours (CMHs) in Ethics.

After completion of academic course work and practica, graduates must pass the national examination adopted by ASHA (i.e., PRAXIS) for purposes of certification in speech-language pathology. The student must also successfully complete a 36-week

Table 3–2. *ASHA Standards for Speech-Language Pathology, Standard IV-C (2020)*

Std. IV-C: The applicant must have demonstrated knowledge of communication and swallowing disorders and differences, including the appropriate etiologies, characteristics, anatomical/physiological, acoustic, psychological, developmental, and linguistic and cultural correlates in the following areas:

"Big Nine" Clinical Areas	
Clinical Area	**Descriptor**
Speech sound production	To encompass articulation, motor planning and execution, phonology, and accent modification
Fluency	Fluency and fluency disorders
Voice/resonance	Voice and resonance, including respiration and phonation
Language	Receptive and expressive language to include phonology, morphology, syntax, semantics, pragmatics (language use and social aspects of communication), prelinguistic communication, paralinguistic communication (e.g., gestures, signs, body language), and literacy in speaking, listening, reading, and writing
Hearing	Including the impact on speech and language
Swallowing/feeding	Including structure and function of orofacial myology, oral, pharyngeal, laryngeal, pulmonary, esophageal, gastrointestinal, and related functions across the life span
Cognitive aspects of communication	Including attention, memory, sequencing, problem solving, and executive functioning
Social aspects of communication	Including challenging behavior, ineffective social skills, and lack of communication opportunities
Augmentative and alternative communication modalities	Augmentative and alternative communication modalities

Source: Council for Clinical Certification in Audiology and Speech-Language Pathology of the American Speech-Language-Hearing Association. (2018). *2020 Standards for the Certificate of Clinical Competence in Speech-Language Pathology.* Retrieved from https://www.asha.org/certification/2020-SLP-Certification-Standards. All rights reserved. Adapted with permission.

Speech-Language Pathology Clinical Fellowship (CF). Upon successful completion of the CF, the clinical fellow is awarded the Certificate of Clinical Competence (CCC) in Speech-Language Pathology by the CAA (2017).

Although the credential issued by ASHA is the CCC professional certification, licenses issued by governmental agencies are usually required for SLPs who work in settings such as schools or health care agencies. ASHA's Certificate of Clinical Competence in Speech-Language Pathology (CCC-SLP) is a nationally recognized professional credential that serves as a mark of excellence in the SLP profession and a standard licensing requirement in a number of states. Even in states where the CCC-SLP is not a requirement for licensure, it is still considered the gold-standard credential for speech-language pathologists in all practice settings. Maintenance of the CCC requires that the licensee participate in continuing education to maintain currency and continues to uphold the standards of practice acceptable to the profession. To facilitate continuing professional development, ASHA publishes a number of scholarly journals and newsletters, offers continuing education opportunities (e.g., annual convention, seminars, webinars, self-study), has 19 special-interest divisions representing specific areas of practice, maintains a website (http://www.asha.org), and offers ASHA members and/or certificate holders the Award for Continuing Education (ACE) by the Continuing Education Board (CEB) in recognition of continued professional study.

To ensure that the standards for practice are followed, ASHA requires that every individual who is (a) a member of the American Speech-Language-Hearing Association, whether certified or not; (b) a nonmember holding the Certificate of Clinical Competence from ASHA; (c) an applicant for membership or certification; or (d) a clinical fellow seeking to fulfill standards for certification abide by the ASHA Code of Ethics (ASHA, 2016b, 2016c). Adherence to the standards ensures the welfare of the consumer and protects the reputation and integrity of the professions. Ultimately, SLPs must be knowledgeable about the Code of Ethics and scope of practice, as these are essential for professional development and practice. ASHA's Practice Policy Documents, along with other important documents of the association, provide SLPs with direction on best practices and standards in the profession (Davidson & Denton, 2010).

ASHA Practice Policy Documents

ASHA has published a multitude of documents and policy statements that outline the competencies associated with the various needs (disorders or conditions) of persons being served. These documents detail the scope of practice, the necessary precautions (educational and training), and the knowledge and skills needed to meet the unique needs of individuals with communication disorders across settings and the life span. ASHA has drafted many practice policy statements and standards that provide (or have provided) the SLP with guidelines for practice across populations and settings. For example, with the ever-increasing diversity in schools, SLPs are required to work with other professionals to ensure that all students receive quality, culturally competent services. In various ASHA professional issue statements on the role and responsibility of SLPs in the schools, SLPs are required to "provide quality, culturally competent services, develop competencies to distinguish a language disorder from a language difference, address the impact of language differences and second language acquisition on student learning, and, provide support to teachers in promoting efficient and effective outcomes for students" (ASHA, 2010a, 2016c).

The advent of groundbreaking research on culturally and linguistically diverse (CLD) populations in the early 1980s marked the beginning of the distinction between communication differences and disorders (Saad & Polovoy, 2009). As the difference versus disorders research increased, a series of ASHA position papers, guidelines, and technical reports specific to providing culturally and linguistically appropriate services were developed (e.g., *Social Dialects Position Paper* [ASHA, 1983]; *Clinical Management of Communicatively Handicapped Minority Language Populations* [ASHA, 1985]; *Bilingual SLPs and Audiologists: Definition* [ASHA, 1989]; provision of instruction in English as a second language by speech-language pathologists in school settings [ASHA, 1998a, 1998b]; *Knowledge and Skills Needed by Speech Language Pathologists and Audiologists to Provide Culturally and Linguistically Appropriate Services* [ASHA, 2004b]; The Clinical Education of Students with Accents [ASHA, 1998c, 1998d, 2011b]). To date, several of these guidelines have been rescinded (e.g., *Bilingual SLPs and Audiologists: Definition* [ASHA, 1989]; *Knowledge and Skills Needed by Speech Language Pathologists and Audiologists to Provide Culturally and Linguistically Appropriate Services* [ASHA, 2004b]), but ASHA maintains a Practice Portal that contains information on professional and clinical issues and evidence maps pertaining to working with bilingual client/patient populations (see https://www.asha.org/practice-portal). The evidence maps (organized by disorder) provide a summary of clinical research from systematic reviews and guidelines.

Additionally, ASHA's Office of Multicultural Affairs (OMA) became responsible for (a) addressing cultural and linguistic diversity and inclusion issues related to professionals and persons with communication disorders and differences, (b) disseminating information and providing expert information on current events and resources, and (c) promoting quality service to historically underrepresented, bilingual, and other culturally diverse populations (age, gender, sexual orientation) and persons with disabilities.

Knowledge and Competencies for SLPS Who Work with ELs

The growing population of ELs in U.S. schools has been well documented. Nearly one in five Americans speaks a language other than English at home, and almost 45% of U.S. teachers have at least one student designated as an EL in their classrooms. There is a critical shortage of school SLPs prepared to meet the specialized needs of ELs with disabilities (Rosa-Lugo, Mihai, & Nutta, 2017; Roth, 2015). Students learning English are disadvantaged by lack of skilled personnel to conduct linguistically and culturally relevant educational assessments (Bedore, Peña, Garcia, & Cortez, 2005; Hammer, Detwiler, Detwiler, Blood, & Dean Qualls, 2004; Kimble, 2013; Klingner et al., 2005; Mattes & Saldana-Illingworth, 2009; National Association for Bilingual Education & ILIAD Project, 2002; Pieretti & Roseberry-McKibben, 2016). There is also a critical need to incorporate effective pedagogical strategies for university students in communication sciences and disorders to address ELs' language and disability-related needs simultaneously (Caesar & Kohler, 2007; Guiberson & Atkins, 2012; Kohnert, 2008; Rosa-Lugo & Fradd, 2000; Rosa-Lugo, Rivera, & McKeown, 1998).

In Chapter 2, we discussed the diversity among EL students and the heterogeneity within the EL population. Research on fair, valid, and effective assessment has brought into question existing classification policies and practices for determining which students require English language services and which students have speech and language disorders (Abedi, 2008; Goldstein, 2004; Kayser, 2002; Kohnert, 2008). We indicated that English learners with communication disorders belong to the broader categories of English learners and students with special needs. Determining the population of children and adults with speech and language disorders among ELs remains challenging. SLPs continue to have difficulty distinguishing between a language difference and an underlying language impairment (Collier, 2011; Guiberson, Rodriguez, & Dale, 2011; Roseberry-McKibbin, 2018) in part due to the lack of appropriate assessment instruments and the tasks inherent in the assessment process (Caesar & Kohler, 2007; Guiberson & Atkins, 2012; Hammer et al., 2004).

Research continues to demonstrate that SLPs rely on the use of standardized assessment instruments to assess the language abilities of EL students and determine disability despite their limitations (Kimble, 2013; Kritikos, 2003). Often, administration of these tests is most likely only in English or requires the use of an interpreter; therefore, the knowledge and skills in all the students' languages are not measured. As a result, critical data from which to make sound educational decisions are not available and can lead to over- or under identification of ELs with disabilities. Thus, decisions to determine eligibility for special education must be based on the presence of a speech-language impairment in L1, not the child's limited English proficiency (Ireland & Conrad, 2016).

Approximately 20 years ago, ASHA adopted a resolution that "encouraged undergraduate, graduate and continuing education programs to include specific information, course content and/or clinical practica that address the communication needs of individuals within socially, culturally, economically and linguistically diverse populations" (ASHA, 1987). In response to the need to serve an increasingly diverse population, ASHA mandated that, as of January 1, 1993, accredited graduate programs in communication sciences and disorders must offer course content pertaining to culturally diverse groups (ASHA, 1992). The goal was to ensure that SLPs develop the knowledge and competencies to identify and serve ELs with communication disorders and clients who speak nonstandard dialects (ASHA, 1983, 2003a; Edwards et al. 2014; Evans, Munson, & Edwards, 2018; Horton-Ikard, Munoz, Thomas-Tate, & Keller-Bell, 2009), as well as to continue to increase the percentage of ASHA professionals from underrepresented groups, which to date continues to remain low (ASHA, 2019d). Embedded in the ASHA standards and scope of practice is the requirement to utilize culturally and linguistically appropriate assessment protocols and provide culturally and linguistically appropriate services (ASHA, 2016b, 2016c).

The roles and responsibilities of school-based SLPs have changed over the years in response to legislative, regulatory, societal, and professional influences. Schools are striving to meet the various mandates and current revisions of leaving no child behind, despite the challenges associated with teaching students from multiple cultural, linguistic, and experiential backgrounds, including those who are new to the English language. The responsibility of determining whether a student's academic difficulties stem from learning a second language, the presence of a disability, or both requires that SLPs have the expertise to facilitate the necessary changes that would move the profession "from past practice patterns to those that reflect current legislation, research, and practice guidelines" with respect to practice in the school setting, specifically with underrepresented populations (ASHA, 2010a, 2016e; Caesar & Kohler, 2007; Rosa-Lugo & Champion, 2007; Roseberry-McKibben, 2015).

The current educational context of speech-language services calls for SLPs to provide support to students with disabilities and, as appropriate, to learners who are at risk for school failure. This requires that SLPs are knowledgeable about general curricular goals and benchmarks and skilled in more educationally relevant approaches that support and reflect content-area learning for ELs (ASHA, 2001; Mihai, 2010; Nutta, Bautista, & Butler, 2010; Watson & Bellon-Harn, 2013).

In 1998, ASHA issued a position statement and technical report entitled *Provision of Instruction in English as a Second Language by SLPs in School Settings* (1998a, 1998b). This position paper noted that, increasingly, SLPs are being requested to work in a role traditionally assigned to instructors of ESOL. Due to the growing population of students who are ELs and the increasing requests for SLPs to function in this role, SLPs requested clarification on their role in working with ELs in the school setting. ASHA's position statement clearly indicates that ESOL instruction should be provided *only* by professionals with appropriate training and experience. ESOL instruction requires academic preparation and experience in such areas as second language acquisition theory, comparative linguistics, ESOL methodologies, assessment, and practica. ASHA recognized that the required knowledge, skills, and competencies for providing such service may extend beyond those provided in CSD preservice educational training program; thus, they recommended that SLP and ESOL professionals work collaboratively in the preassessment, assessment, and intervention stage of service in the language and academic development of ELs with communication disorders. This paper set the stage for SLPs to self-reflect on their knowledge and competencies to work with EL students and particularly CDEL students. It also emphasized the importance of collaboration with professionals with expertise in working with EL students.

Interestingly, in 2007, Teachers of English to Speakers of Other Languages (TESOL) issued a position statement on *The Identification of English Language Learners with Special Educational Needs*. This position paper acknowledged that identifying ELs with special needs is a complex and difficult process and requires culturally responsive expertise and purposeful collaboration (TESOL, 2007a). In this age of changing demographics, SLPs are not exempt from the possibility of being asked to provide services to ELs. As a result, SLPs and ESOL professionals are being tapped to respond to the call for new collaborative roles and responsibilities in identifying and serving ELCDs (Pawan & Ortloff, 2011; Rosa-Lugo & Champion, 2007; Rosa-Lugo & Fradd, 2000; Rosa-Lugo, Mihai, & Nutta, 2017; Roseberry-McKibben, 2003, 2008a).

Service Delivery Models for ELCDs

The choice of effective service delivery is a major challenge for school-based SLPs. In general, one of the greatest challenges of school-based SLPs is how to deliver speech-language services in a way that results in the most change in students within the daily schedule and logistics of the school environment (Flynn, 2010). A service delivery model is often conceptualized as an organized configuration of resources to achieve a particular educational outcome. It must address questions such as: Where will the service be delivered? Who will deliver the service? How frequently will the service be provided? And for how long?

Service delivery in the schools (Blosser & Kratcoski, 1997; Moore & Montgomery, 2008; Paul, Blosser, & Jakubowitz, 2006; Peters-Johnson, 1998; Throneburg, Calvert, Strum, Paramboukas, & Paul, 2000; Whitmire, 2002) has evolved over the years and dramatically influenced the role of school-based SLPs. In 1997, Blosser and Kratcoski chronicled speech-language delivery models over three decades and posed a framework for decision making and service delivery that would take into consideration the provider, the activities, and the context (PACs) necessary to meet the needs of individuals with a communication disorder. With changes in education and health care reform and advances in technology, the role of the SLP and in-service delivery has broadened. There is a call for (a) more consumer involvement in planning and implementing treatment, (b) increased account-ability and use of evidence-based practice, (c) expanded alter-nate service delivery options, (d) use of telecommunications technology to deliver speech-language services remotely, and (e) clarification of the competencies and skills needed to be a qualified service provider, especially in working with ELCDs.

In 2001, a national survey of speech-language pathologists across the United States was conducted to determine current conditions regarding service delivery to ELCDs. The SLPs identi-fied several concerns. Specifically, they noted that inappropri-ate assessment instruments were major constraints in providing effective services. Unfortunately, many experienced SLPs as well as recent graduates noted that they had limited opportunities to work with ELs or their families and were not prepared to collaborate with interpreters (Roseberry-McKibben, Brice, & O'Hanlon, 2004). A primary concern expressed by SLPs was that they were not able to communicate with the student because they didn't speak the language of the student (Pham, Kohnert, & Mann, 2011; Roninson, 2003; Roseberry-McKibben, O'Hanlon, & Brice, 2004). This has major implications for SLPs who are expected to provide educational programs and clinical services for ELCDs. A key question often expressed by practitioners is "in what language do I provide treatment?"

Currently, there continues to be a lack of consensus regarding language choice in intervention with bilingual children (Gutierrez-Clellan,1999; Summers, Smith, Mueller, Alexander, & Muzza, 2017). Some scholars advocate the use of a variety of bilingual approaches (often known in the literature as "additive bilingualism") (Bruck, 1985; Cummins, 1991; Krashen, 1994), while others subscribe to the use of English only in intervention (also referred to as "subtractive bilingualism") (Karniol, 1992). Although the literature examining the effects of bilingual approaches with ELs is extensive, there is limited research on the effectiveness of these approaches with ELCDs. Nonetheless, the studies that have examined outcomes of bilingual approaches with children with special needs suggest that intervention approaches may be most effective when they are designed to broaden, rather than reduce, the child's linguistic resources (Gutierrez-Clellan, 1999).

Speech-language pathologists have traditionally provided services to school-age children in the public schools using a variety of service delivery mechanisms (Moore & Montgomery, 2017).

One of the most common service delivery method used by speech-language pathologists is the pull-out model. In this model, speech-language pathologists often work independently as they pull students out of their regular classrooms for individual or small-group treatment sessions. While several alternate direct (e.g., itinerant services, such as the traditional pull-out model; the resource room model, or several types of classroom-based approaches) and indirect service delivery models (e.g., consultative/collaborative) have been discussed in the literature (Archibald, 2017; Brandel & Loeb, 2011; Cirrin et al., 2010; Flynn, 2010; Friend & Cook, 2010; Giess & Serianni, 2018; Katz, Maag, Fallon, Blenkarn, & Smith, 2010; Moore & Montgomery, 2008; Pershey, & Rapking, 2003; Suleman, McFarlane, Pollock, Schneider,

Leroy, & Skoczylas, 2014; Schooling, Venediktov, & Leech, 2010), there continue to be few changes in service delivery options. This can, in part, be due to the lack of evidence-based research that can provide SLPs with guidance on the most effective service delivery models, dosage, and intensity for speech and language interventions (Cirrin et al., 2010). To date, most research has provided theoretical frameworks to guide SLPs (ASHA, 2000; Ukrainetz et al., 2009), but very few studies have reported on the efficacy of particular service delivery and/or intervention practices with bilingual children. While no single model is appropriate for all students, it is important that SLPs understand the range of service delivery models and the advantages and limitations of each model (Nippold, 2012). Applying research methods to systematically document treatment outcomes is sorely needed to establish empirical evidence for best practice with ELCDs (Brandel & Loeb, 2011; Kohnert & Derr, 2004; Kohnert & Medina, 2009).

The two primary goals of providing services to ELCDs are to (a) to conduct appropriate assessments and (b) to design culturally responsive intervention approaches to minimize the extent of the functional impact of the disorder (ASHA, 2016b). Ideally, bilingual clinicians who have native or near-native proficiency in the target language and the clinical expertise should be the service provider for ELCDs. However, the number of languages used and the number of individuals who require services in a language other than spoken English far exceed the capacity of bilingual service providers to accommodate them. In the absence of a bilingual SLP, it is acceptable to use an interpreter who has the skills to work with the clinician to provide language support for services appropriate to the client's communication disorder (ASHA, n.d.-b). However, it is critical that SLPs be familiar with the policies and procedures for accessing interpreters in their work setting, as well as the protocols and best practices for the use of their services (ASHA, n.d.-e; Langdon & Cheng, 2002; Langdon & Saenz, 2016; Rosa-Lugo & Abreu, 2017). For example, Langdon and Saenz (2016b) discuss the importance of their "briefing, interaction, and debriefing (BID)" process in the preparation of interpreters to collaborate in the assessment or treatment of ELs or ELCDs.

Thus, to specifically serve ELCDs, service delivery models will have to incorporate culturally and linguistic appropriate approaches that are evidence based. SLPs will have to consider the use of nonbiased assessment, the role of the native language, the use of interpreters in intervention, accents and dialects spoken by ELs, evidence-based interventions, and ways to successfully collaborate with professionals and families who are culturally competent and/or culturally and linguistically diverse (Moore & Montgomery, 2008; Ortiz & Yates, 2001; Thordardottir, 2010).

Given the many activities that school-based SLPs are required to accomplish (i.e., diagnostic assessments, intervention, in-class collaboration, supporting literacy, consultation with other school professionals), the issue of caseload and workload has also been considered (Moore & Montgomery, 2008). The term "workload" refers to all activities required and performed by school-based SLPs and other professionals (ASHA, 2002a). Caseload (or the number of students served) is just one part of the SLP's workload and typically refers to the number of students with Individualized Education Programs (IEPs) or Individualized Family Service Plans (IFSPs) that school SLPs serve through direct and/or indirect service delivery options. Several methods and strategies have been recommended for developing a workload approach to service delivery to ensure that SLPs can engage in the required workload activities and implement best practices in school speech-language pathology to meet the individual needs of students (ASHA, 2002a, 2003b; Giess, 2010).

The Individuals with Disabilities Education Improvement Act of 2004 also allows services for students who are having academic difficulties but are not identified as having a disability. This initiative, known as response to intervention (RtI), is an alternative to the use of a discrepancy model to assess underachievement. This model, also known in the literature as a prevention model (Schraeder, 2008), uses a multitiered approach to provide a seamless system of instruction and interventions to struggling learners at increasing levels of intensity guided by child outcome data. RtI and dynamic assessment (DA) are examples of early intervening approaches that have been recommended for use to determine if speech and language patterns are the result of a normal phenomenon of second language acquisition or the result of a communication disorder (ASHA, 2016e; Rosa-Lugo & Esparza-Brown, 2011; Rosa-Lugo, Rivera, & Rierson, 2010)

Esparza-Brown and Doolittle (2008) proposed an RtI model for use with ELs that calls for collaboration among professionals and increased opportunities for professional dialogue. They outlined a three-tiered framework that considers students' ecologies and cultural and linguistic needs in addition to the skills that professionals must possess when working with an EL student. Rinaldi and Samson (2008) support the use of a three-tiered RtI model with ELs and suggest that professionals use a data-driven decision-making process to inform assessment and implementation of evidence-based interventions and to determine disability in ELs. Ultimately, SLPs play an important role in using RtI to identify ELs with disabilities and to provide instruction to students who are struggling in the general education setting. These roles have required some fundamental changes in the way SLPs engage in assessment and intervention activities (Ehren, Montgomery, Rudebusch, & Whitmore, 2006) and in particular with EL students (Esparza-Brown & Sanford, 2011).

The current climate of accountability requires SLPs to apply evidence-based practice (EBP) when making assessment and intervention decisions. Specific to ELs, SLPs must identify and execute the most ethical and appropriate services. However, making clinical decisions for ELs and their families can be challenging. Selecting the language of instruction (Gutierrez-Clellan, 1999; Nixon, McCardle, & Leos, 2007; Schiff-Myers, 1992), using interpreters (Langdon & Cheng, 2002), acknowledging accents and dialects (ASHA, 2003b; Langdon, 1999; Wilkinson & Payne, 2005), and working with families are all factors that influence service provision to ELs (Caesar & Kohler, 2007; Moore & Montgomery, 2008; Roseberry-McKibben, 2018). A decision-making framework to assist the SLP select and implement a culturally and linguistically appropriate service delivery model has been recommended by Chabon, Esparza-Brown, and Gildersleeve Neumann (2010). This systematic approach proposes that SLPs should (a) examine relevant evidence and clinical expertise; (b) consider the perspectives, values, and beliefs of the individuals involved; and (c) evaluate all data in relation to the ASHA Code of Ethics (2010a) in order to identify and implement the most ethical and appropriate services.

Although a number of recommendations have been provided within the discipline of communication sciences and disorders, Cirrin et al. (2010) concluded that clinicians had little research evidence on which to base decisions about service delivery options for ELs with CDs. Furthermore, as highlighted in Kangas's (2014) ethnographic study on the delivery of services to EL students with disabilities, ESL and disability-related services were in tension with one another specifically in four factors: scheduling, school culture, teacher expertise, and ESL program models. Within the school day, there were challenges scheduling ESL services to ELs with disabilities due to the complex school schedules of children who required related services such as occupational counseling and speech-language therapy in addition to other general education classes. Interestingly, findings suggested that although practitioners were expected to provide ESL services through accommodations in the general education classroom, many practitioners were not aware of the importance of ESL education or did not possess adequate knowledge of ESL to provide appropriate support to ELs with disabilities. The findings of this study shed light on the importance of instruction that addresses both disability and L2 educational needs of ELs with disabilities. The researcher concluded that ESL services were somehow less legally significant when compared to special education; that is, when ESL and special education are in conflict, "special education legislation apparently trumps ESL legislation" (Kangas, 2014). Nonetheless, when one service was prioritized over the other—regardless of the service—ELs with disabilities' needs were not being fully met. This study concluded that there was a critical need to consider how schools can provide services to ELs with disabilities that adequately addressed both their linguistic and disability-related needs.

In the absence of conclusive data on providing services to ELs with CDs, it is imperative that we look to other disciplines such as general and special education, linguistics, and bilingual education or English as a second language (ESL) to provide us with additional data and resources. Specifically, the 1998 ASHA position paper on the role of SLPs working with ESL professionals in school settings set the beginning groundwork for a collaborative process for both professionals to merge their skills and knowledge to facilitate learning outcomes and language proficiency in ELs (ASHA, 1998a, 1998b). Therefore, it is critical that SLPs understand this discipline and the skills and competencies of the ESOL professional.

English Learners—Perspectives of the ESOL Professionals

The field of English for Speakers of Other Languages (ESOL) is grounded in the discipline of second language acquisition (SLA). This area of study combines research and theory in a variety of fields to address how languages other than the native (first) language are learned. Linguistics has historically been the foundation of SLA research and theory. This is fitting as SLA examines language, specifically language acquired after acquisition of the native tongue. Scholars in the areas of applied linguistics, psycholinguistics, and sociolinguistics have been the primary developers of SLA theory, but disciplines such as cognitive psychology, literacy studies, and critical pedagogy, among others, have also influenced the direction of SLA. Second language acquisition encompasses not only ESOL but also any other language learned after the first. In other words, researching how an American exchange student learns Spanish in Colombia or a German high school student learns French in Berlin is also the focus of SLA. However, there are specific issues that pertain to the context of teaching ESOL.

Like any other subject matter, ESOL has an abundance of jargon and acronyms. Just as ELs must learn new vocabulary to communicate in English, professionals need to know the language of ESOL. The term "ESOL" refers to both a subject and an instructional approach. ESOL as a subject is a sequence of increasingly complex linguistic competencies, involving both comprehension and expression. The aim of the subject of study is to become fully proficient in listening, speaking, reading, and writing the language. In other words, the target is to be nativelike in proficiency. For example, being able to understand the question, "What is your name?" and being able to state an appropriate response would be a typical early competency. Furthermore, being able to correctly use comparative and superlative adjectives such as "more advantageous than" and "the most advantageous" would be a more advanced competency in an ESOL course. School districts also treat ESOL as an instructional approach or intervention, meaning that common types of accommodations and modifications of instruction for English learners may fall under the terms "ESOL services" or "ESOL strategies."

ESOL is not the only accepted acronym for this field. Other common terms include English as a second language (ESL), English as an additional language (EAL), and English as a new language (ENL). The term "ESOL" is most frequently used in K–12 school settings, whereas ESL is used more in postsecondary environments, although this is not always the case. English as a new language and English as an additional language are less frequently used and were developed to more precisely describe the field. In other words, nonnative speakers who are learning English may already know two or three languages, so calling English a second language is inaccurate for many students. English for speakers of other languages does not necessarily convey that these speakers are not proficient in English (they could have been brought up bilingually or English could be their first of two or more languages acquired). As evident by the variety of terms to refer to the field, no term has been coined that is perfectly descriptive of the diverse conditions that comprise ESOL.

Professional Association—TESOL

The professional organization that represents ESOL specialists is Teachers of English to Speakers of Other Languages, or TESOL (https://www.tesol.org/about-tesol). Although ESOL is part of the acronym TESOL, it is interesting to note that the preposition that is bounded by the E and S differs between the two acronyms. The subject area or field is English *for* Speakers of Other Languages, but the profession is Teachers of English *to* Speakers of Other Languages.

TESOL International Association, formerly Teachers of English to Speakers of Other Languages (TESOL), began in 1966, supported by five existing professional organizations in related fields: (1) the Center for Applied Linguistics, (2) the Modern Language Association, (3) the National Association for Foreign Student Affairs, (4) the National Council of Teachers of English, and (5) the Speech Association of America (Alatis, 1987). The mission of this organization is to "advance the expertise of professionals who teach English to speakers of other languages in multilingual contexts worldwide." This is accomplished through "professional learning, research, standards, & advocacy" (TESOL, n.d.-b). Its values include "professionalism learning and excellence in standards, research, and practice that enhance English language teaching and learning; respect for equity, diversity . . . and individuals' language rights; inquiry and lifelong learning" (TESOL, n.d.-b).

As of August 2018, there were approximately 10,000 members (TESOL, n.d.-c) representing 170 distinct countries. The top five countries were as follows: 74% of TESOL members are from the United States, 2.7% from Japan, 2.7% from Canada, 2.2% from China, and 1% from Ecuador. In the United States, the state with the most members was California (8.6%), followed by Illinois (7.9%), New York (6.1%), Michigan (4.1%), and Texas (4%).

Although ASHA began developing position statements on issues affecting children in K–12 in the 1980s, TESOL did not issue position papers on these topics until the 1990s. As of spring 2019, TESOL has approximately 57 position statements, with recognition of all varieties of English, including dialects, creoles, and World Englishes; acquisition of academic proficiency in English at the postsecondary level; recommendations for the reauthorization of the Elementary and Secondary Education Act in the United States; immigration policy and reform in the United States; and language and literacy development for young ELs.

TESOL Position Statements

A number of TESOL's position statements address issues pertaining to teaching ELs in the K–12 setting. For example, in 2010, TESOL issued a position statement on language and literacy development for young ELs, ages 3 to 8. It made six recommendations regarding language and literacy development for young children. In addition, TESOL developed position statements that focused on students with special needs. One position paper addressed the rights of deaf students to become proficient in sign language or written or spoken languages, such as English (TESOL, 2009a), while another position paper concentrated on the identification of ELs with special needs. In this position paper, it emphasized the disproportionate number of CLD students in special education and argued that in some cases, ELs with special needs were incorrectly identified due to confusion over the characteristics of second language acquisition versus a communication disorder (TESOL, 2007b). The statement cites IDEA (2004), which specifies provisions for assessing EL students for special education services. TESOL believes that multiple means of assessment must be used for identifying learning disabilities in ELs. Moreover, it highlights the need to conduct assessments in the EL's strongest language and to consider the student's level of proficiency in English, the native language, and/or dialect. Similar to ASHA (n.d.-e), TESOL position statements accentuate the knowledge and competencies ESOL professionals must have in order to work with ELs and ELs with special needs.

Competencies for Teachers of ELs—Specialists and Generalists

TESOL and the Council for the Accreditation of Educator Preparation (CAEP) have clearly defined the knowledge base and skill set for ESOL professionals who focus entirely on teaching ELs. These performance-based standards, used in the preparation and licensing of ESOL professionals, are often referred to as the TESOL/CAEP Standards for P–12 Teacher Education Programs or the TESOL Professional Teaching Standards (Fenner, 2012; TESOL, 2010a, 2019). These standards were originally approved in 2001 for P–12 ESL teacher education programs and revised in 2010 and again in 2018. The 2018 *Standards for Initial TESOL Pre-K–12 Teacher Preparation Programs* outline the professional expertise needed to prepare effective PreK–12 TESOL educators in the United States (TESOL, 2019). These performance-based standards are designed to be used by PreK–12

TESOL preparation programs to ensure that candidates have the content, pedagogical knowledge, and skills to serve PreK–12 ELs and qualify for their initial TESOL credential. Institutions wishing to become nationally recognized must align their programs to the standards and submit a program report to CAEP in order to become accredited.

The 2018 TESOL/CAEP standards consist of five essential domains: *language, culture, instruction, assessment,* and *professionalism,* which remain constant. All five standards cover generally the same topics and include updates related to current research in the fields of TESOL and second language acquisition. The first domain, *language,* includes the ability to describe language and the process of acquiring it. The second domain, *culture,* focuses on its nature and role as well as cultural groups and identity. The third domain, *instruction,* focuses primarily on planning for standards-based EL and content instruction, managing, and implementing instruction through the effective use of resources and technology. The fourth domain, *assessment,* includes general assessment issues, assessing language proficiency, and classroom-based assessment. In addition, recommendations for collaboration with other professionals, to include the SLP, are noted to specifically determine differences among normal language development, language difference, and learning problems. The final domain, *professionalism,* encompasses research and history of the field, partnerships and advocacy, and professional development and collaboration. To sum up, the 2018 TESOL/CAEP Standards are less prescriptive about how teachers should proceed and describe the general required knowledge and applications that are necessary to provide appropriate instruction to EL students.

In contrast to the TESOL/CAEP standards, reports and studies on building teacher capacity to serve ELs (Ballantyne, Sanderman, & Levy, 2008; Boyle, Golden, LeFloch & Day, 2014; Samson & Collins, 2012) focus on general information and skills that mainstream teachers who have one or more ELs in their regular classrooms should possess. They divide essential competencies into language acquisition and communicative competence, academic language, curriculum and instruction, content assessment, culture and education, and school and home communities. Assuming that the SLP or other professionals (e.g., regular classroom teacher, special education teacher, bilingual education teacher) will collaborate with an ESOL specialist as necessary, they maintain that mainstream teachers and/or other professionals require a less specialized and in-depth skill set and knowledge base to accommodate one or more ELs in the regular classroom.

Many states have set requirements for professionals who work with ELs. For example, in Florida, the Consent Decree (also known as the META or ESOL Consent Decree) of 1990 is the framework for compliance with federal and state laws and jurisprudence regarding the education of ELs (FLDOE, n.d.). The Consent Decree outlines specific requirements and competencies for personnel who instruct and interact with ELs and monitors compliance to ensure that ELs have equal access to comprehensible instruction. The Florida Department of Education (FLDOE), Bureau of Student Achievement through Language Acquisition, has set requirements for state certification and competencies and skills for professionals who work with ELs (FLDOE, 2010). The SLP who is working with ELs with communication disorders is one of the professionals required to complete prescribed professional development to ensure that they are able to provide appropriate services to ELs.

Who Are ESOL Students?

Even more intricate than the terms for the field of ESOL are the terms that describe the students. At one time, students were described by the subject they were taught—ESOL students. However, not all students who are not proficient in English are ESOL students. Some may be in bilingual programs, whereas others may be mainstreamed with in-class support. Therefore, a term was needed that reflected the nature of the students rather than the subject. As discussed in Chapter 2, the federal term that became prevalent in the 1980s was "limited English proficient," or LEP. This term troubled many in the field because it emphasized the students' limitations. Equally troubling was the unspoken assumption that having a native language other than English and developing as a bilingual was a limitation. On the contrary, developing fluency in more than one language is an asset that most native speakers of English would like to attain.

As federal terms are difficult to change, some states referred to the acronym of LEP as "language-enriched pupil," but over time that acronym has fallen into disfavor. Subsequently, the term "English language learner" (ELL) has become the most common descriptor, with the term now being shortened to "English learner" (EL). Some take issue with this term because its precision in describing these students is lacking. One could make the case that an EL is any student in an English-speaking environment, even native speakers of English, as they are learning to read and write in English. Although the term "EL" has this shortcoming, it is currently the term used to describe students who are identified as needing ESOL support services or ESOL instruction (OELA, 2016).

The field of ESOL is unique in its varied emphases in different parts of the world. In Europe, ESOL is currently termed "English language teaching," with origins that reach back to the 15th century (Howatt & Widdowson, 2004). Because of British colonialism, English language instruction spread throughout the British Empire as a language of trade or lingua franca. In the United States, however, ESOL focused on the instruction of immigrants. The Naturalization Act of 1906 required English proficiency to become a naturalized citizen. Citizenship and "Americanization" classes emerged in response to the immigrant influx at the turn of the 20th century. Job sites and community organizations began to teach English along with citizenship classes. After World War I, immigration rates declined, with the lowest period of immigration during the 1930s. In subsequent decades, immigration continued to increase. During the U.S. civil rights movement, language minority issues were raised by Latino populations in Arizona, California, and Texas (Roos, 1978). In 1964, the Civil Rights Act established a basis for equal access to educational programming and freedom from segregation and discrimination for ELs. The Bilingual Education Act of 1968 followed, opening the door to instruction in the native languages of ELs. In 1974, the Supreme Court ruling *Lau v. Nichols* declared that to abide by civil rights laws, public schools were required to accommodate the linguistic needs of ELs. To meet the spirit of the *Lau v. Nichols* ruling, schools have a variety of options for service delivery (Garcia, 1991; Gibbons, 2002; Montone, 1995;

Rennie, 1993). In the next section, we will survey the most common service delivery options for ELs in the United States.

Instructional Program Models for English Learners

ESOL programs differ in multiple ways. The literature often discusses two approaches used with ELs, "English as a second language (ESL)" and/or "bilingual" approaches. Each of these varies primarily in terms of the use (or nonuse) of a student's native language (L1) during instruction that targets development of English as a second language (L2). Typically, ELs in ESOL or bilingual programs are taught by specialists who hold certification or endorsement in ESOL or bilingual education. Various instructional models are subsumed under each approach (U.S. Department of Education, 2012) (Table 3–3).

The use of an ESOL approach focuses on instruction in English as the primary means to help ELs acquire the language and ultimately meet high academic standards. In an ESOL approach, students often learn and are taught in English exclusively or primarily. Instructional materials or instructional techniques may make use of basic L1 vocabulary but only as a means to transition the students to the use of English. Models that follow the ESL approach may include both language instruction, wherein English language is the instructional content itself, and content-based instruction, in which academic content is the object of instruction, but it is delivered in such a way as to support ELs' acquisition of English as well.

The bilingual approach to educating ELs is built on the increasing body of research indicating that L1 skills contribute positively to students' acquisition of a second language (L2) and that L1 instruction does appear to promote gains in English achievement (August & Shanahan 2008; Cook, 2001; Cummins, 2000; Cummins & Corson, 1997; Perozzi, 1992; Short & Fitzsimmons, 2007). The bilingual approach is based on a commitment to the understanding that instruction in students' L1 will help them to meet the goals of attaining English proficiency and meeting high academic achievement standards. Beyond this common trait, bilingual models vary in their details and orientation—some see L1 development as an important goal in itself, while others see it as a scaffold or steppingstone to English fluency.

Table 3–3. Instructional Program Models Used with ELs in K–12 in the United States

	Instructional Program Models for EL Students	
	English-Only Program Models	Dual-Language Program Models
Goal	The goals are proficiency and literacy in English. Focus is on English language development.	Goal is bilingualism and biliteracy in English and a partner language. Focus is on developing literacy in two languages simultaneously.
Description	ESL programs (rather than bilingual programs) are likely to be used in districts where the language minority population is very diverse and represents many different languages. ESL programs can accommodate students from different language backgrounds in the same class, and teachers do not need to be proficient in the home language(s) of their students.	Two-way immersion:* Native English speakers and native speakers of the target language are taught in the same classroom, with the goal of helping both sets of students become bilingual and biliterate by splitting instruction between the two languages. Also known as two-way bilingual, dual-language immersion, developmental bilingual, or maintenance bilingual or late exit.
		Stand-alone program with its own specially trained teachers.
Examples of English-Only Models		**Examples of Dual-Language Models**
English as a Second Language (ESL) Instruction (also known as English language development (ELD)		**Total Immersion**
Instruction focuses on development of proficiency in the English language, including grammar, vocabulary, and communication skills.		Native English speakers are taught almost exclusively in the target language. Also known as one-way immersion or transitional bilingual or early-exit bilingual.
		Mainstream teachers must have training in sheltered instruction.

82

English-Only Program Models	Dual-Language Program Models
Sheltered English or Content-Based Programs These programs place language minority students from different language backgrounds together in classes where teachers use English as the medium for providing content area instruction, adapting their language to the proficiency level of the students. Teachers may also use gestures and visual aids to help students understand. Although the acquisition of English is one of the goals of sheltered English and content-based programs, instruction focuses on content rather than language. **The Sheltered Instruction Observation Protocol (SIOP)** is a specific version of the SI model with a considerable research base and specific strategies associated with it. **Structured English Immersion (SEI)** These use only English, but there is no explicit ESL instruction. As in sheltered English and content-based programs, English is taught through the content areas. Structured immersion teachers have strong receptive skills in their students' first language and have a bilingual education or ESL teaching credential. The teacher's use of the children's first language is limited primarily to clarification of English instruction. Most students are mainstreamed after 2 or 3 years.	**Partial Immersion** Only a portion of academic subjects is taught in the target language.

continues

Table 3–3. *continued*

English-Only Program Models	Dual-Language Program Models
English as a Second Language (ESL) Pull-Out	
Students leave the classroom to meet with the ESL specialist. Although it is difficult to coordinate schedules around specials and lunch times, this type of model may allow the ESL specialist to group students across classrooms or grade levels who are at a similar level of English proficiency for ESL support. This program model is especially effective for beginning ELLs who need to develop "survival" English skills. As students advance in their English language proficiency, the ESL specialist may take responsibility for teaching a specific subject area, providing background information for upcoming lessons or reviewing difficult content. However, grouping intermediate ELLs across grade levels or even across several classrooms from the same grade level for instruction bring challenges in effectively supporting students in content area learning.	

English-Only Program Models	Dual-Language Program Models
English as a Second Language (ESL) Inclusion or "Pull-In" Model Rather than pulling students out of their grade level classroom, this program model brings the ESL specialist into classrooms. The specialist may work with students individually at their seats or as a group someplace in the classroom. The specialist may assist ELLs with the same lesson that the rest of the class is doing or modify the lesson or assignment in some way. The ESL specialist could also assist while the classroom teacher instructs the whole class by displaying pictures, key words, or providing other aids to comprehension. In this type of model, the ESL specialist can sometimes even provide an extra set of hands in a way that is useful for the entire class.	

continues

85

Table 3–3. *continued*

English-Only Program Models	Dual-Language Program Models
Team Teaching Model The ESL specialist may spend several hours a day in an elementary classroom when this model is implemented. As the name implies, when team teaching approaches are used, the ESL specialist and grade-level teacher work as a team both to plan and deliver instruction to all students in the class, the classroom teacher as the content expert, and the ESL specialist as the expert on effective strategies for ELLs. Though they could work together to teach the entire class at once or break up the class into two flexible groups, in this model, all students receive the same high-quality instruction. It is important that team teaching occurs in the curriculum areas in which ELLs would need the most language support. Because this model involves so much time in one classroom, it is most often used in schools with large populations of ELLs. **Newcomer Programs/High-Intensity Language Training** EL students who are recent immigrants from various language backgrounds and typically have low literacy and are new to formal education receive intensive ESL training the majority of the day to prepare for mainstream classes. Schooling is designed to acclimate them to U.S. school settings.	

Source: Adapted from Moughamian, Rivera, & Francis, 2009; Rennie, 1993; Lindholm-Leary & Genesee, 2010; Sugarman, 2018.

Several service delivery models have been discussed in the literature that range from a continuum of English-only models to bilingual models (U.S. Department of Education, 2012).

For example, one common service delivery model for ELs is the *pull-out ESOL model*. Pull-out ESOL programs remove ELs from one or more class periods per day to gather with other ELs for language development and subject matter support. Often, pull-out ESOL sessions replace 1 or more hours of English language arts instruction. ESOL teachers may use a special language arts curriculum for ELs, or they may work with the classroom teacher to identify vocabulary and grammar related to the content taught in the mainstream class.

Another model of service delivery for ELs is the *push-in ESOL model*. In contrast to the pull-out ESOL model, the push-in ESOL model involves coteaching with the classroom teacher and ESOL specialist. The ESOL specialist and classroom teacher collaborate in planning, delivering, and evaluating lessons for ELs who are integrated in the regular classroom. When the classroom teacher is leading a lesson, the ESOL specialist may sit in the back of the room with the ELs, using supplemental materials and targeted language to reach the ELs at their levels of English proficiency. Sometimes a bilingual aide may be the push-in specialist, working with ELs in both English and their native language to improve comprehension and performance.

Another model of service delivery is the *self-contained ESOL class*. Self-contained ESOL classes are offered where and when there is a critical mass of ELs at the same grade level. English learners are grouped with other ELs and are taught using "sheltered" instruction. Sheltered instruction has a long history in teaching ELs, and most recently it has come to mean teaching regular academic content at the level and pace appropriate for ELs (Echevarria, Vogt, & Short, 2008). Teachers of self-contained classes are ESOL specialists who have completed a state-approved teacher preparation program for initial licensure in ESL as well as certified in the subjects and/or grade levels they teach. In some instances, the teacher of the self-contained class is a content-area expert who might have added an ESL certification/add-on endorsement to an existing state teaching license. Variations on self-contained classrooms are newcomer schools. Newcomer schools typically are provided at the secondary level for ELs who are at beginning to intermediate levels of proficiency. By grouping ELs together at a high school dedicated entirely to these students, teachers can provide intensive English instruction while teaching academic content at the students' level of English proficiency or even in the native language. Typically, students remain a year in newcomer schools before transitioning into a mainstream environment.

In many areas, there are not enough ELs to warrant hiring specialists who provide ESOL services and classes. This situation often leads to another option in the schooling of ELs, *mainstreamed education (inclusion)*. If mainstream (meaning regular classroom) teachers have appropriate training, ELs can be successful. In general, the smaller the gap between the EL's level of English proficiency and the language demands of the grade level/subject, the better chance of the EL's success in the mainstream. When the mainstream teacher has also learned about second language acquisition and instructional and assessment accommodations and modifications for ELs, successfully bridging the English proficiency/language demands gap is more likely. For example, an intermediate-level EL in a kindergarten class, where the language demands are simple and supported by a great deal of extralinguistic context, has a smaller gap to navigate than an intermediate EL in a 10th-grade social studies class, where students are expected to read the textbook and discuss and write about abstract concepts. As a rule of thumb, in the upper grades, ELs need much more content comprehension support and English language development instruction than ELs in lower grades.

In the past, mainstreamed instruction for ELs has also meant a "sink or swim" approach to learning (Ovando, 2003). Children with low levels of English proficiency were placed in regular classrooms and were expected to catch up on their own. However, current research has indicated that mainstreamed ELs will achieve greater gains if their teachers use appropriate strategies for their comprehension of content and English language development.

Bilingual/Dual-Language Instruction

Often an area of controversy and misunderstanding, bilingual education has been part of the American educational system since the 1800s. Interestingly, German was the first language other than English used as a medium of instruction in the United States, but with the dawn of World War I, an anti–bilingual education movement ended the practice. The current national debate on the merits of bilingual education ignores a great deal of empirical evidence that supports its effectiveness. We will look at the evidence in the following section; before we examine the research, it is important to define the many types of options for bilingual education.

According to the Center for Applied Linguistics (Rennie, 1993), there are three main categories of bilingual education programs: early exit, late exit, and two-way. Sugarman (2018), in her description of EL program models in K–12, uses the terms "dual language," "transitional bilingual education," and "English only." Despite the variation in terminology, another option to serve ELs in the school setting is through *bilingual/dual-language instruction* (Calderon, Slavin, & Sanchez, 2011; Cloud, Genesee, & Hamayan, 2000; Collier & Thomas, 2004). Dual-language education refers to programs that provide grade-level content and literacy instruction to all students through two languages—English and a partner language.

Early exit programs typically conclude by the end of the second grade. Their purpose is to support reading skills in both languages through reading instruction in the first language (L1) and to phase out L1 instruction quickly. Late exit programs typically transition students into full English instruction over a longer period of time, usually lasting throughout the elementary school years. For either program, the transition period usually involves reducing the percentage of instruction in the native language and increasing the amount of instruction in English. Late exit programs typically progress to 60% English instruction prior to mainstreaming the students in instruction conducted entirely in English.

Two-way bilingual programs have a very different purpose —they are designed to develop full proficiency in two languages in English-speaking and EL students. Typically, two-way bilingual programs involve combining English speakers with English learners of one native language and offering instruction in the two languages. The definitive split is half of instruction in each language, but this ratio can vary according to community and school needs and resources. A more recent term for two-way bilingual programs is dual language, which offers a range of options for dividing instruction in two languages.

In one-way dual-language programs, the partner language is the native language of all of the students in the class. In two-way programs, approximately half the students are native speakers of the partner language and the other half are native speakers of English. Dual-language programs typically begin in kindergarten or first grade and continue for a minimum of 5 years and have the goals of promoting bilingualism and biliteracy, high levels of academic achievement, and cross-cultural competence (Lindholm-Leary & Genesee, 2010; Thomas & Collier, 2012).

There are two basic but highly important decision points in dual-language program design: the allocation of instructional time in each program language and the determination of which content areas are to be taught in each program language at each grade level. For example, a 50:50 Program Model is a commonly adopted approach to allocating instructional time in the two languages (e.g., initial literacy instruction is provided 50% in English and 50% in the partner language). Some programs allocate language in kindergarten as 70:30 or 60:40 (instruction in L1/instruction in L2), with a gradual increase in time devoted to instruction in English until achieving a balance of 50:50, typically around Grade 3 or 4 (Howard et al., 2007; Kennedy & Medina, 2017).

Although school districts choose different service delivery options based on multiple factors, including parental preference, the philosophical perspectives of administrators and board members, access to qualified teachers and other personnel, and cost, research on the impact of the program model on EL achievement is clear. In *A National Study of School Effectiveness for Language Minority Students' Long-Term Academic Achievement*, Thomas and Collier (2002) found compelling differences among program models. Results from this study showed differences in English and Spanish achievement, and achievement in different subject matters such as math based on the type of program ELs completed. ELs who received no ESOL and bilingual education services had substantial decreases in reading and math scores by the fifth grade compared to ELs who received the services. In addition, the greatest number of dropouts came from this category. Spanish-speaking students in bilingual programs scored higher in reading in their native language than English-speaking students did in English in Grades 1 through 5, 7, and 8. They also scored higher than English-speaking students when tested on math in their native languages. In general, this study documents the academic achievement of ELs over the long term (4–12 years) and across content areas. It offers a much-needed overview of programmatic successes in the education of ELs for policy makers.

Sugarman (2018) provides an updated view of the different models currently used with EL students in U.S. school settings. Noting the similarities and variations in several models, she points out that EL students may experience different models at different points during the day as educators teach grade-level academic content and make every effort to address the students' language proficiency. Current trends have emerged over the past two decades that emphasize the responsibility of all professionals (e.g., ESL specialist, general education teacher, speech-language pathologist) to plan instruction that facilitates English language development and acquisition of state standards. Professionals must support EL students not only during "ESL instruction time" but also indirectly by partnering with content teachers to plan instruction that supports English language development within the general education setting in major content areas (e.g., English, Math, science, and social studies).

Summary

This chapter detailed the roles and professional preparation characteristics of the SLP and ESOL professional. When both professionals serve the same students, ELs, it is critical to understand the professional preparation and competencies of each, their respective roles and responsibilities, and how they influence educational decisions and student language and learning outcomes. This chapter also discussed EL students from the perspective of each of the disciplines. For the ESOL professional, the EL student is in various stages of second language acquisition and needs support to develop oral, reading, and writing skills in English while challenged with meet core curriculum standards. For the SLP, the EL student has been referred due to a possible speech-language delay or disorder and might also be in the process of second language acquisition. It is the role of the SLP to provide appropriate intervention (e.g., prereferral activities or Response to Intervention strategies or intervention) and assessments to make that determination. Both professionals must be familiar with the service delivery models used by the SLP and the instructional models used by ESOL professionals in educating ELs in order to facilitate intervention planning and implementation. More important, SLP and ESOL professionals must share a knowledge base to better prepare to work with ELs, and specifically ELCDs.

Thus, the next chapter provides information on first language development and the normal processes of second language acquisition to provide a framework for distinguishing a language difference from a language disorder.

4

First and Second Language Acquisition: Theoretical and Practical Considerations

Introduction

Professionals who are directly and indirectly involved in the instruction of ELs, in general, and ELCDs, in particular, have two goals: to address the language development and instructional and literacy needs of ELs (ASHA, 2001a, 2001b, 2010a; TESOL, 2001a, 2001b) and to use evidence-based approaches to facilitate the academic success of school-age ELs and ELCDs. SLPs and K–12 teachers, as well as K–12 administrators, must understand first (L1) and second (L2) language acquisition theories and the stages of second language acquisition that EL students go through in order to appropriately identify, instruct, and assess ELs with communication disorders. They need to know the difference between naturalistic and instructed second language acquisition, the basic constructs of language proficiency, and the influences culture might exert on the acquisition of a second language. Last, SLPs and classroom teachers need to be able to distinguish between a communication difference and a communication disorder when working with ELs (Antunez, 2002; Battle, 2002; Rosa-Lugo, Mihai, & Nutta, 2017; Roseberry-McKibben, 2007). We begin with an overview of first language acquisition.

First Language Acquisition

First Language Acquisition Theories

Although there is general agreement on the description of the typical process of acquiring a first language, there are differing theories of how and why the process happens. Three theories are discussed in particular: behaviorist, innatist, and interactionist.

Behaviorist Theory

An early perspective on first language acquisition comes from the school of psychology known as behaviorism. Behaviorists believe that language learning is no different from learning anything else. In this view, all learning results from a process of stimulus and response (Freeman & Freeman, 2014). Children reproduce language, or approximate imitations of what they hear, and are reinforced by rewards, such as attention or response. A child produces an utterance (for example, "milk"), and the parent understands and responds affirmatively by fulfilling the request. Hence, the utterance was rewarded and reinforced. If the utterance is unintelligible or incorrect, the parent corrects the child and the child uses the correct form (or approximation) to obtain the intended outcome. B. F. Skinner, the most well-known of the mid-20th-century behaviorists, hypothesized about first language acquisition in his book *Verbal Behavior* (1957), which was subsequently critiqued by Noam Chomsky (1965), the developer of a linguistic model of first language acquisition that stemmed from a cognitive psychology perspective.

Innatist Theory

Cognitivists view language learning as a more innate process, where children apply inborn rules to language input they receive, forming hypotheses about grammar structures (Clark, 2016). This theory, also known as innatism or nativism, contrasts with the behaviorist view that new structures are learned by imitating what adults say. Chomsky (1965) refuted this view with the example "goed," which English-speaking children normally say while acquiring the past tense. Clearly, he noted that children did not learn that term through imitating an adult, since adults do not say "goed" rather than "went." Instead, he advanced this as evidence that children apply the rule "-ed" for the past tense to the verb stem "go" rather than use the irregular form "went." Interestingly, this process is actually U-shaped, because children often first acquire the irregular form as an unanalyzed chunk, and then once they acquire the "-ed" past-tense marker, they apply it to "go" to regularize the irregular verb, and finally they make the distinction that "go" uses an irregular past-tense form (Figure 4–1).

The innatist view sees correction of such grammatical errors as unnecessary and ineffective, because children move through the same process with or without correction. Another example of how children apply rules to language is offered by psychologist Jean Berko Gleason's (1958) exploration of children's pluralization of nonsense terms. When shown a cartoon figure and told it was a wug, the children were instantly able to name two of the figures wugs, adding the plural "-s" marker to the nonsense noun. Again, that plural form could not have been an imitation of an adult's use of the plural noun, as it is an invented word (Pinker, 1999). Innatists attribute children's capacity to analyze and construct language forms to an inborn mental facility they term the "Language Acquisition Device" (LAD) (Chomsky, 1965). Chomsky has developed the construct of LAD into a theory

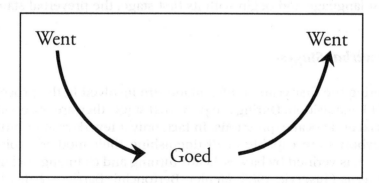

Figure 4–1. *The U-shaped process that children undergo when learning the irregular past-tense form of "go."*

called Universal Grammar (UG). UG is considered to be innate and contains a theoretical system of categories, operations, and principles shared by all human languages (Chomsky, 2005; Yang, Crain, Berwick, Chomsky, & Bolhuis, 2017).

Interactionist Theory

A more recent perspective on first language acquisition is the interactionist position. Interactionists believe that the give-and-take between an adult caregiver and a child is a critical factor in language development. Through what is termed "child-directed speech," adults adjust their language to engage and communicate with children. The characteristics of this speech include slow expression, high pitch, exaggerated intonation, pauses, simple syntax, repetition, comprehension questions, paraphrasing, and a focus on the concrete aspects of the immediate surroundings at the present time (Brown & Attardo, 2014). This position emphasizes the interaction between the learner and the environment as a primary factor in language acquisition.

Stages of First Language Acquisition

The process of normal L1 acquisition goes through predictable stages. In this section, we briefly examine the process of acquiring first language and begin with its first stage, the preverbal stage.

Preverbal Stages

During the first years of life, infants are involved in the process of L1 acquisition. During the preverbal stage, they are observing facial and vocal expressions. In fact, only a few days after birth, newborns are capable of distinguishing their mother's voice, which is verified by babies' heads turning and changing sucking patterns (Jusczyk, 1985; Mehler, Bertoncini, Barriere, & Jasski-Gerschenfeld, 1978). From birth to 8 weeks, they cry, burp, and cough. At 8 to 20 weeks, they laugh and coo, and their crying differs based on their needs. From 16 to 30 weeks, they repeat vowel or consonant sounds (/o/, /o/, /o/ or / m/, /m/, /m/). The reduplicated babbling stage begins with the repetition of vowel and consonant combinations (/ma/ /ma/ /ma/ /ma/) and continues until infants are approximately 1 year old. Somewhere around 9 months, infants begin the 9-month-long process of un-reduplicated babbling, which incorporates more consonants as well as stress and intonations (Brown & Attardo, 2014).

Verbal Stages

Children go through predictable stages in acquiring the building blocks of languages: phonology (sounds), morphology (the form of words and units of meaning, such as the addition of "s" to a noun to denote plurality), syntax (word order in phrases and sentences), and semantics (the meaning of an utterance). In phonology, children tend to acquire stops (consonant sounds such as /p/, /t/, and /k/ in English) before liquids (consonant sounds such as /l/ and /r/ in English). Replacing the later-acquired sounds with ones that have already been acquired is a common feature of "baby talk," such as saying "weeawee" instead of "really" (Parker & Riley, 2010).

When babies are about 12 months old, they begin to form words. According to Pinker (1994, 2007), children begin using the same types of words, half of which are terms for familiar objects, such as "bottle." However, one word can have different meanings. For example, if a child at this stage states "bottle," this could mean "get my bottle" or "fill my bottle." Their vocabulary grows by adding simple adjectives and adverbs and eventually what are called function words, which have a specific grammatical purpose, such as prepositions and articles. Children acquire these grammatical morphemes in a predictable order. In English, the following morphemes are acquired in a regular sequence (Brown & Attardo, 2014):

1. "-ing in the present continuous (smiling)
2. the preposition "in"
3. the preposition "on" (some children acquire "on" before "in")

4. "-s" for plural nouns (dogs)
5. irregular past (had)
6. "-'s" for possessive (Mary's)
7. the verb "be," not in contraction form (I am playing.)
8. articles (a, the)
9. "-ed" for regular past (walked)
10. "-s" for third-person simple present-tense verbs (she walks)
11. third-person present irregular (He marches to bed every night.)
12. auxiliary (also known as helping) verbs, not in contraction form (I have played Go Fish.)
13. the verb "be" in contraction form (She's laughing.)
14. auxiliary verbs in contraction form (I've been to London.)

At about 18 months, children assemble two-word utterances, which is the beginning of eventual sentence formation (syntactic development). "Daddy gone" or "tummy hurt" are examples of such two-word utterances. Pinker (1994, 2007) identifies 18 months as a point of rapid vocabulary growth, followed by a period of rapid syntactic growth from the late twos to late threes (Freeman & Freeman, 2014).

Next comes the multiword stage, termed "telegraphic speech" (Brown, 1973; Yule, 2016), because it lacks many function words. An example is "Mommy make cake," meaning "Mommy is making a cake." The most common word order, subject/verb/object, is typically acquired early, whereas questions, negatives, and the passive voice are acquired later. Developing the proper word order for questions and negatives typically involves a predictable process of simplification and word order errors that gradually and finally acquire the proper form. In questioning, for example, children typically use rising intonation to designate a question before they master the correct word order. For example, "Grammy going?" with rising intonation is a common way young child use to express "Is Grammy going?" For questions using interrogative terms (who, what, etc.), children also go through stages. For instance, "Where Grammy going?" precedes "Where Grammy's going?" which precedes the proper form, "Where is Grammy going?" Similar to questions, negative sentences follow a developmental pattern: (1) "no go," (2) "I no go," and (3) "I won't go" (Parker & Riley, 2010).

How children begin to understand the meaning and boundaries of words or sentences is known as semantics. The meaning of words is called lexical semantics and the meaning of sentences is called sentence semantics. A common feature of developing lexical semantics is called under- and overextension (Brown & Attardo, 2014). Underextension involves children's assumption that the meaning of a word denoting a concept or category is specific to an item that is part of or possesses a possible characteristic of the concept or category. For example, the verb "fly" applies only to birds (but not airplanes or bumblebees, etc.). Overextension is the opposite of underextension and means overgeneralizing a specific word to include all terms in its class or category. An example would be using the word "dog" to refer to any four-legged mammal. In general, overextension involves categories ("daddy" for all men) or analogies ("wheel" for anything round) (Brown & Attardo, 2014).

This section briefly presented the theories of L1 acquisition and emphasized the predictable stages children go through in its development. The goal is to establish a basic foundation to be able to compare L1 and L2 processes. Next, the construct of language proficiency, the theories of second language acquisition, stages of second language acquisition, and the similarities and differences between L1 and L2 are discussed.

Second Language Acquisition

Second Language Acquisition and Second Language Proficiency: Defining the Constructs

The term "second language acquisition" (SLA) encompasses many concepts and assumptions. Although the word "second" is used, SLA can incorporate the second, third, fourth, and so forth language learned. In other words, "second" refers to any language learned after an individual starts learning the first. In its broadest sense, SLA denotes learning language in different contexts and ways, although there are technical distinctions used for narrower purposes. For example, learning a language where it is the native language of the area, such as English in the United States or French in the Canadian province of Quebec, is known as second language learning, but learning a language that is not the native language of the area, such as Japanese in the United States, is known as foreign language learning; the latter is typically what high school students engage in when they fulfill a foreign language requirement. However, "second language acquisition" is also the umbrella term that includes second and foreign language learning, as well as the academic discipline or field of study of these phenomena. This means that those who conduct research and develop theories on how people learn second or foreign languages are called "second language acquisition scholars."

Similar to the technical distinctions for the word "second" in SLA, the word "acquisition" has multiple meanings. In its broadest definition, acquisition refers to any way that a learner develops proficiency in a second language. We can consider two different approaches to learning a second language as being opposite ends of a continuum: On one end is the study of the rules and features of the language, and at the other end is "picking up" the language by immersion in a community that speaks a particular language. Undoubtedly, there are many variations and combinations of the two extremes.

The study of bilingual development explores second language acquisition in infants and children. According to Letts (1999) and Letts and Sinka (2013), bilingual development complicates the study of second language acquisition due to the variety of factors that lead to the attainment of proficiency in two or more languages. For example, bilingual learners may have parents who speak different languages, they may live in areas where two languages are spoken, or they may be immigrants in a community that speaks a different language than their home language. Letts (1999) and Letts and Sinka (2013) describe a rudimentary categorization of two major modes of bilingual development, termed "simultaneous" and "sequential" bilingualism. Simultaneous bilinguals are exposed to both languages in rather equal proportions, beginning at birth. Sequential bilinguals begin acquiring one language before they are exposed to another.

For simultaneous bilinguals, there are three stages of development: (1) one lexical (vocabulary) system for both languages, (2) two lexical systems but a simplified and combined syntactic (sentence structure) system, and (3) two separate lexical and syntactic systems (Rodina, 2018; Silva-Corvalán, 2018; Volterra & Taeschner, 1978). For sequential acquisition, Letts (1999) and Letts and Sinka (2013) suggest that younger children go through a process of acquiring an L2 that is similar to acquiring their L1, but that L2 acquisition in older children may be facilitated by formal instruction. Research indicates that children who have had significant input in two languages before the age of 3 seem to experience minimal interference between the languages (Asaad Daana, 2018; Patterson & Pearson, 2004) and that those who are exposed to L1 during infancy and learn an L2 at a later time show greater diversity in rates and stages of acquisition (Kan & Kohnert, 2005; Kayser, 2002; Proietti Ergün, 2018).

An important question to examine at this point is what dimensions define second language proficiency. Cummins (1992, 2000, 2008) described two models of language proficiency, the Separate Underlying Proficiency (SUP) and Common Underlying Proficiency (CUP) models (Figure 4–2).

In the SUP model, language proficiency in the first language is viewed as entirely separate from proficiency in the second language. Thus, one ramification of this model is that skills learned in the first language will not transfer to the second language. Supporters of this viewpoint suggest that language development activities in the first language will not enhance learning of a second language and often recommend use of English only. Interestingly, there is little evidence to support the SUP model. Roseberry-McKibben (2014) points out that:

> As children learn their first language, they acquire concepts and strategies that will facilitate the learning of a second language. Concepts are acquired through interaction with the environment. High-quality exposure enhances the learning of concepts that are important for cognitive and linguistic development. As children hear and use their native language in a variety of contexts, they develop the conceptual knowledge and cognitive strategies necessary for success in acquiring new information and linguistic skills. (p. 229)

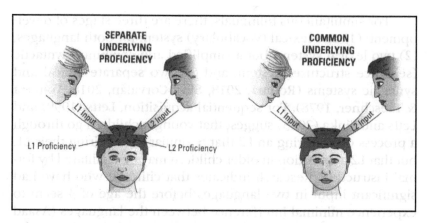

Figure 4–2. *Separate Underlying Proficiency (SUP)* (left) *and Common Underlying Proficiency (CUP)* (right) *models. Adapted from "The Role of Primary Language Development in Promoting Educational Success for Language Minority Students," by J. Cummins, in* Schooling and Language Minority Students: A Theoretical Framework, *by California State Department of Education (Ed.), 1984, Los Angeles: California State University, Evaluation, Dissemination, and Assessment Center.*

Cummins (1992, 2008) suggests that in the course of learning one language, a child acquires a set of skills and implicit metalinguistic knowledge that can be drawn on when working in another language. This CUP, as he labels such skills and knowledge, provides the basis for the development of both the first language and the second language. It follows that any expansion of CUP that takes place in one language will have a beneficial effect on the other language(s).

The CUP model, then, has major implications for SLPs working with ELs. If a student is not provided with opportunities to strengthen the foundation of the first language, the conceptual foundation necessary for academic success will be underdeveloped. Using the second language for instruction when the first language has not yet been fully developed can provide an unstable foundation and result in low language and literacy competence in both L1 and L2 (Chamberlain, 2005; Cummins, 2000; Cummins, Chow, & Schecter, 2006; Walker & Barry, 2018). This limited performance can at least in part be attributed to limited skills in the first language and lack of opportunities for continued development of skills in that language. However, often this limited performance leads professionals to suspect a language learning disability and the need for special education intervention.

Cummins (1980) introduced two important concepts that have been used to define second language proficiency. They arise from his early work in which he demonstrated his ideas about second language development in a simple matrix. These terms are known as Basic Interpersonal Communication Skills (BICS) and Cognitive Academic Language Proficiency (CALP). The distinction between BICS and CALP was introduced to make educators aware of the very different timetable required by immigrant children to acquire conversational fluency in their L2 as compared to grade-appropriate academic proficiency in their L2. Cummins (2000, 2017) describes these skills as being on a continuum instead of being discrete and separate entities.

Basic Interpersonal Communication Skills (BICS), or conversational English, are language skills that ELs need to have in order to fully function in social situations. These are cognitively undemanding, context-embedded forms of communication. In context-embedded communication, participants can actively negotiate meaning and they have a shared reality. For example, ELs can be observed to use BICS on the playground, in the lunchroom, on the school bus, at parties, playing sports, and talking on the telephone. These language skills usually develop within 6 months to 2 years after arrival in the United States. BICS typically occur in meaningful social contexts and the required language is not specialized. A word of caution for SLPs and K–12 teachers: Many problems arise when educators and administrators think that ELs are proficient in English because they demonstrate good social English language skills or BICS.

Cognitive Academic Language Proficiency (CALP), or academic English, refers to formal academic learning. CALP refers to the cognitively demanding, context-reduced forms of communication and does not assume a shared reality. This type of proficiency includes listening, speaking, reading, and writing about subject area content material. CALP is essential for ELs to succeed in school and usually takes from 5 to 7 years to develop. However, research by Collier and Thomas (1995, 2017) has shown that if an EL has no prior schooling or has no support in native language development, it may take 7 to 10 years for ELs to catch up to their peers. It is also important to note that academic language acquisition goes beyond the mere understanding of content-area vocabulary. It often includes skills such as comparing, classifying, synthesizing, evaluating, and inferring (Alvear, 2018; Ovando & Combs, 2018). Table 4–1 summarizes the characteristics of the two concepts that are the foundation of Cummins's (1980) L2 language proficiency framework.

EL-Specific Difficulties Related to Academic Language

Academic language, an essential component of CALP, can generate comprehension problems to ELs in the areas of vocabulary or syntax (Mihai, 2017). First, vocabulary knowledge is critical for ELs who want to communicate well in academic settings. One way to classify academic vocabulary is to use the Three Tier Model (Beck, McKeown, & Kucan, 2002; Sibold, 2011) that places vocabulary words into three categories. Tier 1 consists of

Table 4–1. *Characteristics of BICS and CALP*

Basic Interpersonal Communication Skills (BICS)	Cognitive Academic Language Proficiency (CALP)
• Conversational fluency: social language	• Academic proficiency: school language
• Includes "silent period" when ELs don't produce oral language but are able to comprehend spoken/written language.	• Lasts 5 to 7 or up to 10 years
	• Refers to cognitively demanding, context-reduced forms of communication
• Lasts 6 months to 2 years	
• Involves cognitively undemanding, context-embedded forms of communication	• Vocabulary:
	a. 1–5 years: 6,000 words
• Vocabulary:	b. 5–7 and even 10 years: 7,000 words +
a. 0–1 year: 1,000 words	
b. 1–2 years: 3,000 words	

Source: Adapted from "The Construct of Language Proficiency in Bilingual Education," by J. Cummins, in *Georgetown University Round Table on Languages and Linguistics,* by J. E. Alatis (Ed.), 1980, Washington, DC: Georgetown University Press.

basic or common words such as sight words, function words, or words that name objects. Examples of Tier 1 words are "often" and "empty," which are nonspecialized and are used across all academic subjects. Tier 2 is represented by academic words that are both specialized and nonspecialized and can be used across content areas. These can be difficult for ELs: An EL might know the everyday meaning of "table" but might be unfamiliar with the meaning of *table* when used in math or science. Finally, Tier 3 is content-specific vocabulary. In science, examples of Tier 3 words are "neutron" and "covalent," which are field-specific terms for science, while "feudalism" and "republic" are content-specific words for social studies.

ELs who have an excellent command of social English or BICS might have problems comprehending academic materials or assessments when academic language or CALP is involved. An example of vocabulary confusion was provided by a K–12 teacher who was surprised to see her EL draw a picture in the response box during a test. According to the test directions, that particular test item required test takers to draw a conclusion. The EL took the social English meaning into account and started drawing the answer to the question. Nevertheless, in academic-language-based assessments and instructional material, the phrase *draw a conclusion* has nothing to do with the actual act of drawing (Mihai, 2017).

In addition to vocabulary difficulties, the academic language contains syntactical structures that are not frequently used in everyday social language or BICS. For example, conditional sentences represent another problematic aspect of academic English. ELs might have problems solving the math problems when problems are stated using *if* as a marker for a hypothetical situation (Accurso, Gebhard, & Purington, 2017; Mihai, 2017; Turkan & Schramm-Possinger, 2014). Let's consider the following word problem: *If you can run a lap in 2 minutes, how much time does you need to run 10 laps?* The same EL might be able to solve the same problem if it is stated as follows: *Tommy can run a lap in 2 minutes. How much time does he need to run 3 laps?*

Second Language Acquisition Theories

The road to acquiring a second language is long and arduous and has been the matter of much theoretical debate, especially over the last half of the 20th century. Even now, there is no commonly accepted theory of second language acquisition that clearly explains how all learners in all circumstances acquire any language. The second language acquisition community has adapted and proposed various theories to explain second language acquisition; four are presented below.

Behaviorism

In the 1950s, when behaviorism was popular, it was applied to second language learning. Behaviorist theory stems from the works of Skinner (1957) and Thorndike (1932). As previously noted, behaviorists view language learning as a result of habit formation (Johnson & Johnson, 1999). Theorists following this approach believe that we are born with a tabula rasa, or blank slate, and that language is learned through a series of stimulus-response behaviors and repeated reinforcements (Brown, 2014). Through imitation, practice, and reinforcement, language learning can be achieved (Lightbown & Spada, 2013). Behaviorism helped introduce the idea of contrastive analysis to the field of second language learning. Contrastive analysis is the comparison of two languages to identify similarities and differences (Johnson & Johnson, 1999; Sehlaoui, 2018). According to behaviorists, the differences between two languages can hinder the development of the second language (Lightbown & Spada, 2013).

For behaviorists, second language learning was believed to be about habits. In the learning situation, learners were expected to memorize parts of scripts, which they frequently practiced with a partner. The learners also listened to audiotapes, which were used to help them form habits. The learners did not have to know what their lines or their partners' lines meant, as long as they memorized the words (Ausubel, 1968; Bloomfield, 1942; Lightbown & Spada, 2013). However, others, including Noam Chomsky (1965), perceived language learning differently. He conceived of another way to explain second language acquisition.

Comprehension Hypothesis

As mentioned previously, Chomsky (1965, 2005) believed that all people are born with the ability to learn a language. Children are innately predetermined to learn languages, and he observed them doing this within a few short years. Chomsky created the theory of universal grammar, which alleges the existence of a set of basic grammatical elements that are common to all-natural human languages and that predetermine how people organize the input. Although Chomsky did not directly address second language acquisition, his L1 theory has had a profound influence on SLA scholars. One such scholar is Stephen Krashen (1981, 1987), who developed the comprehension hypothesis. In his view, first and second language acquisition are similar.

Krashen's Comprehension Hypothesis (1981, 1987, 2003, 2017), previously known as the Monitor Model or Input Hypothesis, is one of the most influential and widely accepted explanations of how we acquire a second language. This view on second language acquisition consists of five hypotheses in which Krashen offers a comprehensive explanation of the SLA process: the acquisition versus learning, the natural order, the monitor, the input, and the affective filter hypotheses (Table 4–2).

Krashen (1987, 2003) looked at the differences between acquisition and learning to explain what he believed are two independent systems for developing knowledge of a second language. The first system is through acquisition, which, in non-technical terms, is the "picking up" of a language. Acquisition is subconscious and does not really address grammar rules. The second system of developing second language competence in a language is through the learning system, which is concerned with grammar rules and being aware of them (Krashen & Terrell, 1983). Each system has different functions. The acquired system is used to produce language. The learned system acts as an evaluator of the acquired system to make sure that what the acquired system is producing is correct. Krashen also looked at the natural order of acquisition, which supported the idea that the rules of language were acquired in a predictable order. This claim is based on the morpheme studies of second language acquirers (Dulay & Burt, 1974). The order is the same regardless of whether the language is learned (through instruction or not). The natural order is part of the acquired system, which is not interfered with by the learned system (Krashen & Terrell, 1983).

The third component, the monitor, is related to the important difference between learning and acquisition. According to

Table 4–2. *Krashen's Theory of Second Language Acquisition*

Natural Order Hypothesis	Acquisition-Learning Hypothesis	Monitor Hypothesis	Input Hypothesis	Affective Filter Hypothesis
Language is acquired in a predictable order.	Acquisition is the product of a subconscious process very similar to the process children experience when they acquire their first language. Learning is the product of formal instruction resulting in conscious knowledge about the language	This hypothesis explains the relationship between acquisition and learning. The monitor is an internal editor and is a product of conscious learning. The monitor plans, edits and corrects L2 when learners have time, focus on form and know the grammar rule	Humans acquire language in only one way — by understanding messages or by receiving "comprehensible input"	Affective factors, such as high motivation, good self-confidence and low anxiety can facilitate second language acquisition. Low motivation, low self-esteem, and debilitating anxiety can contribute to the prevention of comprehensible input being used to prevent second language acquisition

Source: Adapted from *Principles and Practices in Second Language Acquisition*, by S. D. Krashen, 1987, New York, NY: Prentice-Hall.

Krashen (1987, 2003), the sole function of learning is to act as an editor, or monitor, for language use. In other words, the learned system is responsible for monitoring the output of the acquired system. Krashen claims that the monitor could only be used under certain conditions. The learners need time to consciously think about and utilize the appropriate rule. The learner must also be able to pay attention to what is being said and be able to focus on form. Finally, the learner must know the grammar rule in order to apply the rule appropriately (Krashen & Terrell, 1983).

In the discussion of his fourth component, the input, Krashen (1987) theorized that learners need compelling comprehensible input in order to move through the natural order of acquisition. Learners acquire a second language by "understanding messages, or by receiving 'comprehensible input'" (Krashen & Terrell, 1983). A message that contains structures and vocabulary unknown to the learner can be made comprehensible through the additional support of nonverbal input. As the learner's L2 proficiency increases, less nonverbal input is needed. In order to advance the learner's current knowledge, the language used by the teacher has to include structures and vocabulary at one level higher than what the learner has already acquired. Thus, acquisition for learners with language knowledge level of "i" can only take place if they are exposed to comprehensible input at a slightly higher level, which Krashen describes as level "i + 1." For example, if "i" is the current acquired linguistic competence, then ELs progress from "i" to "i + 1" by comprehending input that contains "i + 1." The "+1" is symbolic of the new language structures and knowledge that the learner is ready to acquire. In addition to being comprehensible, the input is also compelling, meaning that the input learners receive is so interesting they forget it is in another language (Bland & Krashen, 2014; Krashen, 2011, 2017).

Krashen's final component, the affective filter, explains differences in individual learners. The affective filter can be a potential barrier to second language acquisition. Negative responses to one's environment, such as self-doubt, anxiety, boredom, and any other process, may interfere with the process of learning a second language. This hypothesis accounts for the failure of language acquisition through insufficient input of the appropriate kind or a high affective filter. In other words, the theory states that obstacles to learning a second language can be reduced by providing a low-anxiety environment, sparking the learner's interest, and boosting the learner's self-esteem. In summary, learners must receive comprehensible input and must have a low affective filter for acquisition to take place (Krashen, 2017; Krashen & Terrell, 1983).

In summary, these five hypotheses work together to explain second language acquisition. The process starts with the input hypothesis, which provides the information that the learner needs in order to acquire the language. As the input becomes intake, it makes its way into the developing system, which is the acquisition part of the first hypothesis. The rules that students are taught about the language, metalinguistic knowledge, make up the learning part of the learning-acquisition hypothesis. The learning-acquisition hypothesis has two separate functions. The metalinguistic knowledge of the learning part of the hypothesis becomes the monitor, which corrects output that the learner produces. Any difference that may exist between language learners is explained through the final hypothesis, the affective filter. In order for input to get through to the learner, the affective filter must be low. All of these hypotheses function in concert to produce the language of the learner.

Interactionist Theory

Similar to Krashen (1987), interactionists also believe in the importance of comprehensible input, but they believe that modified interaction is necessary to make language comprehensible. According to Long (1983), modified interaction includes, but is not limited to, linguistic simplification, conversational modifications such as comprehension checks (efforts made by the L2 native speaker to make sure that the L2 learner understands the meaning of the utterance), clarification requests (efforts made by the L2 learner asking the L2 native speaker to clarify an aspect of the conversation that has not been understood), and self-repetition or paraphrase (efforts made by the L2 native speaker to repeat or paraphrase aspects of the conversation either partially or entirely).

Speakers engaged in conversations negotiate meaning. Negotiation of meaning leads to modified interaction, which consists of various modifications (i.e., linguistic simplification). Long (1983) claims that negotiation for meaning that triggers interactional modifications by the L2 native speaker facilitates acquisition because it connects input; internal learner capacities, particularly selective attention; and output in productive ways. In other words, interactional modifications make input comprehensible, and comprehensible input promotes acquisition.

Sociocultural Theory

Related to the interactionist view, which places a great deal of importance on language interaction as a facilitator of second language acquisition, is the concept of the *zone of proximal development (ZPD)* developed by Lev Vygotsky, a Russian theorist and researcher in child development. He viewed language learning as a dynamic process in which external knowledge and abilities in children become internalized. To help explain the way that this social and participatory learning took place, Vygotsky (1962) developed the concept of the zone of proximal development, defined as the difference between what learners can do without help and what they can do with assistance (Figures 4–3 and 4–4).

The ZPD is where learning can most productively take place. It is the domain of knowledge or skill where the learner is not yet capable of independent functioning but can achieve the desired outcome given relevant scaffolded help (Mitchell & Myles, 2013). Other theorists have expanded the concept of the ZPD and conceptualized learning as distributed, interactive, contextual, and the result of the learner's participation in a community of practice. Essentially, it is the difference between the child's current level of independent problem solving and the higher level of potential development they gain through problem solving with adult guidance or in collaboration with peers. This learning can take place in any situation and does not only apply to language learning.

Also, it is important to note that the learning can take place with anyone, as long as that person is more knowledgeable and utilizes scaffolding in order to take learners to the next level in

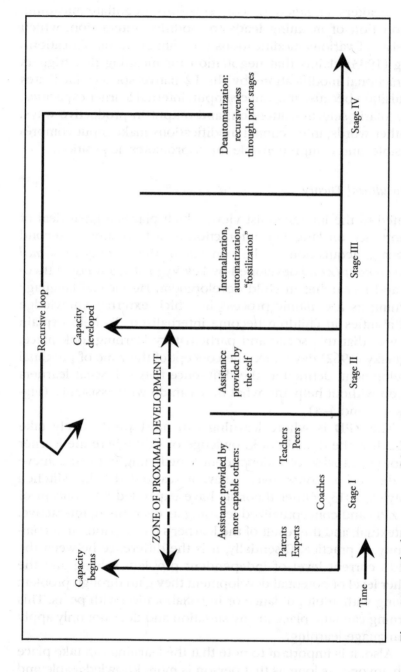

Figure 4–3. *The four-stage model of ZPD. Source: Rousing Minds to Life (p. 35), by R. G. Tharp and R. Gallimore, 1988, New York, NY: Cambridge University Press. Copyright 1988 Cambridge University Press. Adapted with permission.*

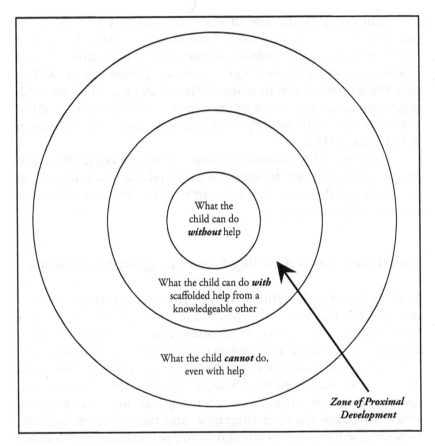

What the
child can do
without help

What the child can do *with*
scaffolded help from a
knowledgeable other

What the child *cannot* do,
even with help

*Zone of Proximal
Development*

Figure 4–4. *The zone of proximal development.*

their learning. The applicability of this theory can be easily demonstrated, whether the tasks are language based or not. For example, a teacher may assign a task to a group of students in a class. One student may demonstrate some difficulty in answering a question in the assigned task. One of his more knowledgeable peers explains the question to the student and both students decide on an appropriate answer for the problem. This situation highlights one of the key aspects of Vygotsky's ZPD theory, in that one's present ability is taken to the next level with the help of a "knowledgeable other." The example cited above utilized the process of scaffolding.

Scaffolding is the use of dialogue and direction to point out key steps in a process or environment. Also known as "other regulation," scaffolding is one of the key methods that a teacher, caregiver, or peer can use to teach someone a skill to take the learner to the next level. The ultimate goal of scaffolding, however, is to achieve self-regulation, the ability to function autonomously with no help (Mitchell & Myles, 2013; VanPatten & Williams, 2015).

The previously discussed theories have all been offered to explain how a second language is acquired. Further information on additional theories can be found in Ellis (2008a) and VanPatten and Williams (2015).

Individual Factors Affecting Second Language Acquisition

Multiple factors affect the development of second language proficiency. For example, individual differences in learners are a significant factor that has been studied in the field of second language acquisition (Ellis, 2008a). Six major categories believed to be associated with second language acquisition have been discussed in the literature (Walqui, 2000). These include personality, language aptitude, motivation, learning and cognitive styles, language learning strategies, and other factors (anxiety, creativity, willingness to communicate, self-esteem, and learner beliefs) (Dornyei, 2005). Ellis (2008a) identifies four "core" areas of individual differences: language aptitude, motivation, personality, and anxiety. A closer examination of these four areas is necessary to understand individual variations in second language acquisition.

In the area of *language aptitude*, Skehan (1989) notes three abilities: auditory, linguistic, and memory. Studies (Harley & Hart, 1997; Horwitz, 1987; Skehan, 1986a, 1986b, 1990) indicate that language aptitude is a significant factor in second language acquisition, whether the language task is grammar or communication focused.

Motivation has also been studied extensively. Two major types of motivation, integrative and instrumental motivation, were identified by Gardner (1980, 2001). Integrative motivation is divided into three main areas, including the degree to which an individual wants to integrate in the L2 language community, attitudes toward the learning context, and the desire to learn the language. A meta-analysis conducted by Masgoret and Gardner (2003) found that integrative motivation is a significant factor in second language acquisition. Complementary to the construct of integrative motivation is Gardner's notion of instrumental motivation. In this case, motivation is determined by the learner's sense of the utility or positive outcomes of learning the second language. Various research studies show that instrumental motivation is a less significant factor in second language acquisition than integrative motivation (Ellis, 2008a).

In the area of *personality*, the concepts of extroversion and introversion have been the subject of study in SLA. Extroversion appears to correlate positively with the development of social language, or BICS (Strong, 1983). This may be due to extroverts' willingness to participate in speaking activities in the classroom (Robson, 1992).

The last individual difference core factor, *anxiety*, affects second language learners in various situations and ways. There are multiple triggers for anxiety regarding listening and speaking a second language. Ellis (2008a) reports that anxiety affects learners differently and to greater or lesser extents, and this is affected by other individual factors such as motivation and personality.

Stages of Second Language Acquisition

Similar to L1 acquisition, L2 acquisition has predictable stages. In their seminal work about the natural approach, Krashen and Terrell (1983) name these stages and provide a rich description of their characteristics. Depending on learners' first language backgrounds, there may be substages within the sequence. All ELs progress through these four stages but not at the same rate. Some learners may progress at slower or faster rates due to a variety of factors, including native language, age, and affective factors. Moreover, outcomes vary according to learner characteristics, and the stages are fluid and not discrete. The natural approach divides SLA into four basic stages: preproduction, early production, speech emergence, and intermediate fluency (Table 4–3).

Table 4–3. *Stages of Second Language Development*

1st Stage: Preproduction	2nd Stage: Early Production	3rd Stage: Speech Emergence	4th Stage: Intermediate Fluency
Characteristics	**Characteristics**	**Characteristics**	**Characteristics**
• 10 hours to 6 months of exposure to English • language skill—listening (receptive) level • BICS development • English vocabulary—500 receptive words	• 6 months to 1 year of English • language skill—continued, mainly listening • BICS development • English vocabulary—1,000 receptive words	• 1 to 3 years of English • Student speaks in phrases and short sentences • BICS development • English vocabulary—7,000 receptive words	• 3 to 4 years of English • Student engages in dialogue • CALP development • English vocabulary—12,000 receptive words
Sample student behaviors	**Sample student behaviors**	**Sample student behaviors**	**Sample student behaviors**
• "silent period" • Has minimal comprehension • Points to or provides other nonverbal responses • Responds to commands	• One-word responses • Has limited comprehension • Produces one- or two-word responses or short utterances • Participates using key words and familiar phrases • Uses present-tense verbs	• Has good comprehension and demonstrates comprehension in a variety of ways • Can produce simple sentences • Makes grammar and pronunciation errors • Participates in small group activities	• Has excellent comprehension • Makes few grammatical errors • Participates in reading and writing activities to acquire new information

Source: Adapted from *The Natural Approach: Language Acquisition in the Classroom,* by S. Krashen and T. Terrell, 1983, Oxford, UK: Pergamon Press.

Other researchers have described the various levels of acquisition, proposed additional stages (i.e., advanced intermediate fluency, advanced fluency), and noted the length of time it takes an EL to achieve the indicated levels of acquisition (Collier, 2008, 2011; Hoover, Klingner, Baca, & Patton, 2008). TESOL (2006) has also identified five language levels that overlap somewhat with the Krashen and Terrell (1983) levels: Level 1 (Starting), Level 2 (Emerging), Level 3 (Developing), Level 4 (Expanding), and Level 5 (Bridging). The TESOL levels apply to oral and written language, whereas the Krashen and Terrell levels apply only to oral language. We focus on the stages presented by Krashen and Terrell (1983).

Stage 1—Preproduction

Learners at this stage have experienced 10 hours to 6 months of exposure to English and are beginning to comprehend the language. Most ELs at this level need time to listen and absorb the language before they are required to speak it. This is sometimes referred to as the "silent period." As they move through this stage, ELs' vocabulary includes approximately 500 receptive words (words they can understand but don't use in speaking or writing), and they are beginning to develop BICS (Cummins, 1980). In order for the language learner at this stage to comprehend speech, communication should include lots of pantomime, body language, facial expressions, and gestures. Second language learners can show comprehension nonverbally. For example, they can point to an item, nod to answer simple yes/no questions, and carry out simple commands (e.g., put the apple on the table).

Stage 2—Early Production

At this stage, learners have been exposed to 3 months to 1 year of English. They can now begin to produce some language, in one- to two-word responses, along with similar nonverbal responses used in Stage 1. Their receptive vocabulary consists of about 1,000 words, and as at any other level, about 10% of their receptive vocabulary is expressive (words they regularly use). Learners at this stage can answer yes/no questions, "what" questions that elicit one- to two-word responses ("What is this?"), "who" questions ("Who has the red ball?"), "either/or questions" ("Is this an apple or an orange?"), and "where" questions that require a simple phrase response ("Where is the Statue of Liberty?"). Learners begin using formulaic chunks of language, with most of the elements of the chunks remaining unanalyzed. For example, they may be able to use the phrase, "Where've you been?" but they may not be able to understand the function of each word and how the words form a sentence.

Because learners develop expressive skills in English at the early production stage, they can communicate in a simple manner with others. Interacting with language learners and native speakers to solve problems, develop projects, and/or discuss issues provides opportunities for ELs to develop language skills. Once students have developed basic vocabulary and syntax in English, their progress accelerates. This limited vocabulary and syntax forms the basis on which to build their proficiency, and by understanding and using a few words and phrases, ELs can increase their receptive and expressive abilities in English more independently.

Stage 3—Speech Emergence

Typically, learners' proficiency increases exponentially after 1 to 3 years of exposure to the second language. They use phrases and sentences, and their receptive vocabulary grows to nearly 7,000 words. Questions they can answer include "how" and "why," which require fairly complex responses. They can understand a great deal and can express themselves fairly effectively, although they tend to simplify more complex grammatical structures or produce them with developmental errors. At every stage, when communication breaks down, learners should employ the same strategies as those used in the beginning stages, such as showing a picture, consulting a bilingual dictionary, gesturing and acting out, and so forth.

Stage 4—Intermediate Fluency

After about 3 to 4 years of exposure to L2, a shift occurs. English language learners begin to develop CALP (Cummins, 1980). Having mastered the knowledge and skills required for social language (BICS), ELs have accumulated approximately 12,000 receptive words. They have gone beyond speaking in phrases and simple sentences to being able to engage in extended discourse. They can answer complex questions that require them to synthesize and evaluate information because they possess adequate academic language proficiency to do so in English. This means that they can write essays, solve complex problems, research and support their positions, and critique and analyze information. Although it may seem that they are able to perform the same activities as native speakers, they continue to need special support until their CALP in the second language is fully developed.

These four stages represent the foundation for TESOL and WIDA standards-based language proficiency levels. WIDA is a 39-state consortium established with the purpose of promoting educational equity and academic achievement for ELs. In 2004, WIDA produced a set of standards for English language proficiency (ELP), which were revised in 2007, and then in 2012 revised to English language development (ELD) standards (WIDA, 2012). Table 4–4 illustrates the language performance definitions for listening and reading, the two receptive language skills, while Table 4–5 details the language performance definitions for speaking and writing, the two productive skills.

Differences Between First and Second Language Acquisition

Although first and second language acquisition have many commonalities, there are distinct differences. We can consider the degree of commonalities on a continuum, with virtually identical processes for birth through infancy, followed by gradually differing elements that increase incrementally from age 3 to adulthood. In other words, an infant learning two languages simultaneously goes through the same processes for each, but a 3-year-old beginning to learn a second language employs strategies and uses information from the already acquired first language to build the second. The more mature and proficient the learner, the greater the differences in the processes employed to acquire a second language.

Table 4–4. WIDA Performance Definitions Listening and Reading, Grades K–12

At each grade, toward the end of a given level of English language proficiency, and with instructional support, English language learners will process . . .

	Discourse Level	Sentence Level	Word/Phrase Level
	Linguistic Complexity	Language Forms and Conventions	Vocabulary Usage
Level 6—Reaching Language that meets all criteria through Level 5, Bridging			
Level 5 Bridging	• Rich descriptive discourse with complex sentences • Cohesive and organized related ideas	• Compound, complex grammatical constructions (e.g., multiple phrases and clauses) • A broad range of sentence patterns characteristic of particular content areas	• Technical and abstract content-area language • Words and expressions with shades of meaning for each content area
Level 4 Expanding	• Connected discourse with a variety of sentences • Expanded related ideas	• A variety of complex grammatical constructions • Sentence patterns characteristic of particular content areas	• Specific and some technical content-area language • Words and expressions with multiple meanings or collocations and idioms for each content area
Level 3 Developing	• Discourse with a series of extended sentences • Related ideas	• Compound and some complex (e.g., noun phrase, verb phrase, prepositional phrase) grammatical constructions	• Specific content words and expressions

	Discourse Level	Sentence Level	Word/Phrase Level
	Linguistic Complexity	Language Forms and Conventions	Vocabulary Usage
Level 3 Developing *continued*		• Sentence patterns across content areas	• Words or expressions related to content area with common collocations and idioms across content areas
Level 2 Emerging	• Multiple related simple sentences • An idea with details	• Compound grammatical constructions • Repetitive phrasal and sentence patterns across content areas	• General and some specific content words and expressions (including cognates) • Social and instructional words and expressions across content areas
Level 1 Entering	• Single statements or questions • An idea within words, phrases, or chunks of language	• Simple grammatical constructions (e.g., commands, Wh– questions, declaratives) • Common social and instructional forms and patterns	• General content-related words • Everyday social, instructional, and some content-related words and phrases
	. . . within sociocultural contexts for language use.		

Source: From 2012 AMPLIFICATION OF THE ENGLISH LANGUAGE DEVELOPMENT STANDARDS, KINDERGARTEN–GRADE 12 by WIDA Consortium. Copyright © 2012 by Board of Regents of the University of Wisconsin System. Reprinted by permission.

Table 4–5. *WIDA Performance Definitions Speaking and Writing, Grades K–12*

At each grade, toward the end of a given level of English language proficiency, and with instructional support, English language learners will produce . . .

	Discourse Level	Sentence Level	Word/Phrase Level
	Linguistic Complexity	Language Forms and Conventions	Vocabulary Usage
Level 6—Reaching	Language that meets all criteria through Level 5, Bridging		
Level 5 Bridging	• Multiple, complex sentences • Organized, cohesive, and coherent expression of ideas	• A variety of grammatical structures matched to purpose and nearly consistent use of conventions, including for effect • A broad range of sentence patterns characteristic of particular content areas	• Technical and abstract content-area language • Words and expressions with precise meaning related to content area topics
Level 4 Expanding	• Short, expanded, and some complex sentences • Organized expression of ideas with emerging cohesion	• A variety of grammatical structures and generally consistent use of conventions • Sentence patterns characteristic of particular content areas	• Specific and some technical content-area language • Words and expressions with multiple meanings or common collocations and idioms across content areas

	Discourse Level	Sentence Level	Word/Phrase Level
	Linguistic Complexity	Language Forms and Conventions	Vocabulary Usage
Level 3 Developing	• Short and some expanded sentences with emerging complexity • Expanded expression of one idea or emerging expression of multiple related ideas	• Repetitive grammatical structures with occasional variation and emerging use of conventions • Sentence patterns across content areas	• Specific content words and expressions (including content-specific cognates) • Words or expressions related to content areas
Level 2 Emerging	• Phrases or short sentences • Emerging expression of ideas	• Formulaic grammatical structures and variable use of conventions • Repetitive phrasal and sentence patterns across content areas	• General content words and expressions (including common cognates) • Social and instructional words and expressions across content areas
Level 1 Entering	• Words, phrases, or chunks of language • Single words used to represent ideas	• Phrase-level grammatical structures • Phrasal patterns associated with familiar social and instructional situations	• General content-related words • Everyday social and instructional words and expressions

. . . within sociocultural contexts for language use.

Source: From 2012 AMPLIFICATION OF THE ENGLISH LANGUAGE DEVELOPMENT STANDARDS, KINDERGARTEN–GRADE 12 by WIDA Consortium. Copyright © 2012 by Board of Regents of the University of Wisconsin System. Reprinted by permission.

If we look at adolescent and adult learners who are fully proficient in their native languages, we find two main differences between them and their younger counterparts: (1) first language transfer and interference and (2) cognitive development.

The concepts of *transfer* and *interference* are derived from the behaviorist view of language development. Both concepts relate to the influence of the first language on the acquisition of the second. Simply put, transfer is the positive influence from the native language to the second language, and interference is the negative influence. For example, if an Italian speaker reads the word "conversation" in English and infers that it means *conversazione* in Italian, his comprehension of the term is facilitated by transfer from his first language. This positively contributes to comprehension and expression in the second language. Conversely, if a speaker of Italian adds a vowel sound to the end of every consonant-final word in English (as in "She's-ah nice-ah"), that is interference from his native language. Because the majority of Italian words end in vowel sounds, Italian speakers transfer this phonological pattern to English. This can be considered a negative impact on the expression of the second language, as it results in a "foreign" accent and can be perceived as a communication disorder instead of a communication difference. The more developed the native language in the second language learner, the more influence transfer and interference have in the acquisition of the second language. Second language acquisition researcher Rod Ellis (2008b) lists four measures of transfer from the first to the second language: (1) learner errors, (2) positive transfer or facilitation, (3) avoidance, and (4) overuse. Certain of these effects are apparent in productive language, including pronunciation, vocabulary, grammar, and discourse, and/or in the receptive language modalities of reading and listening.

In analyzing transfer through learner errors, care must be taken to ascertain whether they are developmental in nature, meaning that they are common to all learners of L2, regardless of L1, or are a result of transfer from L1. Positive transfer is perhaps more clearly identified, as the learner can often articulate how knowledge of the first language enabled comprehension or expression of the second. Transfer may also be evident in avoidance and overuse of language elements in L2 production (Ellis, 2008a). When learners know that there is a substantial contrast in a particular structure in the first and second languages, they may underuse L2 structure. Conversely, if learners perceive that a particular form in L1 is appropriate in L2, they may use it for all contexts and circumstances.

There is a great range of cognitive capacity between the span of infancy and adulthood, so more fully developed cognitive skills can be applied to acquiring a second language. Clearly, toddlers do not possess the reflective ability to compare linguistic features between their first and second languages, but adolescents and adults have this capability. This means that older children can begin to analyze certain aspects of the second language they are learning, such as when to use which pronoun and why (i.e., "Is it Reese and I or me and Reese?"). Paying attention to the rules of language is an effective strategy for learners whose cognitive development permits this type of analysis, and it is a hallmark of instructed SLA.

Naturalistic and Instructed Second Language Acquisition

There are different pathways to becoming proficient in a second language. Most similar to the first language acquisition process is what is called *naturalistic second language acquisition*. A typical case of naturalistic SLA is when an adult immigrates to a country without understanding or speaking the language. In the United States, for instance, certain industries employ immigrants who cannot speak or understand English in entry-level positions. A group of employees who speak the native language of the new immigrant (let's call him Quan, whose native language is Khmer) often help explain the job responsibilities. Over time, Quan comes into contact with English-speaking workers and supervisors and begins to develop a work-related vocabulary. Outside of work, depending on the extent of the community of speakers of Quan's native language, Khmer, he will begin to develop survival English phrases for shopping, going to the doctor, and other routine needs that may be conducted in English. In other words, if there is a large enough community of Khmer-speaking immigrants, services and businesses may be available in Quan's native language, and there would be less urgency to learn English in order to conduct his daily affairs. As he interacts with English speakers, he will begin to acquire necessary vocabulary, gradually developing the ability to string together simple sentences. This is, in simple terms, the process of naturalistic language acquisition.

As can be seen with the examples of Quan, there are many variables that affect naturalistic second language acquisition. Before we examine these variables and their influence on the rate and ultimate level of second language acquisition, let us look at what the process of naturalistic SLA commonly involves.

Second Language Acquisition Phases and Their Relation to L1 Acquisition

Similar to first language acquisition, naturalistic second language acquisition follows a series of predictable phases, particularly in morphology and syntax. Because those who are learning a second language are already verbal in at least one other language, they do not experience a preverbal phase the way infants who are learning their first language do. In particular, the process of acquiring the phonology of a second language is quite different from acquiring the first. Whereas babies babble new sounds to develop competence in using and combining them, adults typically learn sounds as parts of words. So, where a baby will repeat "pa-pa-pa," an adult will learn the word "paper" and will correctly pronounce the sounds that also exist in their native language but will approximate the sounds that do not. This might mean that an Arabic-speaking learner will pronounce it as "baber," /bebr/, because Arabic does not have a /p/ sound, and the /b/ sound is the closest approximation. A Spanish speaker may pronounce the /p/ sounds properly but will "tap" the final /r/ sound, /ɾ/, because this retroflex sound used in English is not a feature of Spanish phonology. Clearly, acquiring the phonology of a second language (either naturalistically or through formal instruction) is heavily influenced by the already acquired phonology of the first language. With babies learning any language, sounds are acquired in an order (i.e., stops before liquids); however, with adults learning a second language, sounds are acquired as the learners are exposed to words that use them, and some sounds that don't exist in the native language or that are used in different combinations or word positions in the native language are not pronounced the way a native speaker would utter them.

Whereas the preverbal stage is limited to first language acquisition, the verbal stages of first and second language acquisition share many commonalities. The acquisition of vocabulary tends to be similar, with frequently used nouns acquired early in first and second language acquisition, probably because of their tangible nature. Of course, nouns used frequently with infants differ from those used frequently with adults. An adult in the workplace will more likely hear the word "paper" before "crib." In addition, adults generally know and understand the concepts for most of the tangible words they learn—if they learn the word "ball," they probably won't assume the moon is also called "ball." However, a concept represented by a word in one language may be represented by two different words in another. For example, the word "know" in English is represented by "conocer" (to know a person) and "saber" (to know a fact) in Spanish, and the word "nipote" in Italian means "grandson" and "nephew." These differences can cause confusion or the misuse of a term.

Morphology acquisition is similar in first and second language acquisition. During the 1970s, researchers attempted to determine the acquisition of second language learners from different first language backgrounds (Brown & Attardo, 2014). A general order was established for grammatical markers and function words:

1. Pronouns
2. Articles
3. Copula (be)
4. Present progressive ("-ing")
5. Plural ("-s")
6. Be + verb + "-ing"
7. Regular past ("-ed")
8. Irregular past
9. Irregular plural ("-es")
10. Possessive ("-'s")
11. Third-person present ("-s")

Knowing that the first language profoundly affects the acquisition of phonology in the second language, it is surprising that despite various native languages, learners follow the same general sequence of morphological development in their second language (English) (Brown, 2014; Dulay & Burt, 1980; Kroll & Tokowicz, 2001). Certain morphemes from the list may cluster together at different points in the process (in stages) rather than be acquired individually in a sequence. Additionally, learners from different first language backgrounds may progress from acquiring one morpheme to another at a different rate. Nonetheless, the general order holds true regardless of the native language.

In the area of syntax acquisition, there are also numerous first and second language similarities (Cook, 2008; Dulay, Burt, & Krashen, 1982; Krashen, 1987; Krashen, Scarcella, & Long, 1982; Paradis & Genesee, 1996; Paradis, Genesee, & Crago, 2011). Second language learners begin with one- and two-word statements, often focusing on nouns and verbs and omitting function words. As they develop more competence in the grammar of the second language, their sentences become longer, adding prepositions and other function words as well as connecting phrases with conjunctions. Throughout this process, learners produce grammatical errors that are gradually replaced by the correct form in most cases. Questions and negative statements go through the same type of error patterns in SLA as they do during their acquisition in the first language. For example, "How could she have done that?" might be stated, "How she can did that?" or in an attempt to avoid making an error in question phrasing, a learner may make a statement with a rising intonation, such as "She came to school late?" With negative statements, second language learners often use "no" when "not" is correct and omit or improperly form the particle "do," such as "I no work on Mondays" instead of "I do not work on Mondays," or state words out of order without the proper grammatical (morphological) markers, such as "She no did laughed at my joke" instead of "She didn't laugh at my joke."

Because learning a second language naturalistically is in many ways similar to the way one learns a first language, many of the same processes and stages occur. Just as first language learners acquire new vocabulary through exposure to real objects and actions and their associated words and phrases, so do L2 learners in naturalistic language learning settings. In addition, the need for communicating different real-life functions, such as requests, providing information, and other communication functions, creates a need for first and second language learners to develop comprehension and expression ability through negotiation of meaning.

Naturalistic Second Language Acquisition

Understanding the nature of both naturalistic and instructed second language acquisition has important implications for SLPs. For ELs enrolled in elementary, middle, and high schools in the United States, both naturalistic and instructed second language acquisition are involved. Depending on the grade level and instructional model, ELs may be immersed with native speakers of English, studying subjects such as math, science, and social studies. Under these circumstances, most of their language acquisition is a result of naturalistic learning, where they acquire new vocabulary and structures by understanding academic content that includes multiple means of conveying information, not just language alone. In some schools, ESOL professionals work separately with ELs, providing more focus on the language of instruction to improve comprehensibility as well as to accelerate language development. For example, the ESOL professional might work on science vocabulary and cause-and-effect sentences to help ELs progress more quickly. This approach comes closer to formal instruction. In a preK–12 learning context where English is the language of instruction, it is reasonable to assume that whatever program model that an EL is enrolled in, much more time is spent learning in a naturalistic rather than an instructed way. This includes not only subject area classroom instruction but interaction with native speakers of English, in and out of the classroom.

One way to describe the necessary conditions for learning a second language naturalistically is through the information-processing concepts of input, interaction, and output (Ellis, 2003; Skehan, 1998; Swain, 1985). Second language acquisition research has demonstrated the importance of each verbal element for language development. Input refers to the information directed toward the learner. The key issue is whether the verbal input is comprehensible to the learner (Krashen, 1981). In other words, if the learner understands the meaning of the input, then she can add the new words and phrases to her linguistic repertoire. For example, if a teacher told you "siediti" and you did not know Italian, the verbal input would not be comprehensible. However, if the teacher modeled the action of sitting down or gestured by extending and lowering her palm facedown, you would comprehend the term "siediti" as "sit down." After hearing the term a few times and seeing others responding to the command, you would learn the new phrase.

Comprehensible input is necessary but not sufficient for developing proficiency in a second language. A language learner has to do more than just understand—the learner must also express meaning. The expression of information is called output. Although it is normal and even beneficial for second language learners to focus on listening through what is termed a "silent period" (Krashen & Terrell, 1983) in the beginning stages of acquisition, learners in naturalistic settings will often prolong this nonverbal response phase for fear of making pronunciation and grammatical errors. In order for learners to develop speaking skills, it is necessary for them to express meaning in the second language (Swain, 1995).

Communicating in any language requires input (received through listening and reading) and output (produced through speaking and writing), but in real communication, input and output do not happen independently. We don't hear input and then speak unrelated output. For example, if you are asked, "What is your name?" (input) you don't state, "It's very hot outside." Input and output in communication are connected. If you sit down with a friend and she asks you if you would like some tea, her question is the input that you need to comprehend. Your answer, "Yes, I would," is your output. The connected exchange of information that occurs in the back and forth between input and output is called interaction, and it is absolutely critical to acquiring a second language. If it was a hot day and you would love a cold drink, you might want to clarify the offer, "Would you like some tea?" with a question of your own, "Is it iced or hot?" Your friend could then provide the necessary detail for you to make your decision. Similarly, those communicating in a second language may not understand a word and can ask for elaboration or explanation, such as "What is a saucer?" to which a native speaker may either point to a saucer or state that it is a dish that goes under a teacup.

Second language learners attempting to use new vocabulary and put together more complicated sentences may make an error that impedes comprehension, at which point the listener can ask for clarification. For example, if an L2 learner states, "Have you shizzor?" and the English speaker replies, "What do you mean? I don't understand what you're asking." The English learner could then reply, "Shizzor, for cutting," while opening and closing his extended index and middle fingers. "Oh, you mean scissors!" would be a likely reply, confirming the correct word. The give-and-take in these two examples is known as *negotiation of meaning* (Pica, 1994), and its function is critical to language development. Through confirming comprehension of and trying out new ways to express meaning, language learners build their vocabulary and grammar.

Instructed Second Language Acquisition

Depending on the learning environment, instructed SLA can be the sole means of learning a foreign language or a complement to learning a second language naturalistically. Some learners in foreign language contexts have no other means of developing communication skills in the language other than in a formal classroom setting. These language learners' SLA developments would then result primarily from instruction, although the proliferation of Internet technologies has broadened the types of opportunities for exposure to a foreign language beyond the classroom. In a second language learning context where the learner is immersed in a community of speakers of the new language, one can learn entirely naturalistically but can benefit from the addition of instructed SLA to the process (Ellis, 2008b). As a rule of thumb, formal instruction in the second language becomes more important at later ages and grade levels. In a preK–12 learning context, language awareness activities that begin in elementary school and progress to formal study of grammar in middle and high school can be very beneficial for English learners.

There are many variations on the approach to instructed SLA, but the vast majority of approaches involve some focus or emphasis on grammar. Ranging from studying grammar rules and practicing examples of the rules to learning dialogues that are organized by grammar points, instructed SLA offers benefits for both the rate of acquisition and ultimate level of attainment. For adults, instructed SLA can speed the process through the various stages of language acquisition. In addition, grammar instruction can help avoid the establishment of errors in the speaker's production. Research shows that learners who study specific grammar points are more likely to acquire the correct form without *fossilizing* an incorrect form (Ellis, 2008b; Pica, 1994; Rowe & Levine, 2006). For example, if Quan learned English without grammar study, he might never move past a particular phase of syntactic errors in questions (e.g., "Why you no come?"), thereby fossilizing.

Fossilization (Selinker, 1972) has also been termed "stabilization" (Long, 1990) to emphasize the possibility of moving beyond the plateau of a non-target-like grammatical form. The notion has important implications for those who work with ELs because when a form becomes fossilized, the learner cannot spontaneously utter it following correction or instruction. Let us look at Quan's question error as it relates to fossilization. If an English speaker corrected Quan and explained how to form the question properly, Quan might understand the rule, but 30 minutes later in conversation with a coworker, Quan would make the same error without realizing it. For SLPs, the important issue is to recognize that some morphological and syntactic errors can hit a plateau that may or may not be overcome with instruction.

Social and Affective Variables in Second Language Acquisition

Second language acquisition occurs in very rich contexts that go beyond linguistic input. In his seminal study, Schumann

(1978) proposed that acculturation, defined as the integration of the L2 learner with the target language group, can explain second language acquisition in adults who are learning English in naturalistic settings. Because his acculturation model intends to explain the context of naturalistic SLA for adults who are immigrants or want to reside in the target language country for an extended period of time, it does not directly apply to L2 curriculum design or methodology, especially in the case of children who are bilingual or learning another language. However, the social and affective factors that are the basis of Schumann's model affect children just as they affect adults, albeit in different ways and with different degrees of intensity. Therefore, it is very useful to explore the social and affective variables that are related to aspects of second language acquisition.

Schumann's model looks at acculturation as a result of the clustering of two groups of variables: social factors and affective factors. Social factors involve the relationship between two linguistically different groups of people who are in contact: One group consists of people who are learning an L2, and the other group is made up of the native speakers of L2 or the target language group. A number of social factors can, in Schumann's opinion, either promote or hinder contact between two groups with consequences on whether or not the L2 learning group acculturates and consequently acquires L2. Table 4–6 lists and explains the eight social variables that are an integral part of Schumann's acculturation model.

Table 4–6. *Social Factors in Acculturation*

Variable	Characteristics
Social Domination Patterns	• If the L2 learning group is dominant, it will tend not to learn L2.
	• If the L2 learning group is subordinate, they will tend to resist acculturation and not learn L2.
	• If the L2 learning group and the L2 group are equal, the contact is likely more extensive with positive influences on L2 acquisition.

continues

Table 4–6. *continued*

Variable	Characteristics
Integration Strategies	• Assimilation: The L2 learning group adopts the values of the L2 group, maximizing contact and L2 acquisition. • Preservation: The L2 learning group rejects the values of the L2 group, minimizing contact and L2 acquisition. • Adaptation: The L2 learning group adapts to the values of L2 group but maintains its own values for intragroup use, with various degrees of contact and L2 acquisition.
Enclosure	• Refers to the degree to which secondary social institutions (school, churches, professions, etc.) are shared by both groups. • Low enclosure: they share many of these institutions, enhancing contact and L2 acquisition. • High enclosure: they have different secondary social institutions, limiting contact and L2 acquisition.
Cohesiveness	• If the L2 learning group is cohesive, there will be separation limiting contact and L2 acquisition.
Size	• If the L2 learning group is large, the intragroup contact will be more prevalent than intergroup contact, limiting L2 acquisition.
Cultural Congruence	• If the two group cultures are similar, then contact is more likely facilitating L2 acquisition
Attitude	• If the two groups have positive attitudes toward each other, this will likely facilitate L2 acquisition.
Intended Length of Residence	• If the L2 learning group intends to reside for a long time in the L2 group area, more contacts are possible with positive influences on L2 acquisition.

Source: Adapted from "The Acculturation Model for Second Language Acquisition," by J. H. Schumann, in *Second Language Acquisition and Foreign Language Learning,* by R. C. Gingras (Ed.), 1978, Washington, DC: Center for Applied Linguistics.

Although the social factors discussed above and in Table 4–6 appear to facilitate second language acquisition, individual variables represented by affective variables might impede the learning of a second language. In the acculturation model, the important affective factors are language shock, culture shock, motivation, and ego permeability, discussed in Table 4–7.

Table 4–7. *Affective Factors in Acculturation*

Variable	Characteristics
Language Shock	• The L2 learners might fear criticism and ridicule when they attempt to speak another language. • Even for young learners, there is wide individual variation in the willingness to tolerate the frustration when trying to use another language in a variety of school activities.
Culture Shock	• Culture shock is the anxiety resulting from entering a new culture. • Adults experience this more than children, but even young L2 learners may be affected by various degrees of culture shock affecting their parents and other members of their community.
Motivation	• Integrative: L2 learners want to learn another language in order to become like the speakers of the other language. • Instrumental: L2 learners want to learn another language for utilitarian purposes. • Integrative motivation is seen more powerful because the L2 learner wants to integrate with L2 speakers, with positive effects on L2 acquisition.
Ego Permeability	• Each person has a language ego that establishes as sense of language limits and boundaries, which are flexible in the early stages of development and become more rigid later. • L2 learners with more permeable language egos will have more success in L2 acquisition.

Source: Adapted from "The Acculturation Model for Second Language Acquisition," by J. H. Schumann, in *Second Language Acquisition and Foreign Language Learning,* by R. C. Gingras (Ed.), 1978, Washington, DC: Center for Applied Linguistics.

The social and affective factors discussed in Schumann's acculturation model work together in determining the success of learning another language. The social factors emphasize the collective distance between two language communities, whereas the affective factors look at perceptions regarding the two languages within individuals. Of the two sets of factors, Schumann suggests that the affective factors may be more important in the success of second language acquisition. L2 learners who perceive a vast psychological distance between themselves and L2 would not likely seek opportunities to develop their proficiency in L2 and might attain an incomplete mastery of the target language.

It is true that Schumann's model was designed with adult immigrants who are learning L2 in a naturalistic way in mind. His model has no direct instructional application. Nevertheless, the social and affective factors that are the basis for his model have an influence on learners engaged in formal language learning as well as on their second language acquisition. It is reasonable to suggest that these factors interact with instructional programs and settings in ways that influence the success of second language teaching, either positively or negatively.

Following a general overview of first and second language acquisition, this chapter now turns to one of the challenging tasks faced by SLP professionals: how to determine whether ELs have a communication disorder or whether they are simply displaying behaviors that are typically associated with normal second language development.

Communication Difference or Disorder?

To distinguish between a communication difference and a communication disorder, it is important to revisit what constitutes a communication disorder. Communication disorders embrace a wide range of conditions that generate challenges in effective communication. They include speech disorders, which affect the articulation of speech sounds, fluency, and voice, and language disorders, which include impairments in the use of the spoken, signed, or written system. In general, communication disorders are typically classified by their impact on a child's receptive skills (i.e., the ability to understand what is said or to decode, integrate, and organize what is heard) and expressive skills (i.e., the ability to articulate sounds, use appropriate rate and rhythm during speech, exhibit appropriate vocal tone and resonance, and use sounds, words, and sentences in meaningful contexts).

Communication differences are behaviors that are commonly observed among second language learners. For example, ELs at the beginning stages of language proficiency normally produce shorter and less elaborate sentences than their native English-speaking peers, have an underdeveloped vocabulary due to their limited L2 exposure, and have a limited capacity for understanding L2 (Paradis, Genesee, & Crago, 2011). Some students, when learning a second language, go through a silent period where they use their receptive skills only; however, this does not mean they do have not expressive skills (Paradis, 2007). When a child is learning a new language, he or she will demonstrate differences in sentence structure, speech sound production, vocabulary, and pragmatics. Unfortunately, children with language differences that result from limited experience in using a language are often misidentified as having a communication disorder and are labeled "language learning disabled" (Roseberry-McKibben, 2014). Table 4–8 presents the common conditions that are associated with receptive and expressive communication challenges (Prelock, Hutchins, & Glascoe, 2008). If we examine the challenges associated with the last category in Table 4–8, *specific language impairment,* we can easily see how processes typically associated with normal second language acquisition, or language differences, might be interpreted as signs of a communication disorder.

One of the more difficult tasks for SLPs is to determine whether a child is displaying characteristics of normal, typical behaviors for those who are not yet proficient in English or if the child is displaying characteristics of a language disorder. Factors such as language loss, code-switching, and/or interference can confound the issue. For example, code-switching, the practice of switching between a primary and a secondary language or discourse, is a phenomenon that occurs when bilingual speakers substitute a word or phrase from one language with a phrase or

Table 4–8. *Disorders Commonly Associated with Receptive and Expressive Communication Problems*

Condition	Expressive Communication Problems	Receptive Communication Problems
Autism	Variability in speech production Use of language in social situations is more challenging than producing language forms Difficulty selecting the right words to represent intended meaning	Difficulty analyzing, integrating, and processing information. Misinterpretation of social cues
Brain Injury	Difficulty in using language appropriately across contexts	Difficulty making connections, inferences and using information to solve problems. Challenges in attention and memory which affect linguistic processing. Challenges in understanding symbolic language and words with multiple meanings.
Hearing Impairment	Limited oral output depending on degree of hearing loss. For oral communicators, vocal resonance, speech sound accuracy, and syntactic structure often affected.	Difficulty with sound perception and discrimination, voice recognition, and understanding of speech.
Intellectual Disability	Production is often below cognitive ability; similar but slower developmental path than typical peers.	Comprehension of language is often below cognitive ability. Difficulty organizing and categorizing information heard for later retrieval.

Table 4–8. *continued*

Condition	Expressive Communication Problems	Receptive Communication Problems
Intellectual Disability *continued*	Tendency to use more immature language forms. Tendency to produce shorter and less elaborated utterances.	Difficulty with abstract concepts.
Specific Language Impairment	Shorter, less elaborated sentences than typical peers. Difficulty in rule formulation for speech sound, word, and sentence productions; ineffective use of language forms in social contexts sometimes leading to inappropriate utterances. Poorly developed vocabulary	Slower and less efficient information processing. Limited capacity for understanding language.

Source: Adapted from "Speech-Language Impairment: How to Identify the Most Common and Least Diagnosed Disability of Childhood," by P. A. Prelock, T. Hutchins, & F. P. Glascoe, 2008, *Medscape Journal of Medicine, 10*(6).

word from another language. The sentence "I want a bicycle roja" is an example of code-switching. In this sentence, the English word "red" is replaced with its Spanish equivalent.

Understanding that L2 learners go through predictable stages of language development with clear characteristics is critical in determining if the child has a communication difference or disorder. The diagnosis of "language learning disabled" should only be used to identify students who have a relatively poor ability in language that cannot be attributed to differences in the child's cultural, linguistic, or educational experiences (Kohnert, 2008). To determine if ELs with communication disorders are eligible to receive services, the Individuals with Disabilities Education Improvement Act regulations published in the *Federal Register* in 2006 (U.S. Department of Education, 2006) stipulate that the speech and language evaluation of ELs must assess both (all) languages, include the use of culturally appropriate assessment instruments and practices, be conducted by professionals who are familiar with the current best practices literature, and understand the cultural, social, cognitive, and linguistic norms of the child's speech community.

Specifically, in order for ELs to be diagnosed with a communication disorder, they must demonstrate delays or difficulties in both (across) languages, demonstrate that the disorder has an adverse effect on their educational performance, and the linguistic behaviors must meet the definition and eligibility requirements of a particular state to be designated as having a "language disorder." For example, in the state of Georgia, language impairment is defined as the "impaired comprehension and/or use of spoken language which may also impair the written and/or other symbol systems and is negatively impacting the child's ability to participate in classroom environment. It may involve, in any combination, the form of language, the content of language, and/or the use of language in communication that is adversely affecting child's communication performance." In the state of Georgia, "language impaired" does not include children who:

◆ are in normal stages of second language acquisition,
  unless it is determined that they have a language
  impairment in their native language;
◆ have regional, dialectic, and/or cultural differences;
◆ have auditory processing disorders not accompanied by
  a language impairment; and
◆ have anxiety disorders (e.g., selective mutism), unless it
  is also determined that they have language impairment.

What, then, do SLPs and ESOL professionals need to consider when assessing ELs to ensure they do not mistake a communication difference for a communication disorder? SLPs and ESOL professionals must consider L2 normal processes (i.e., the "silent period," the BICS-CALP gap, and code-switching) and determine if the child is demonstrating behaviors that are characteristic of the normal processes of second language acquisition. The student's performance needs to be compared to the performance of other children who come from a similar cultural, linguistic, and economic background. In diagnosing ELs, extensive information about their home, school, and community needs to be examined alongside test data (Ortiz & Yates, 2002). Professionals who work with the child can provide crucial information about his or her language and literacy competence. Although the focus of this text is on the role of the SLP and ESOL professional as collaborative partners, it is critical to acknowledge the role of all professionals (i.e., general education teachers, bilingual education teachers, and special education teachers) in native and second language assessment and intervention of ELs (Archibald, 2017; ASHA, 1998; Peercy & Beltran, 2011; Rosa-Lugo & Fradd, 2000; Watson & Bellon-Harn, 2013).

Next, it should not be assumed that all EL children have the same language experiences. Some ELs experience language loss or arrested development of their primary language after exposure to English. Language loss occurs as the dominant language (usually English) tends to displace the mother tongue (Brice, Brice, & Kester, 2010). Arrested development occurs as the child ceases to develop L1 while trying to learn L2 (Schiff-Myers, 1992). These two processes, arrested development or language loss, can occur when ELs do not use their primary language. Interestingly, the loss of L1 can occur even in instances when L1 is still used in the home for social interaction by other family members. This may occur when L1 is not valued by the EL or when EL parents encourage the children to become speakers of L2. It is not uncommon for second-generation ELs to become predominantly passive users of their first language. These ELs may respond to their elders in English rather than in their native language.

Language loss has also been attributed to the lack of programs or instructional activities that focus on building conceptual knowledge in the first language (Crawford, 2003). Currently, there are many schools that do not have programs for bilingual students or have transitional programs where the focus is on transitioning into English as quickly as possible. Scholars have discussed some of the deleterious effects of language loss on the development of academic language skills in English (Collier &

Thomas, 2014; Thomas & Collier, 1997) and transfer of language skills from L1 to English (Cummins, 1984, 1998). Often, language loss may resemble a language learning disability.

Given the length of time it takes to develop academic language proficiency in English, it would seem beneficial for ELs to introduce the learning of L2 as early as possible. However, for many children, the early teaching of subjects in L2 is not preferable. It seems that the more proficient a child is in L1, the easier it will be to learn L2. The level of development of L2 may be influenced by or limited to the level of development of L1 when L2 was introduced. For example, many ELs have never formally developed their L1 and cannot read and write in their home language (i.e., Spanish). Many of these ELs may be dominant in English but have deficits in school performance in English. For many of these children, accessing and mastering the curriculum will be a challenge.

The third consideration for understanding a communication difference from a communication disorder is related to the challenges in assessment of ELs in their primary language. There are only a few formal assessment instruments in languages other than English. In addition, some of the assessment instruments are direct translations from English versions, a fact that poses serious threats to the validity of the scores obtained. Moreover, some languages or dialects are spoken only by a minority; therefore, interpreters must be used to assist in the assessment process. However, this is not always a possibility. Interpreters are bilingual individuals who translate written information or who facilitate communication between speakers who do not speak the same language (ASHA, n.d.-a). Parents are often used as interpreters; however, this is not considered a best practice. Criteria to select and use interpreters in the assessment and/or intervention process have been described by several scholars and should be used as guidelines in the assessment of ELs (Langdon & Cheng, 2002; Langdon & Saenz, 2015).

SLPs and ESOL professionals assessing ELs must keep in mind that there is a great deal of diversity in languages. Additionally, information concerning code-switching and the dialectal variations that the EL hears in the home must be evaluated (Gutierrez-Clellen, Simon-Cereijido, & Leone, 2009). A formal and informal evaluation of the primary language requires not only fluency in the language of the EL but also knowledge about cultural similarities and differences and linguistic variations.

Summary

To provide common ground for understanding the fundamental issues in the language acquisition of ELs with a communication disorder, this chapter provided an overview of first and second language acquisition theories and the developmental stages involved in L1 and L2 acquisition. Additionally, recognizing that second language learning is influenced by many non-language-related variables, we examined several nonlinguistic factors and discussed how these might affect L2 acquisition. The practical application and the importance of second language acquisition processes were made evident in the discussion of whether observable second language behaviors are indeed examples of communication disorders for ELs or simply normal language differences all ELs go through during their acquisition of English.

To increase accuracy in disability determinations, professionals must be informed about the possible challenges faced by ELs. These students are required to acquire proficiency in English for both social and academic purposes, learn to read and write English, and obtain background knowledge of mainstream culture to integrate and function effectively in school and achieve the curriculum standards (Cloud, Genesee, & Hamayan, 2009). The next chapter will provide a definition of literacy and an overview of literacy development in ELs.

5

Literacy Development in a Second Language

Introduction

Regardless of specialization or academic preparation, all teachers and professionals who work with students are "teachers" of literacy. Literacy development provides the perfect venue for collaboration between SLPs and ESOL professionals. Language is the foundation of literacy and plays a very important role in the academic achievement of ELs, with or without communication disorders. In order for ELs with communication disorders to be successful, it is imperative that SLPs and ESOL professionals collaborate fully in developing language and literacy skills of ELs with communication disorders (ASHA, 1998, 2001a, 2001b, 2010a; Rosa-Lugo, Mihai, & Nutta, 2017). Their collaboration will ensure that ELs with communication disorders are appropriately identified and that evidence-based interventions are provided for the purpose of decreasing the "at risk for literacy development" likelihood for the student (ASHA, 2002a).

ESOL professionals are first and foremost literacy teachers because the ESOL curriculum strongly emphasizes the development of English language and literacy for ELs (TESOL, 2001a, 2001b, 2010a). In the era of standards-aligned instruction and language practices required by the Standards, ESOL professionals need to ensure that K–12 EL students with varying levels of first language literacy, background knowledge, and English language proficiency are prepared for postsecondary education and careers (TESOL, 2013a).

In the area of EL literacy, the academic preparation of ESOL teachers makes them aware of the differences between literacy (i.e., reading and writing) in L1 and literacy in L2 (de Jong & Harper, 2005; TESOL, 2007a, 2013b; Valdés, Kibler, & Walqui, 2014). Some of the key issues in L2 literacy are language transfer, background knowledge, affective factors, and the importance of oral language in literacy development.

The importance of oral language development underlines the pivotal role of the SLP-ESOL collaboration. In this partnership, SLPs can provide critical information and support ESOL professionals when they have ELs with communication disorders in their classrooms (ASHA, 1998). ESOL teachers have a very good knowledge of the English literacy issues and challenges pertaining to the EL general student population, but they might not be as prepared to address specific issues linked to the literacy development of ELs with communication disorders (Kangas, 2018, 2019). This is where the contribution of the SLP is invaluable. In 2001, the American Speech-Language-Hearing Association (ASHA) published several documents addressing literacy and the roles and responsibilities of SLPs in the development of reading and writing among children and adolescents, particularly for younger children who have communication disorders (ASHA, 2001a, 2001b, 2002a). These documents specified the role of SLPs in literacy in the areas of prevention, identification, assessment, collaboration, and advocacy (ASHA, 2002a) and noted their unique contributions to literacy instruction. Within this framework, specifically in the area of prevention, the response to intervention (RtI) process and its focus on optimizing student performance prior to being declared a special education student provides the SLPs with an excellent opportunity to make greater use of their expertise in language and literacy (Ehren, 2005; Ehren, Montgomery, & Whitmire, 2006).

SLPs have acquired a great deal of information in their academic training about English literacy challenges related to communication disorders. Their knowledge of language and its subsystems (phonology, morphology, syntax, semantics, and pragmatics), their training in language development and acquisition, and communication processes and disorders, combined with their skills in using diagnostic-prescriptive approaches to assessment and intervention, are particularly valuable in the educational context (Ehren & Murza, 2010; Ehren, Nelson, Staskowski, & Davis, 2012; Spracher, 2000). Depending on the educational placement of the EL student, the ESOL professional might have the primary role of facilitating oral language skills and the general education teacher for teaching reading and writing. An SLP can complement and augment the skills and knowledge of these and other professionals, who also have unique perspectives, knowledge, and skills (ASHA, 2010a). These professionals can include general education teachers, bilingual education teachers, ESOL professionals, reading specialists, literacy coaches, and special education teachers. For example, SLPs are able to provide a solid analysis from their perspective of the English language demands present in the textbooks, language of instruction in the classroom, and grade- and age-level curriculum expectations for ELs (Powell, 2018).

If we are to describe the role of each element of the SLP-ESOL pair as it relates to ELs with communication disorders, we can say that SLPs have detailed knowledge about communication disorders and general EL knowledge, whereas ESOL professionals have detailed EL knowledge and general knowledge about communication disorders. The SLP-ESOL collaboration vis-à-vis ELs with communication disorders encompasses the entire educational cycle of this student population. This collaboration starts with the correct identification and appropriate placement of ELs with communication disorders, a process that should determine whether the student demonstrates normal characteristics and processes found in students acquiring English as a second language or a communication disorder. The very nature of this fundamental question points out that an accurate identification and placement is not possible without the full involvement of SLPs and ESOL professionals, as well as other school professionals (ASHA, n.d.-a, 2016a; Girolametto, Weitzman, & Greenberg, 2012; Rosa-Lugo & Fradd, 2000; Zygouris-Coe & Goodwiler, 2013).

Once EL students with communication disorders are identified and placed in appropriate programs to include English language development programs, the SLP-ESOL team should work together in providing the best instruction and intervention strategies (Collier, 2010; Echevarria, Richards-Tutor, & Vogt, 2015; Herrell & Jordan, 2020). These strategies should target the specific literacy challenges of ELs with communication disorders and should incorporate evidence-based literacy development practices during ESOL classes and speech and language therapy sessions. Finally, the SLP-ESOL team should work closely in the assessment of ELs with communication disorders. Classroom-based and large-scale assessments should measure the literacy development of this student population to determine whether the intervention has proven effective and to routinely monitor progress (Hoover, Mendez Barletta, & Klingner, 2016). The importance of measuring academic and English language development for all students is a critical and unavoidable requirement of the Every Student Succeeds Act (ESSA), making the collaboration between SLPs and ESOL professionals crucial.

Literacy: Definition and Attributes

The definition of literacy has evolved over the past century. Literacy has traditionally been defined as the ability to read and write. Today the definition has been expanded. The Workforce Investment Act of 1998 defines literacy as "an individual's ability to read, write, speak in English, compute and solve problems at levels of proficiency necessary to function on the job, in the family of the individual, and in society" (ASHA, 2008b). This is a broader view of literacy than just an individual's ability to read. As new information and technology have increasingly shaped our society, the skills needed to function successfully have gone beyond reading and literacy and have come to include the skills listed in the current definition of literacy (National Institute for Literacy, n.d.). The relationship between language and literacy and the connection between spoken and written language are addressed in ASHA's position statement *Roles and Responsibilities of Speech-Language Pathologists Related to Reading and Writing in Children and Adolescents* (ASHA, 2001a) and subsequent paper on written language disorders (ASHA, n.d.-a). Specifically, these documents establish the connection between spoken and written language and point out that:

A. Spoken language provides the foundation for the development of reading and writing abilities.

B. Spoken and written language have a reciprocal relationship, such that each build on the other to result in general language and literacy competence.

C. Instruction in spoken language can result in growth in written language, and instruction in written language can result in growth in spoken language (ASHA, n.d.-a, 2002a).

One possible way of operationalizing the construct of literacy is by examining literacy attributes. Walmsley (2008) defines literacy attributes as what students should know, do, understand, and have experienced. In other words, *knowing* means that students should "know what" (e.g., knowledge of vocabulary, background knowledge, etc.) and "know how" (e.g., strategies of inferring meaning of an unknown word). *Doing* means that students should have constant engagement in literacy behaviors, such as independent reading, and *understanding* means that students should be able to make sense of many types of texts, either literary or informational. The last part of the definition, *have experienced*, means that students should accumulate literacy and continue to increase these experiences over time. Literacy attributes are based on the Communication Triangle, a concept developed by Kinneavy (1969) (Figure 5–1).

The Communication Triangle illustrates the basic relationships between the encoders, or those who originate communication; the decoders, or those who receive the communication; and the reality, or the knowledge shared by the encoder and decoder. Central to the entire triangle is the medium used to convey the message, or the signal. It is important to note that these relationships occur in a social context and have a crucial role in defining and sometimes constraining the types of communication that typically take place, the ways language is used, and the perceived appropriateness and correctness of the conveyed message. Using the Communication Triangle, literacy attributes are defined in three major areas: receptive language, expressive language, and background knowledge (Walmsley, 2008). Receptive language focuses on understanding meaning that is read, heard, or viewed. Expressive language focuses on creating meaning through writing, speaking, and/or drawing. Finally, background knowledge is the knowledge that is necessary

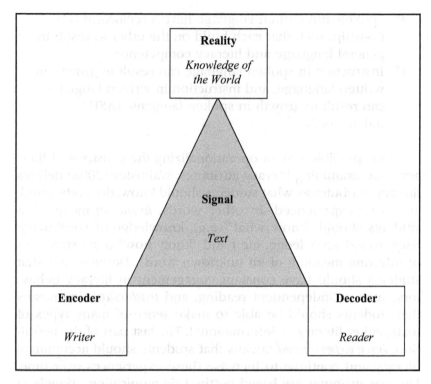

Figure 5–1. *The Communication Triangle.* Source: *Adapted from "The Basic Aims of Discourse," by J. E. Kinneavy, 1969,* College Composition and Communication, *20(5), 297–304. Published by National Council of Teachers of English.*

to understand and create meaning (Table 5–1). Because of the importance assigned to reading and writing, we will concentrate our attention on these two domains and the importance of background knowledge for reading and writing in a second language.

Receptive Language: The L2 Reading Domain

Reading: Definition and Purpose

Reading is a cognitive process that involves the comprehension of written messages. During this process, the reader not only

Table 5–1. *Literacy Attributes*

Area	Domains
Receptive Language	Reading—can make sense of what it is read – *understands what is read* – *decodes fluently* – *understands different types of text* – *understands big ideas* – *understands vocabulary* – *applies comprehension strategies* – *reads extensively* Listening—can make sense of what it is heard – *is a critical and responsive listener* Viewing—can make sense of what is observed – *is a critical and responsive viewer*
Expressive Language	Writing—can express ideas in written form – *communicates ideas effectively* – *demonstrates effective language/style* – *organizes and develops writing adequately* – *uses appropriate mechanics* Speaking—can express ideas in spoken form – *communicates ideas effectively* Representing—can express ideas in a variety of media (drawing, photography, etc.) – *communicates ideas effectively*
Background Knowledge	Knowledge of the world – *understands the world around and beyond himself/herself*

Source: Data from *Closing the Circle: A Practical Guide to Implementing Literacy Reform, K–12,* by S. A. Walmsley, 2008, San Francisco, CA: Jossey-Bass.

receives but also interprets language that is encoded in print. It is very important to emphasize the interdependence of the three literacy attributes as noted by Walmsley (2008). Reading comprehension takes place when the reader decodes the information contained in the text in written form and utilizes background knowledge to integrate and interpret the decoded information.

Why do readers read? There are many purposes for reading. Readers read for enjoyment, to locate specific information, or to learn new information. Let us focus on two other important purposes of reading: reading for comprehension and reading to learn. When readers read novels or newspaper articles, they read for enjoyment or pleasure. In that case, readers read for general comprehension or to get the "gist" of the text. Readers who read for pleasure are not preoccupied with remembering all the important details for a later recall task.

To develop proficiency in casual reading and related comprehension takes time, but this type of reading and comprehension is usually an effortless process. It does not mean that reading for comprehension is easy; rather, fluent readers have achieved reading fluency as a result of considerable (in both time and quantity) extended reading, which ultimately leads to automaticity of reading processes, such as word recognition, meaning formation, and strategies for constructing meaning for unknown words. Reading for comprehension is essential and provides the foundation for other reading purposes, such as reading to learn. In academic contexts, probably the most important purpose for reading is reading to acquire new information. However, it is not the only purpose of academic reading. Many times, EL and non-EL students read to search for specific information. In that case, they skim and scan through texts to find out, for example, a specific date a historical event occurred, the name of the person who wrote a famous novel, or the researchers who created a life-saving medicine. Nevertheless, most of the time, students read to learn new information with the purpose of using it in a related academic task either immediately following the reading or in the near future (Fang, Schleppegrell, & Cox, 2006).

Reading to learn involves not only the comprehension of the main themes or ideas presented in a text but also to recall critical supporting ideas and details. The need to process all this information in an attempt to learn results in a slower rate of reading fluency in comparison to reading fluency associated with general comprehension. When students read to learn, in addition to reading for understanding the main idea of a text, they use supporting information, create outlines that organize information by cause and effect and/or compare and contrast, and use their prior knowledge consciously.

Reading in L1 and L2: Similarities and Differences

Early literacy development in a first language is well documented for young children. We have information about young children's early literacy development in English, Spanish, and other languages (Peregoy & Boyle, 2016). However, there is a need for research that documents early literacy development in English as a second language (Alfano & Douglas, 2018; Lesaux & Siegel, 2003). Specifically, information is lacking about students who have never had literacy instruction in their first language (Freeman, Freeman, & Mercuri, 2002; Potochnick, 2018). In the past, literacy experts claimed that both English learners and native English speakers go through similar reading and writing development processes (Edelsky, 1981; Hudelson, 1984). Although many aspects of reading and writing development are basically similar for English learners and native English speakers, there are important differences. To obtain information about reading in L1 and L2 literacy, research has posed the following questions: Is reading in L1 similar to reading in L2? Do ELs go through the same processes when they read as non-ELs?

Several researchers have supported a reading universal hypothesis, which affirms that reading processes in L2 are very similar to reading processes in L1 (Bialystok, Luk, & Kwan, 2005; Goodman & Goodman, 1994; National Reading Panel, 2000). Reading processes are very much the same in all languages, and variation occurs simply due to specific characteristics of the writing system particular to one language or perhaps its grammatical structure (Goodman, 1979; Perfetti, 2003). There are, indeed, universals of reading abilities, as identified by Grabe (2009). The first one relates to the cognitive nature of reading. All readers utilize pattern-recognition skills, working memory, and long-term memory. Therefore, reading in L1, as well as reading in L2, is a cognitive process.

Second, all writing systems are based on spoken language, and phonological decoding is an essential element of reading in all languages, including those that do not use alphabetical script.

Research that has focused on reading in Chinese has shown that phonological awareness is a predictor of Chinese abilities. For example, one aspect of phonological awareness in Chinese, syllable awareness, seems to be very strongly related to the ability to read Chinese characters (Chow, McBride-Chang, & Burgess, 2005; Lin, Cheng, & Wang, 2018). When comparing alphabetical and nonalphabetical languages, ELs whose L1 is alphabetical (e.g., Spanish or French) seem to be better at acquiring the letter-to-sound correspondence of English than ELs whose first language is nonalphabetical (Bialystok, 2001; Oschwald, Schättin, von Bastian, & Souza, 2018). Alphabetical languages have a much stronger letter-to-sound correspondence. After ELs acquire an alphabetical system in their L1, their phonological awareness will transfer to an alphabetical L2, even when the sound-to-letter relationship is not clear, as is the case in English.

The third universal of reading abilities is the extent to which transfer in L2 reading is facilitated by the similarities between L1 and L2. When L1 and L2 share similar linguistic properties, L2 reading comprehension is vastly improved. For example, in a research study conducted by Muljani, Koda, and Moates (1998), Indonesian students speaking Indonesian Bahasa were faster in English word recognition than Chinese students were because of their previous alphabetical experiences, especially when the English words conformed to the syllable structures of their L1. Finally, reading processes in all languages rely on background knowledge and culture socialization in order to make sense of print and incorporate the new information into existing knowledge and linguistic systems.

There is strong evidence of similarities between reading in L1 and reading in L2, but not an absolute congruence between the two. The fundamental difference between the two processes is revealed in the nature of L2 reading. Reading in L2 involves two languages. They continuously interact and make reading in L2 more complex than reading in L1 (Koda, 2007; Koda & Miller, 2018). In most cases, ELs who start reading in L2 already bring to the reading process their L1 language background. However, L2 reading is not just a transfer of ELs' first language abilities (Durgunoglu, 1998; Leafstedt & Gerber, 2005; Mathes et al., 2007). Although L1 plays an important role in L2 reading proficiency, many issues of L2 reading development are often associated with

L2 language proficiency, L2 language and print exposure, and L2 processing skills development. In fact, these issues are the important differences between reading in L1 and reading in L2.

In a survey of many years of research on L2 reading, the National Literacy Panel on Language-Minority Children and Youth (August & Shanahan, 2006) synthesized nearly 300 studies into a number of important findings on L2 reading. Their review of studies showed that first and second language speakers learning to read can develop word-level literacy (i.e., decoding and spelling) at equal levels. A disparity exists, however, in text-level skills. For example, L2 readers do not attain reading comprehension at the same level as L1 readers. They also found that second language oral proficiency is essential for L2 reading comprehension. This includes vocabulary knowledge, listening comprehension, syntactic skills, and metalinguistic knowledge. The panel determined that second language readers have additional factors involved in reading comprehension in the L2, such as L1 literacy and L2 oral proficiency. Certain errors occur because of differences between L1 and L2; however, research has also demonstrated that literacy skills in L1 facilitate L2 literacy development (Calderon, 2007; Cardenas-Hagan, Carlson, & Pollard-Durodola, 2007; Vaughn et al., 2006). Some language transfer issues are more likely to affect L2 literacy development than others and at certain stages of literacy development. Understanding how the first language of Spanish speakers, the majority of ELs in the United States, is different from English can shed light on this issue.

Contrasting the Spanish sound system with the English sound system illustrates how the native language can transfer to the L2, resulting in errors in reading and spelling (Bear, Invernizzi, Templeton, & Johnston, 2019). For example, there are English vowel sounds that do not exist in Spanish, such as the vowels /æ/, as in the word "man," or /e/, as in "pen." English letters that represent different sounds in Spanish are another area of contrast. For example, the letter "a" as in "cake" is represented by the sound /e/ in Spanish and, similarly, the letter "e" as in "bean" is the sound /i/ in Spanish.

In addition to L1 transfer, sociocultural variables have an effect on reading (August & Shanahan, 2006). Six variables were identified in their review of studies: immigration status;

discourse/interactional characteristics; other specific sociocultural variables; parent and family influences; district, state, and federal policies; and language prestige. The research indicated that mediating home/school interaction differences improved students' engagement in classroom instruction. In addition, culturally familiar texts facilitated comprehension, although it was a weak predictor compared to proficiency in the language of the text. Moreover, it was found that schools did not take full advantage of parents' potential contributions.

In terms of instructional factors in ELs' literacy development, it appears that the same components of literacy instruction that apply to first language learners apply to second language learners, particularly at the word level. Interestingly, instructional practices that are successful with both L1 and L2 learners do not improve literacy skills for ELs as much as their English-speaking peers. The exception to this finding is vocabulary instruction, which seems to yield greater benefits for ELs than native speakers.

Oral English proficiency is necessary for reading in English, and literacy instruction should include the development of listening and speaking skills. Research has demonstrated this because L2 learners with strong L1 reading skills do not read at the same levels in English as their native-speaking peers. A commonality between L1 and L2 readers is the basic sequence of the development of reading skills, beginning with decoding and moving to comprehension at later stages. Throughout this sequence, vocabulary instruction is critical. Taking advantage of ELs' native language oral proficiency has been shown to benefit their L2 reading development—specifically, instructing ELs to read in their native language leads to better outcomes in reading in English at both the elementary and secondary levels (August, Carlo, Dressler, & Snow, 2005).

Learning to Read and Reading to Learn: A Key Distinction

There are more differences than similarities between reading in L1 and reading in L2 (Anderson, 2008; National Reading Panel, 2000). Although the National Reading Panel (2000) report did not focus on preventing reading failure in ELs, they did identify effective practices in five areas of reading instruction: phonemic awareness, phonics, fluency, vocabulary, and text comprehension. Related to the findings identified by the National Literacy Panel, Anderson (2008) identified six key factors that influence L2 literacy for ELs: literacy in L1, oral language proficiency in L2, age of arrival in the United States, expectations of the school experience, types of L2 readers, and parents' educational levels. Language professionals need to know how literate ELs are in L1 and their level of oral fluency in English. Oral proficiency, discussed later in this chapter, is an asset in developing reading proficiency.

Anderson and Nunan (2008) depict the learning/reading continuum as Beginning → Intermediate → Advanced. For L1 readers, Grades K–3 mark the "learning to read" period, starting with the Beginning and ending around Intermediate reading levels; once L1 readers are in fourth grade and beyond (or beyond Intermediate), they are "reading to learn." For years, teaching practices have been influenced around the dichotomy of "learning to read and reading to learn" (Chall, 1983; Chall & Jacobs, 2003). However, researchers now caution that this view is not sufficient to provide adequate instruction in reading to L1 students. Scholars adamantly note that "reading to learn" is a lifelong process (Catts & Kamhi, 2017; Kamhi & Catts, 2012; Moats, 2010; Scarborough, 2001). Studies have indicated that while middle and high school students may have mastered the basic tools of reading, they still continue to need support "learning to read" increasingly complex texts across the content areas (Goldman, Snow, & Vaughn, 2016).

In particular, for L2 readers, we can't assume that reading has been fully developed in K–3. Findings from several studies indicate that although ELs often master foundational skills of reading prior to Grade 3, they often demonstrate "late-emerging" reading difficulties after the fourth grade (Kieffer, 2008, 2010; Mancilla-Martinez, Kieffer, Biancarosa, Christodoulou, & Snow, 2011). At the secondary level, EL students are often challenged with the double task of increasing their proficiency in English and meeting the literacy demands across content areas (e.g., history, science, math, and literature) (de Schonewise & Klinger, 2012; Echevarría, Vogt, & Short, 2010; Garcia & Godina, 2004; Short & Fitzsimmons, 2007). The need for ELs to develop disciplinary literacy and meet common core goals (Shanahan & Shanahan, 2012) requires that professionals use evidence-based strategies to deliver instruction that is comprehensible to ELs (Zygouris-Coe, 2012). In particular, for ELCDs, instruction must be provided by professionals who have "an in-depth knowledge of language" (Ehren, Murza, & Malani, 2012, p. 89), a fundamental theoretical understanding of the variation in language proficiency that ELCDs bring to school, and the supports and accommodations that are necessary to provide students with disabilities with meaningful learning opportunities to access core content (de Schonewise & Klingner, 2012). Therefore, it is critical that all professionals involved in facilitating literacy with ELs at various ages and levels of language use effective reading instruction that extends throughout the curriculum and a student's academic career (Davis & Bistodeau, 1993; Robb, 2002; Vacca, Vacca, & Mraz, 2016; Vacca et al., 2018).

According to Anderson (2009), there are four similarities and 10 differences in L1 and L2 readers. Similarities in L1 and L2 reading processes include the involvement of:

- ◆ the reader, text, and context;
- ◆ metacognitive strategies;
- ◆ bottom-up (for example, decoding) and top-down (for example, inferential reasoning) strategies; and
- ◆ language systems with systematic and rule-governed structures.

Differences include:

- ◆ specific language system contrasts;
- ◆ vocabulary knowledge in L1 and L2;
- ◆ language awareness in L1 and L2;
- ◆ the amount of time necessary to learn to read;
- ◆ reading rate (L2 readers read more slowly);
- ◆ motivation;
- ◆ oral English proficiency;
- ◆ background knowledge;
- ◆ learning context; and
- ◆ position on the literacy continuum.

The general characteristics of first and second language learners are summarized and contrasted in Table 5–2.

We have noted the importance of literacy in L1 and language proficiency in L2 reading research. Given the importance of the relationship between these two necessary key components, this chapter explores that relationship; however, it asserts that these components are not sufficient for EL reading proficiency in L2.

Table 5–2. *Differences in Learning to Read Between L1 and L2 Readers*

L1 (English-speaking) Literacy Learners	L2 (English learners) Literacy Learners
Developing communicative competence in one-language system	Developing communicative competence in two-language systems
Can comprehend and express information orally in language of literacy development	Different degrees of ability to comprehend and express information orally in language of literacy instruction
May already possess precursor literacy skills in language of literacy development	May already possess precursor literacy skills in L2 that can be transferred to L1 literacy
Use a set of strategies to improve comprehension in language of instruction	Use a set of strategies that may include L1 to improve comprehension in language of instruction
Knows only one language system	May experience negative transfer (interference) from the native language when it contrasts with the L2; may experience positive transfer from native language (e.g., cognates) or may be more sensitive to language issues due to knowledge of two systems

Source: From *Reading in a Second Language: Moving from Theory to Practice*, by W. Grabe, 2009, New York, NY: Cambridge University Press, pp. 648–650. Copyright 2009 by Cambridge University Press. Adapted with permission.

L2 Reading: Language Problem (Short-Circuit/ Threshold Hypothesis) or Reading Problem (Interdependence Hypothesis)?

There are important differences between reading in L1 and reading in L2. To address the relationship between L1 and L2 readings, scholars have posed the following question: When ELs struggle with reading in a second language, is that due to a language problem or a reading problem? In other words, do EL readers have comprehension problems when reading in English because of low proficiency in English or because of poor reading skills in their first language?

ELs who have been exposed only to English instruction have experienced low academic achievement and literacy levels in both languages. In contrast, ELs who have been exposed to instruction in both their L1 and English have demonstrated high academic and cognitive achievement. Additionally, instruction in ELs' native language has positively influenced ELs' academic development in English and has facilitated transfer of academic skills and knowledge across languages (Alderson, 1984; Freeman, Freeman, & Mercuri, 2002; Valenzuela & Rubio, 2018).

To address whether a difficulty with L2 reading is a language problem or a reading problem, two hypotheses have been proposed: the short circuit hypothesis or linguistic threshold hypothesis (Clark, 1980; Cummins, 1976; Lee & Schallert, 1997) and the linguistic interdependence hypothesis (Cummins, 1979). The short circuit hypothesis or linguistic threshold hypothesis identifies language proficiency as the key factor in determining the success of reading tasks in L2. This hypothesis suggests that EL readers must achieve a certain level of English proficiency in order to be able to comprehend what they read in L2. Even if EL readers have strong literacy skills in their first language, those skills do not necessarily translate to reading skills in English. Thus, a lack of English language knowledge will hinder access to English language reading knowledge. Several studies are summarized in Table 5–3 and have explicitly investigated the influence of second language proficiency on second language reading.

Although there is evidence to support a relationship between language proficiency in L2 and reading ability in L2, there are

Table 5–3. *Research Evidence for the Linguistic Threshold Hypothesis*

Study	Description
Yamashita (2002)	241 Japanese students participated in the study, which examined L1 literacy, L2 language proficiency, and L2 reading. L1 literacy and L2 language proficiency accounted for 40% of reading ability in L2. Additionally, the L2 language proficiency was a much stronger predictor of L2 reading comprehension than literacy in L1.
Schoonen, Hulstijn, and Bossers (1998)	The study, which involved 274 adolescent Dutch students, looked at the relationship among L1 reading abilities, L2 vocabulary, metacognitive knowledge, and L2 reading. The researchers found that, at lower levels of English proficiency, knowledge of English vocabulary is a very strong predictor of English reading ability. At high proficiency levels in English, metacognitive knowledge, which involves awareness of and knowledge one's own thinking processes, was a much stronger predictor of reading ability in English.
Lee and Schallert (1997)	809 adolescent Korean students learning English participated in the study. The study examined the influence of L1 reading proficiency and L2 language proficiency on L2 reading comprehension and found that 56% of L2 reading comprehension was explained by L2 language proficiency and only 30% by L1 literacy. Also, the study revealed higher correlations between L1 and L2 reading and higher levels of L2 proficiency than at lower levels.
Perkins, Brutten, and Pohlman (1989)	The study had 174 Japanese students and looked at the relationship among L1 literacy, L2 language proficiency, and L2 reading. The findings revealed strong correlations between proficiency in L2 and comprehension in L2, and weak correlations between L1 and L2 literacy.

a variety of complicating factors. Reading is a complex process and the concept of linguistic threshold is not easy to operationalize, isolate from other factors, or quantify. To operationalize the concept of linguistic threshold, one has to consider that reading in English is a very dynamic process and differs depending on whether ELs are children, adolescent, or adults. What a young EL is able to transfer from L1 into L2 is very different from what an adult EL can transfer, both in quantity and quality. These considerations require more research that will account for all the aspects of the ever-changing relationship between L2 proficiency and L2 reading.

The second hypothesis is the linguistic interdependence hypothesis (Cummins, 1979). This hypothesis disputes the claim that difficulty reading in L2 is purely a language problem. According to this hypothesis, proficiency in reading in a second language is shared with the reading ability ELs have in their first language. The premise is that when ELs reading in the first language attain a certain level of proficiency, that reading proficiency will transfer to L2 reading (Cummins, 1979, 2000). In other words, ELs who are literate in their first language simply need to learn English words and sentences, because cognitive skills required to be a proficient reader in English will transfer from the first language into English. At the core of this hypothesis is the belief that second language reading skills are fundamentally interdependent or the same as the skills ELs already have as a result of acquiring their L1 reading skills. Table 5–4 summarizes several studies that investigated the relationship between L1 reading skills and L2 reading comprehension.

These two hypotheses can have positive and negative influences on educational decisions made about ELs. If we concur with the linguistic threshold hypothesis and consider language proficiency as the most important factor in achieving reading proficiency in L2, then ELs would need to have a strong command of spoken English prior to initiating reading instruction in English. However, if we agree with the linguistic interdependence hypothesis and consider second language reading simply as a transfer of first language reading skills, then ELs will not need instruction in second language reading because ELs who are literate in their L1 can become literate in English with little effort. To better understand the initial question of whether a

Table 5–4. *Research Evidence for the Linguistic Interdependence Hypothesis*

Study	Description
van Gelderen, Schonnen, Stoel, de Glopper, and Hulstijn (2007)	This study investigated the relationship between reading comprehension development of 389 Dutch adolescents in Dutch and English. Students' reading comprehension, their linguistic and metacognitive knowledge, and processing efficiency were measured. The findings showed a very strong relationship between L1 and L2 reading comprehension, L1 reading proficiency being a much stronger predictor of reading comprehension in English than the other variables assessed.
Durgunoglu (1998)	The study looked at 46 first graders enrolled in two bilingual classes in the United States. The data revealed that 47% of the variance in English (L2) phonological awareness was explained by Spanish (L1) phonological awareness. Additionally, Spanish phonological awareness and letter recognition explained 84% of the variance in English spelling performance. Strong correlations were reported between Spanish word recognition and English word recognition and Spanish spelling and English word recognition.
Verhoeven and Aarts (1998)	188 Turkish-speaking students learning Dutch participated in this study, which examined the relationship between school literacy and functional literacy. The functional literacy assessment was based on newspapers, maps, application forms, letters, etc. The analysis of data showed that the literacy level in Turkish has an effect on literacy level in Dutch.
Umbel and Oller (1994)	This study looked at vocabulary acquisition processes of 102 English-Spanish first, third, and sixth graders who were native speakers of Spanish. The findings showed that Spanish vocabulary knowledge represented 27% of the variance in English vocabulary knowledge, making Spanish receptive vocabulary development the stronger predictor of English receptive vocabulary scores.

difficulty with second language reading is a language problem or a reading problem, Bernhardt and Kamil (1995) reframed the question as follows: How much English language knowledge do ELs have to have in order to make their L2 literacy knowledge work? What should be the extent of EL literacy in L1 so that ELs can make their English language knowledge work? Reframing the question in this way eliminates the potential dichotomy between the two hypotheses and addresses the issue of accountability. The question then is: How much does second language knowledge and (not "or") first language literacy account for EL reading performance in English?

An L2 Reading Model

Restating the second language reading question and focusing on accountability allows us to acknowledge the contribution of each component of L2 reading performance. Research conducted with this focus has suggested that contribution of L2 knowledge to L2 reading is approximately 30%, whereas the contribution of L1 literacy to L2 reading proficiency is between 14% and 21% (Bernhardt & Kamil, 1995; Bossers, 1991; Brisbois, 1995; Carrell, 1991; Hacquebord, 1989; Koda & Miller, 2018; Pae, 2019). Undeniably, these two variables (L2 proficiency and L1 literacy) account for a very important part of the variance in second language reading; however, they do not capture the entire spectrum of the development of second language reading at different proficiency levels. They do, however, emphasize that more research needs to be conducted to account for the remaining 50%. Bernhardt (2005) has proposed a compensatory processing approach that takes these critical considerations into account. His model offers an explanation of how established knowledge sources assist or even take over when other knowledge sources are not adequate or do not exist. Bernhardt's compensatory model has three dimensions. The first element is L1 literacy, consisting of alphabetics, text structure, vocabulary, and word or sentence configuration. The second element is L2 language knowledge, comprising vocabulary knowledge, cognates, and differences and similarities between L1 and L2. The third final element is unexplained variance, which includes comprehension strategies, motivation, content knowledge, interest, and engagement. For emerging L2 readers, the contribution of each element to L2 reading comprehension is almost equal, or about 1/3. However, when ELs move to a more advanced level of L2 literacy and become readers acquiring L2 literacy, L1 literacy contributes 20% to L2 reading comprehension, whereas L2 knowledge contributes 30% to reading comprehension. The remaining 50% consists of unexplained variance, such as interest, motivation, engagement, and so forth.

The Relationship Between Oral Language Proficiency and Reading Proficiency for ELs and ELs with Communication Disorders

In the discussion of Bernhardt's reading model, we noted that L2 knowledge explains a significant part of L2 reading competence. Additionally, the findings of the National Literacy Panel on Language-Minority Children and Youth (August & Shanahan, 2006) revealed the importance of oral language proficiency in developing literacy in the second language. To better understand the relationship between oral language proficiency and reading proficiency for ELs and ELs with communication disorders, this chapter examines the research on oral proficiency in L1 and literacy in L2. Table 5–5 summarizes research on word-level skills (word and pseudo word reading in English), and Table 5–6 lists studies focusing on text-level skills (reading comprehension in English).

Based on the evidence found in Table 5–5, it is important to note that L1 phonological processing skills are closely related to the development of reading skills in English. However, oral proficiency in ELs' native language does not correlate with English reading skills. Most of the studies in Table 5–6 examining the influence of L1 oral proficiency (measured through self-ratings or language use) and English reading comprehension found little or no relationship between the two. However, there have been studies that noted that phonological memory and other components are directly associated with the development of English reading comprehension (Dufva & Voeten, 1999).

Another dimension of oral proficiency worthy of investigation with regard to literacy development in L2 is oral proficiency

Table 5–5. *L1 Oral Proficiency and L2 Word-Level Skills*

Study	Description
Mumtaz and Humphreys (2002)	The participants were 7- and 9-year-old Urdu-English bilingual students. The study found that rhyme detection and phonological memory in Urdu correlated significantly with word-level reading skills in English.
Gottardo, Yan, Siegel, and Wade-Woolley (2001)	The participants were Cantonese-speaking EL students in grades 1 through 8. Phonemic awareness in Cantonese correlated significantly with word and pseudoword reading skills in English.
Gholamain and Geva (1999)	The participants were Farsi-speaking ELs in grades 1 through 5. Verbal working memory and rapid automized naming, assessed in the first language (Farsi), accounted for significant variance in the students' word and pseudoword reading scored in English, in spite of the orthographic differences between the two languages.
Abu-Rabia (1997)	The participants were Hebrew-speaking tenth grade ELs. The study found that L1 oral language proficiency did not correlate with the ELs' performance on English word reading tasks, such as word attack and word recognition.
Da Fontoura and Siegel (1995)	The participants were Portuguese-speaking ELs attending a Portuguese heritage language program The study found that L1 did not correlate with English word or pseudoword reading.

in a second language. Three studies that focus primarily on speakers of Spanish are used to discuss the relationship between reading in English and English oral language. The first study investigated the relationship between Spanish oral language proficiency, Spanish phonological awareness, and English word and pseudo word reading skills (Durgunoglu, Nagy, & Hancin-Bhatt,

Table 5-6. Oral Proficiency in L1 and L2 Text-Level Skills

Study	Description
Nguyen, Shin, and Krashen (2001)	The study examined the relationship between first language oral proficiency and reading outcomes and did not find a relationship between L1 proficiency and general L2 reading achievement.
Dufva and Voeten (1999)	The study focused on English reading comprehension skills of third grade Finnish-speaking students who were learning English in school. The study reported that the students' listening comprehension skills in Finnish assessed in first grade had an indirect effect on English reading comprehension scores and the students' phonological memory, assessed in second grade, correlated significantly with English reading comprehension.
Royer and Carlo (1991)	The participants were middle school Spanish-speaking ELs in a transitional bilingual education program. The study found no significant correlation between the students' Spanish listening comprehension skills and their English reading comprehension.
Buriel and Cardoza (1988)	The participants were ninth grade Spanish-speaking EL students. The study looked at the relationship between self-reports of L1 proficiency and English reading comprehension. For first- and second-generation Mexican American high school ELs, there were no significant relationships between L1 proficiency and English reading comprehension. For third-generation Mexican American students, there were negative relationships between L1 proficiency and English reading.

1993). English language proficiency was measured in three areas of oral language: morphology, syntax, and semantics. The results of this study revealed that English language proficiency was not a statistically significant predictor of effective English word and pseudo word reading. However, Spanish phonological awareness was significant for beginning L2 readers. Gottardo (2002) also studied the relationship between language skills in L2 (semantic and syntactic processing and phonological awareness) and word reading skills of Spanish-speaking ELs. This study showed that English oral proficiency correlated significantly with ELs' performance on English word reading tasks.

In a different study, Quiroga, Lemos-Britten, Mostafapour, Abbott, and Berninger (2002) examined first-grade Spanish-English bilinguals who had not had systematic reading instruction in Spanish. The study found that there was a modest correlation between ELs' oral proficiency in English and their word and pseudo word reading in English. Moreover, the researcher found a strong correlation between phonological awareness and English word and pseudo word decoding in the case of a phoneme deletion task.

One possible explanation of the discrepancy in the findings presented in the first study and the findings of the second and third study is offered by Geva (2006). In the first study, the children were in a transitional bilingual program and the assumption is that they had fewer opportunities to develop their English language skills. In contrast, the ELs in the second and third studies were taught exclusively in English and presumably had more opportunities to develop their English proficiency.

Studies that focus on the relationship between L2 oral language proficiency and reading ability in L2 in ELs with communication disorders are necessary. It is well known that a large number of ELs are overrepresented in specific special education categories (e.g., learning disabilities, speech and language impairments) because they demonstrate limited English proficiency. It is recommended that professionals who work with ELs be familiar with the characteristics of the second language acquisition process and consider how these often mirror the characteristics of a learning disability (Gonzales, 2007; Hoover, Mendez Barletta, & Klingner, 2016; Kohnert, 2008; Paradis, 2005; Roseberry-McKibben & O'Hanlon, 2005). Professionals should be familiar with the behaviors commonly observed among students learning a second language and students with communication disorders to prevent inappropriate identification and mislabeling of ELs.

It is important to note that ELs' rate of English oral language proficiency differs by the age of introduction to English and their use of English. In general, according to MacSwan and Pray (2005), Spanish-speaking ELs entering kindergarten with little or no English become orally proficient in English by the time they reach fourth or fifth grade. When looking at the length of time required to become proficient in English, Pray (2003) found no statistical differences between bilingual students enrolled in special education and bilingual students enrolled in general education programs. Pray (2009) also looked at oral language use among ELs diagnosed with a learning disability and ELs in general education. All the participants in the study were native speakers of Spanish. The errors in the oral tasks performed by the two groups in both Spanish and English were categorized as syntactic errors ("The car white is going fast"), morphological errors ("ated," "a elephant"), and lexical errors (using the word "can" when the item was a bottle). In the case of oral performance in Spanish, the findings revealed that 95% of all students showed a Spanish morphological error ratio of 5% or less and a lexical error ratio of 2% or less. Error ratio was defined as the ratio of the number of erroneously rendered items to the total number of items. Only one participant who was diagnosed as having a learning disability showed an error ratio of more than 10%. However, that participant made no English lexical errors and had only a 3% morphological error ratio in English. This particular case showed that some children in special education may experience a loss in their first language while making important gains in the second language.

Specific to English oral performance, all students demonstrated an English morphological error ratio of 5% or less and an English lexical error ratio of 3% or less. It is interesting to note that one student diagnosed with a learning disability had an English morphological error rate of 7% (which could be considered within the range of normal performance parameters) but did not have morphological errors in Spanish oral production. This study pointed out that there were significant differences between ELs in special education and ELs in general education: ELs who were diagnosed with a learning disability made proportionally more errors than ELs enrolled in general classrooms. However, 95%

of all ELs regardless of their status showed an English morphological error ratio of less than 6% and a lexical error rate of less than 3%. In other words, according to the data collected on their English oral proficiency, a vast majority of the ELs participating in the study showed they had mastered the fundamentals of English morphology and syntax.

Although there is a paucity of studies that address the language of instruction and the impact on oral L1 in general (e.g., Kan & Kohnert, 2005) or studies that examine the English oral proficiency of ELs with communication disorders, researchers have provided preliminary and essential data on factors to consider when working with students at risk for language and literacy development (Gutierrez, Restrepo, Bedore, Peña, & Anderson, 2000; Restrepo, 1998; Restrepo & Kruth, 2000; Restrepo et al., 2010; Simon-Cereijido & Gutierrez-Clellen, 2007). For example, in a qualitative study conducted by Gutierrez-Clellen and DeCurtis (1999), the Spanish word definition skills of Spanish-speaking children with and without language impairment were compared. Their findings revealed several differences in word definition skills between Spanish-speaking students with and without language impairment (LI). Children without LI had the tendency to use formal definitions more than children with LI. The study also showed a large variation within the groups. Formal definitions represented between 10% and 70% of the word definitions generated by the students without LI, and these were attributed to individual school experiences. Therefore, the limited use of formal definitions by students with LI was proposed to be related to differences in access to educational opportunities that facilitate language development.

This study offers two important recommendations in the area of assessment. First, language tests should include nouns that are concrete and familiar in their word definition tasks. Often tests do not include such words and really are measures of vocabulary knowledge and not vocabulary definition skills. Moreover, many tests emphasize the correctness of the word definition, meaning the focus is on the content of the definition associated with the word to be defined. Instead, tests should take into account the quality or communicative adequacy of the definitions produced by students. There is a need for an evaluation protocol that will consider how well the definitions meet expectations for specificity and relevance, as well as the amount of information contained in the word definitions produced by students. This will help determine whether more emphasis is necessary on definition skill development or content development and which instructional strategy would yield better results with ELs.

Expressive Language: The Writing Domain

Writing: Definition and Purposes

Writing has been defined as the act of creating original text using the individual's intellectual and linguistic resources, rather than using someone else's text, a prepared list of words to create sentences or stories, filling in the blanks, or practicing handwriting. Writing is made of letters or symbols that are imprinted on a surface to represent the sounds of a language (Hudelson, 1988). Writing is a tremendous challenge for ELs. They are required to develop novel ideas and express these ideas using new words that they are often learning in the new language. Current research has provided insight about children's native language writing development (August & Shanahan, 2006; Li & Edwards, 2010). From early childhood, children work to make sense of written language. They make predictions about how written language works and create texts based on these predictions. The text changes as the child's understanding of and predictions about written language evolve (Peregoy & Boyle, 2016). Studies of the writing development of native speakers influenced other researchers to investigate the writing development of ELs. The most general conclusion reached by researchers (Edelsky, 1986; Hudelson, 1984, 1987, 1988; Samway, 1987; Urzua, 1987) is that the process of writing is similar for first and second language writers. Hudelson (1988) offers the following conclusions about writing development in ELs: (1) They can write and create their own meaning as they are learning English; (2) they can respond to the works of others and use another learner's responses to their work to make substantive revisions in their writing; (3) texts produced by ELs are similar to those produced by young native speakers; (4) they approach writing and develop as writers differently from one another; (5) the classroom environment has a significant impact on their development as writers; (6) culture may affect the writers' view of writing, of the functions or purposes for writing, and of themselves as writers; and (7) the ability to write in the native language facilitates ELs' writing in several different ways. Native language writing provides learners with information about the purposes of writing. Writing ability in the native language provides ELs with linguistic and nonlinguistic resources that they can use as they approach second language writing. In addition, ELs apply the knowledge about writing gained in first language settings to second language settings.

Grabe (2001) proposed six purposes of writing. First, we write to learn the mechanical production aspect, to practice motor coordination. For this purpose, minimal fluency is required. Copying sentences from a textbook simply to learn and practice the shape of letters is an example. Second, we write to list, repeat, or paraphrase. This is not composing; it is simply stating knowledge. One example is when we write extended notes to ourselves. The third purpose of writing is to understand, remember, and summarize processes that require composing and recounting. Fourth, we write to solve problems, learn, and synthesize. When we do engage in that type of task, we compose and transform already available text. The fifth purpose of writing is to critique, persuade, or interpret. Academic writing where we use evidence selectively but appropriately is an illustration of this purpose. The sixth purpose of writing is to create an aesthetic experience. Fiction writers and poets adhere to this sixth purpose. They compose in new ways and do not follow writing conventions to the letter; however, the results are effective.

Britton (1975) describes three kinds of writing that are similar to those proposed by Grabe (2001). The three kinds of writing are transactional, expressive, and poetic.

> Transactional writing is used "to get things done." Its purpose is to inform, advise, persuade, or instruct. In short, it is a means to an end. A second category is expressive. This is language "close

to the self," often a kind of "thinking aloud" on paper. It reflects the writer's immediate thoughts and feelings; it is relaxed and familiar rather than formal; and allows the writer to take risk. We frame the tentative first drafts of new ideas . . . where in times of crisis . . . we attempt to work our way towards some kind of a resolution. A third category, the poetic, is language used as an art form, and it exists for its own sake. (p. 88)

Similarities and Differences Between Writing in L1 and L2

Just like reading in a second language, writing in a second language is different from writing in a first language. Scott (1991) articulated a very important distinction between L1 and L2 writing. When writing in L1, we create ideas and then find the words to express them. In a L2 writing process, we do the opposite; we look at the available words in L2 and then we generate ideas based on them. ELs, new to English, usually experience some challenges in expressive written language with vocabulary, syntax, and idiomatic expressions. ELs also may not have had the exposure to written English that comes from reading or being read to. Therefore, they may not understand the way that English conventionally translates into the written form. Some ELs may have experience writing in their native language that can facilitate writing in English. Research has suggested that ELs are able to read and write in the second language prior to having obtained proficiency over the phonological, syntactic, and semantic systems of spoken English (Hudelson, 1984; Peregoy & Boyle, 1991).

At first, the two processes look very similar because writers in both L1 and L2 follow similar protocols in developing their ideas on paper: They all plan, write, and revise. For example, Matsumoto (1995) interviewed four Japanese university professors on the strategies they used when writing a research paper in English. The analysis of data showed that those writers followed the same processes and used the same strategies across L1 and L2 writing. Beare (2000) investigated the inventory of strategies used to plan and generate content for proficient bilingual writers and whether the writing strategies in L1 writing differed from L2 writing in the context of generating content and planning.

Her findings indicated that bilingual writers used the same strategies in L1 as in L2 writing (brainstorming, writing drafts, rereading, etc.). According to Berman (1994), writers transfer their skills from L1 to L2, indicating that writers' thoughts are not restricted to a particular language and are able to transfer across languages. Consequently, because many ELs come with writing skills in their first language, they are able to transfer those skills when they write in English. In an experimental study, Berman (1994) found that ELs' success in transferring writing skills was assisted by their grammatical proficiency in the target language, which was English.

In light of the similarities between writing in L1 and writing in L2, L2 writing practitioners might be inclined to simply adopt practices from L1 writing when teaching L2 writing. However, there are important differences that need to be taken into account so SLPs and ESOL professionals can make sound decisions in adapting practices that work for native English speakers to ELs and ELs with communication disorders.

Silva (1993) examined the distinct nature of second language writing in a meta-analysis of approximately 70 research reports that examined over 27 different first languages. The findings were divided into two categories: the writing process and written text features. In terms of the writing process, Silva's (1993) analysis showed that, overall, when writing in the second language, L2 writers did less planning than L1 writers. More attention was devoted to generating writing material, but it was more difficult and time-consuming. A lot of time was dedicated to understanding the topic, and many of the generated ideas were not found in the final written product. In the actual production of written text in L2, the task was more laborious, less fluent, and less productive. L2 writers spent more time going back to the outline or prompt and consulting a dictionary when it was allowed. L2 writers wrote at a slower rate and generated fewer words of written text. An examination of the last stage in the writing process, "reviewing," revealed that L2 writers did less rereading of and reflecting on the written text. Similar patterns and strategies were reported in L1 and L2 reading, but revisions in L2 were less frequent compared with revisions in L1. The L2 revision was more difficult and focused more on grammar and less on mechanics (e.g., spelling).

The analysis of written text features showed various differences in fluency, accuracy, quality, and structure. For fluency, the majority of research evidence pointed out that L2 writing is less fluent than L1 writing. The research also showed that L2 writers made more errors in their writing, rendering it less accurate than writing in L1. Additionally, a large number of studies reviewed by Silva (1993) stated that L2 writers were less effective and received lower overall scores when their writing was graded holistically by native English speakers. The findings discussing the differences in structure between L1 and L2 writing are summarized in Table 5–7.

In summary, L2 writing research shows that L2 writing is distinct from L1 writing. Although general composing processes are similar in L1 and L2, L2 composing is more difficult and less effective. Writing production in L2 is more time-consuming but less fluent and productive. L2 writers review and reread their writing less and revise more, and such revisions are done with more difficulty. L2 texts are less fluent, contain more language errors, and are not as effective as the texts generated by proficient English writers. Reader orientation of L2 texts is often considered less acceptable and appropriate. In terms of style, L2 writing is simpler in structure and distinct stylistically. The clauses are longer but fewer, and there is more coordination and less subordination. Overall, L2 texts show less lexical control, variety, and sophistication.

The Structure of English Writing: A Contrastive Rhetoric Approach

In his seminal study that set the foundation for the discipline of contrastive rhetoric, Kaplan (1966) described the thought pattern of native and nonnative English writers. He based his assumptions on the comparison and contrast of written samples generated by the two populations. According to Kaplan (1966), the pattern of English rhetorical organization is linear in nature.

English writing is organized around a central idea, or a thesis statement. Every part of the writing is expected to be directly related to the thesis statement and should progress in a straight line from the beginning to the end. Kaplan noted four

Table 5–7. *L1/L2 Differences in Written Structure*

Category	Findings
Argument Structure	L2 writers did not state and support their position fully and had the tendency to develop their arguments by restating their position. L2 arguments had fewer paragraphs and connectors, and contained more errors. Some L2 writers preferred a "situation + problem + solution + conclusion" pattern versus the "claim + justification + conclusion" pattern of native English speakers.
Narrative Structure	L2 narratives often began in the middle of the story, omitted essential elements of the story, had less action and more focus on mental states. Also, many L2 narrative patterns in English were closer to the participants' L1 narrative patterns.
Reader Orientation	L2 writing contained fewer and a smaller range of attention-getting devices. They also used fewer sentences that signaled a following theme, overspecified their themes and underestimated their readers' knowledge by introducing information readers considered obvious.
Stylistic Features	L2 writing was found to be less complex, less mature, and less appropriate from a stylistic perspective. Many L2 writers used a more direct, explicit, and authoritative tone. They also used strong modals (will, should, must), and showed less variety in stylistic devices (fewer interrogative sentences, less analogy, less parallel structure, and more repetition of ideas)
Cohesion	L2 writers used more conjunctive ties and fewer synonyms and collocations.

Source: Data from "Toward an Understanding of the Distinct Nature of L2 Writing: The ESL Research and its Implications," by T. Silva, 1993, *TESOL Quarterly, 27*(4), 657–677.

other organizational patterns very different from the linear English model. These are the Semitic, Asian, Romance, and Russian organizational patterns.

The first pattern discussed by Kaplan (1966) is the Semitic pattern. This pattern is characterized by parallel constructions, as seen from this English example generated by an Arabic-speaking student: "The first problem is that we import many things from other countries and we cannot depend on ourselves in producing the things we need, and we import different kinds of food, electric materials, cars and clothes."

The second pattern, the Asian (called Oriental in Kaplan's study) pattern, is present in Indonesian, Chinese, or Korean, and the writing topic is examined from a variety of points but never directly. Freedom to digress is a characteristic of Romance and German-language writers. Digression introduces extraneous material into the writing, with the purpose of providing additional information, suggesting alternative possibilities in considering an issue, or simply inserting humor in the text. However, English academic writing may consider digression as being irrelevant to the topic or inappropriate to the context, because it violates the linearity of English writing conventions. The last pattern, the Russian rhetorical organization, is similar to the Romance pattern but with more amplification of subordinate elements.

The fact that English rhetorical style is represented by a linear line does not imply it is superior to other rhetorical organizations. It simply emphasizes the idea that each language has its own way of organizing reality, similar to the uniqueness of each culture. Culture is not universal in the sense of uniformity, and each culture views the same reality differently. Rhetorical organization, based on logic, is not universal and varies from culture to culture and sometimes even within the same culture. Even Kaplan has modified his initial position: He no longer views rhetorical patterns as reflective of a certain way of thinking but rather as a result of different writing conventions that are taught (Kaplan, 2000). The idea that writing patterns can be learned is key. Therefore, in the case of Spanish-speaking ELs who are literate in Spanish, they need to learn the new linear convention of English academic writing. This does not mean that they have to abandon their preferred forms of expression, but they should learn when that style of writing is required in specific contexts and necessary for specific tasks. We provide another example of linearity and directness of the English rhetorical style by contrasting it with the Korean language.

Before comparing linearity in English and linearity in Korean, it is essential to operationalize the construct of linearity. In general, linearity is defined as a progression that supports a thesis without digression. This definition needs to be further explored, and more rhetorical parameters need to be added for a more effective contrastive analysis of the rhetorical organization employed by the two languages. Monroy and Scheu (1997) established several guidelines for a linear rhetorical pattern common to the organization of English writing (Table 5–8).

In contrast, the Korean rhetorical organization uses a different, more nonlinear pattern (Eggington, 1987). The nonlinear Korean style originated from the "qi-cheng-zhuan-he" (起承轉合)

Table 5–8. *Guidelines for Establishing Linearity of Discourse*

Thematic Unit	A single thesis connects the whole text together. Multiple theses influence linearity negatively.
Thematic Progression	A direct relationship between all the different thematic sentences that link every paragraph with the main thesis.
Paragraph Unity	Paragraphs have one controlling idea which is developed by expanding, qualifying, and illustrating it.
Personal Tone	The use of one point of view and pronouns that refer to the subject.
Interparagraph Cohesion	Paragraphs are linked to each other in evident ways and they all adhere to the thesis.
Concreteness	The use of concrete words and less reliance on abstract words.
Sentence Simplicity	The presence of simple or coordinated sentences and the lack of overuse of complex or subordinated sentences.

Source: Data from "Reflejo cultural en los estilos de hispanohablantes estudiantes de inglés como LE. Consideraciones pedagógicas," by R. Monroy & D. Scheu, in *Estudios de Lingüística Aplicada y Literatura. Homenaje Póstumo al Prof. Juan Conesa,* 1997, pp. 201–221, Murcia, Spain: Universidad de Murcia.

style in Chinese. A similar pattern can also be found in Japanese writing ("ki-sho-ten-ketsu"). The Korean version, "ki-sung-chon-kyul," has four stages: beginning, development, turn, and end. In Korean, the main idea is presented late in the essay, whereas the thesis in an English essay is expected to be introduced very early. It is important to note that writing conventions might change in time within the same culture. For example, in China, the structure described above is increasingly losing its influence over mainland Chinese students writing in Chinese. A survey of contemporary Chinese textbooks on composition showed that the prescriptive advice given in these texts reflected a linear English rhetorical style more than the traditional Chinese style (Kirkpatrick, 1997).

Korean style is not only nonlinear but also indirect. In other words, the writing is not developed in a straight line proceeding from a statement of the thesis or central idea followed by elaboration. Instead, the subject is looked at indirectly, a process done by examining issues not directly related to the main idea. How do we translate the insights obtained through contrastive rhetoric to the practice of teaching ELs how to write in a second language? Matsuda (1997) proposed a model of L2 writing that goes beyond the background of ELs and accounts for the complexity of factors that contribute to the organization of texts written by ELs in a second language.

Contrastive Rhetoric and the Practice of Teaching Second Language Writing: Matsuda's Dynamic Model

Matsuda's (1997) model emphasizes the dynamic nature of writing in L2. The context of the writing act includes not only the writer but also the reader. The key components of this dynamic model are the backgrounds of the writer and the reader, the shared discourse community, and the interaction of the elements of L2 writing: the EL writer, the EL-generated text, and the EL/native English speaker (NES) reader: *EL Writer* ←→ **EL Text** ←→ *EL/NES Reader*.

The first feature, represented by the writer's and reader's backgrounds, includes more than language, culture, and education

experiences. These sources of influence are undoubtedly important, but there are other influences that might influence a writer's
decisions, such as dialect, socioeconomic status, knowledge of
the subject matter, and membership to various L1 and L2 discourse communities. The background of both the writer and
the reader is a very complex notion and almost escapes a comprehensive definition. However, what is important here is to
understand the complexity of background and the fact that it is
a contributing element to the dynamic nature of L2 writing due
to its flexibility. For example, ELs who have been exposed to the
conventions of English writing and have a good command of the
linguistic aspect of the language might be able to generate L2
writing that is very close to the one produced by NESs who are
proficient writers. From a different background perspective, EL
teachers who have been exposed to a variety of EL-generated
texts might be able to react differently to linguistic and structural
errors in their students' texts than an average NES reader with
limited EL contact.

The discourse community, the second feature of the model,
is shared by both the writer and the reader. Discourse is a construct defining all forms of communication that contribute to a
particular form of thinking. Swales (1990) defines a discourse
community as a community that has an agreed set of common
goals and ways of communication among its members. As a
member of a discourse community in their own native language,
literate ELs share (with their readers) one or more writing genres
and specific languages (i.e., vocabulary) that serve the goals of
that particular discourse community.

To gain access to the L2 discourse community, ELs need to
acquire relevant content and discourse expertise in L2, regardless of their linguistic, cultural, or educational background. For
example, ELs can negotiate their access to an L2 discourse community by learning the rhetorical patterns of English or other discourse conventions specific to the target language. The process
is not unidirectional, though. The EL/NES reader can also help
enlarge the shared aspect of the L1 and L2 discourse communities by becoming more and more accustomed to L2-generated
texts that exhibit different assumptions, experiences, and levels
of L2 discourse expertise.

The last important feature of the model is represented by the bidirectional interaction between the three principal elements of the L2 reading model: the EL writer, the EL text, and the EL/NES reader. The writer influences and is influenced by the participation in the L2 discourse community, an experience that will become part of the EL writer's background. The EL text can be seen as a virtual world in which the writer and the reader meet, building a shared reality. To make L2 writing effective, L2 texts should reflect the EL writer's understanding that acquiring the organizational patterns in L2 is a necessary, but not sufficient, condition for successful L2 writing. Consequently, the text should reflect the fact that the writer knows and understands not only the reader's background but also the writing genres in the discourse community shared by both the writer and the reader. ELs are not solely responsible for gaining membership to existing L2 discourse communities. NES readers might also experience a process of revisiting their own backgrounds as a result of reading an EL-generated English text. The presence of L2 texts may cause the NES reader to gain a new perspective and reevaluate and incorporate new discourse patterns into their own background.

ELs with Communication Disorders and Writing in English: A Focus on Morphology

The majority of studies that examine the acquisition of literacy in a second language have been conducted with typically developing EL students (Bialystok, Luk, & Kwan, 2005; Carlo et al., 2004; Genesee, Lindholm-Leary, Saunders, & Christian, 2005; Paez, Tabors, & Lopez, 2007). As a consequence, there is a very limited body of research exploring the acquisition of language and literacy skills of ELs with communication disorders, specifically in the area of writing (Brea-Spahn & Dunn, 2012). Studies that focus on non-EL students who have communication disorders usually provide us with information on the connection between language and reading disorders, literacy development of students with specific special needs (e.g., deaf and hard of hearing [DHH], specific learning impairment [SLI], or students from low-income backgrounds or high-risk populations; see Catts, 1993; Gillam & Johnston, 1992; Hengst & Johnson, 2008; Roseberry-McKibben, 2008).

In one study focusing on the literacy levels of students who are deaf or hard of hearing (DHH), researchers found that high school graduates were functionally illiterate, with a reading and writing proficiency of a third- or fourth-grade student (Waters & Doehring, 1990). In terms of language usage, studies have found that students who were DHH showed considerable delays in their written language. Their written language was characterized with many nouns and verbs and too few adverbs, pronouns, prepositions, and adjectives (McAnally, Rose, & Quigley, 1994; Simmons, 1962). One study reported that students with hearing loss frequently used the same descriptors at age 18 as they did at age 10 when asked to depict an item (McCombs & McCombs, 1969). In terms of language disorders, most research has been focused on morphological and phonological aspects of second language discrepancies. The importance of phonology and oral language development has been discussed previously in the chapter. The focus now shifts to morphological development, which plays a very important role in the writing domain.

Most of the studies in the area of morphology have looked at ELs with specific language impairment (SLI) and found that ELs with SLI are very similar to their monolingual NES peers with SLI. For example, Paradis, Crago, Genesee, and Rice (2003) investigated the morphological skills of French-English simultaneous bilinguals (bilinguals who are learning two languages at the same time) with SLI and compared them with the skills of French and English monolingual students with SLI. Related to verb tenses and accuracy of tense markers, their findings showed that the bilingual children in their study did not display more profound deficits in the use of these grammatical morphemes than their monolingual peers. They concluded that bilinguals were not more impaired than monolinguals simply because they were simultaneously acquiring two languages.

There are important differences between the language produced by ELs with SLI and ELs without SLI. Jacobson and Schwartz (2002) looked at a number of studies that analyzed the speech of Spanish-speaking ELs with SLI in an attempt to create a profile that could be used for future research or that could be shared among researchers. They reported that conflicting findings in their research and in the literature made it difficult to create a profile of morphological difficulty for that population of students. However, they observed that the morphological problems of Spanish-speaking ELs with SLI included decreased use of function words, such as articles, and difficulty with third-person verb inflections and noun plural inflections. Spanish-speaking children between the ages of 5 and 7 with SLI who were living in the United States used fewer articles than their age-matched control groups. However, no discrepancies in tense marking or increased use of infinitive forms were found. The lack of general consensus on the profile of morphological acquisition of ELs with SLI emphasizes the need for more research in this important area of language acquisition.

An important point that needs to be made here is related to the dilemma SLPs and ESOL professionals face when analyzing EL errors. They must ascertain whether the errors occur as a result of normal language development or if the errors are indicative of language impairment. The presence of morphological errors in writing and speech does not mean that ELs have an SLI, as pointed out by Paradis (2005). Regardless of their L1 background, beginning EL students will make morphological errors, which could extend into their second year of speaking English. Examples of such morphological errors are morphemes that mark the grammatical category tense, such as auxiliary verbs and verb inflections (for example, "-s" for the third-person singular).

As a general characteristic, ELs will interchange the correct use of a morpheme with the omission of a morpheme in their writing and speech, but they will become proficient in using them over time. These characteristics also describe typical English language learning. However, they overlap with the characteristics of monolingual students with SLI. As a consequence, it is challenging to determine whether beginning EL morphological errors are due to second language learning processes or to specific language impairment. Therefore, it is vital that SLPs and ESOL professionals exercise caution in the presence of morphological errors and not consider them a marker of SLI in beginning ELs.

Background Knowledge and Its Contribution to Second Language Literacy

Schema: Definition and Examples

There are several definitions of schema (schemata or schemas in plural form) that can be traced back to Plato, who proposed the theory of ideal types that exist in the human mind, and Kant, who emphasized the importance of background knowledge in comprehending a literary text. However, the origin of the majority of definitions of schema can be traced to Bartlett, who defined schema as an active organization of past responses to past experiences (Bartlett, 1932).

Rumelhart (1980) proposed that schema theory is a theory about how knowledge is represented and how this representation makes possible the use of knowledge in a specific way. According to schema theory, all knowledge is packed into units called schemata. In addition to the knowledge itself, these units also contain information or directions on how these units of knowledge should be used. One example of schema is provided by Davis (1991), as seen in Figure 5–2.

Carrell (1983) identifies two categories of schema: formal schema and content schema. Formal schema, also called textual or discourse schema, refers to the organizational forms and rhetorical structure of the text. It includes syntax, semantics, and all other linguistic knowledge, as well as text genre and background knowledge on how the text should be organized rhetorically. Content schema refers to knowledge beyond the linguistic knowledge. It includes the reader's culture and world knowledge, as well as any kind of information related to a particular topic.

Schema Theory and Reading Comprehension in a Second Language

Research in the area of schema theory and its influence on L2 reading comprehension has concluded that there is a very strong relationship between the reader's schema and the ability

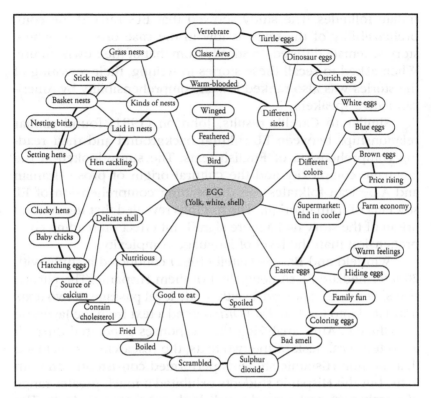

Figure 5–2. *Example of schema.* Source: *Adapted from* Cognition and Learning: A Review of the Literature with Reference to Ethnolinguistic Minorities, *by P. M. Davis, 1991, Dallas, TX: Summer Institute of Linguistics, p. 21. Copyright 1991 by SIL. Reprinted with permission.*

to understand a text. Thus, EL readers may fail to make sense of a text if their schema cannot easily fit within the content of the English text they are reading.

Several studies reviewed by Al-Issa (2006) have shown the influence of content schema on L2 reading comprehension. We previously defined content schema as the degree to which L2 readers are familiar with the subject matter of the text they are trying to understand. Carrell (1981) studied the effect of cultural origin of the reading materials on EL comprehension and recall. Two groups of students, Chinese and Japanese, participated in the study. They were asked to read stories in English that had been translated from Chinese, Japanese, French, and American

Indian folktales. The study showed that ELs ranked the comprehensibility of the texts as low in the case of stories where story schemata differed drastically from that of their own culture. When asked to recall these stories in writing, their rewriting of the stories was also ranked low in comprehensibility by American native speakers.

Similar to Carell's results, Johnson (1981) found similar relationships between EL cultural background and their reading comprehension of English texts. The study looked at the language complexity and the cultural origin of prose (Iranian and American folktales) on the reading comprehension of EL students of Iranian origin. The findings revealed that the cultural origin of the story had a more significant effect on reading comprehension than the level of language complexity.

Winfield and Barnes-Felfeli (1982) conducted a study with 20 intermediate EL students, half of them Hispanic. The participants were asked to read a sixth-grade level passage of two texts translated into English: *Don Quixote* and a text from the Japanese Noh theater. After analyzing ELs' responses generated through a written recall task of the two texts, the researchers concluded that the non-Hispanic students performed consistently on both texts, but the Hispanic students exhibited a much greater range of vocabulary and scored much higher on *Don Quixote*. The researchers proposed that familiar material increases reading fluency in a second language for ELs as a possible explanation for the differences between Hispanic and non-Hispanic students.

The idea of familiar material was expanded by Krashen (1993), who came up with two ways to activate the ELs' content schemata. The first strategy was called free voluntary reading. It referred to an accountability-free (no follow-up comprehension tests) reading activity in which ELs select and read texts that are of interest to them. One important possible result of this strategy was that reading these books would build the familiarity necessary to read more advanced books. The second strategy was to have ELs read school texts in their first language. By doing that, they would construct the knowledge base necessary to understand the material in the second language. If the content of the reading material were familiar in the ELs' first language, the reading selection in English would be easier to understand.

Based on these studies, it is clear that ELs' content schema has a very important influence on their comprehension of English texts. Al-Issa (2006) proposed 12 questions that can be used to guide SLPs and ESOL professionals in selecting reading materials for their EL students and EL students with communication disorders:

1. Will my students be interested in reading such materials?
2. Will these materials be relevant to my students' English proficiency levels?
3. What content knowledge is to be extracted from these materials?
4. Will these materials cause cultural conflicts in the classroom?
5. How can I motivate my students and involve them in reading such materials?
6. What kinds of prereading, reading, and postreading activities and materials can be designed to increase my students' understanding of these materials?
7. Do the reading materials provide students with sufficient background information about the content of the text?
8. How much time and freedom am I giving my students to exercise their understandings of the materials?
9. Am I being sensitive to my students' hidden comprehension problems?
10. Am I helping my students become more aware of the fact that reading is a highly interactive process?
11. Are my students changing their attitudes about reading?
12. Am I allowing my students to become independent, self-directed readers?

Schema Theory and Writing Proficiency in a Second Language

In the discussion on the influence of schema on L2 reading comprehension, this chapter focused on one dimension of schema, content schema. We now turn our attention to another type of schema, formal schema, to determine if it influences the English writing proficiency of ELs. We defined formal schemata as the knowledge about discourse structure, which may include linguistic and rhetorical organization knowledge. In terms of rhetorical organization, we have seen the influences that L1 can have on L2 writing when we compared English rhetorical organization with the rhetorical patterns of several language groups.

Several studies are relevant to the study of form schema in EL writing. For example, Hinds (1990) looked at the differences of rhetorical structures in English and East Asian languages. The analysis of English writing samples generated by Asian students revealed a tendency to use an inductive writing approach, which places the thesis statement at the end of the essay. Because the traditional pattern of English writing is more deductive in nature, it will be more challenging for most English-speaking readers to understand the competent writing of these ELs due to the placement of the thesis statement at the beginning of the essay. The reason for this lack of comprehensibility is not based on lack of language clarity but more likely due to a mismatch between the writers' approach of organizing text and the readers' expectations.

Similarly, a study conducted by Reid (1996) suggested that ineffective EL writers might employ a formal schema in English that was different from that of NESs. The study examined how well NES and EL student readers and writers could predict and produce appropriate second sentences that followed the topic sentence in a paragraph of academic American English. The findings revealed that NES writers were able to predict the second sentences twice as often as EL writers. The researcher attributed this difference to the fact that NESs had more complete formal schemata than ELs. Therefore, NESs were better equipped to identify and fulfill the expectations of U.S. academic readers.

Based on the research done on contrastive rhetoric and on empirical studies that focused on the importance of schema in second language writing ability, the building of formal schema has a very important place in the second language pedagogy. Why should SLPs and ESOL professionals concentrate on teaching the academic English rhetorical form for ELs and ELs with communication disorders? Xiao (2008) provides three reasons. First, form is relatively stable, predictable, and teachable. Even though it has individual variations, it will not change abruptly. Knowing how to organize their academic texts in English will help ELs take control of English literacy in general and make them more effective writers and readers.

Second, the form of textual structure can serve as an advanced organizer for ELs. Once they create the structure of their essay or any other kind of academic writing, ELs will be able to concentrate on selecting the appropriate vocabulary and grammar they need for expressing their ideas on paper. They will not need to worry about organization any longer, thus freeing more cognitive resources for this more linguistic-oriented task. Finally, as was previously noted, second language literacy research has found that many problems that EL writers encounter can be directly related to English academic form. Because writing forms and styles differ vastly across cultures, these differences can have a negative effect on the perceived effectiveness of ELs' writing in English. If the text written by ELs does not contradict the expectations of the English rhetorical style, the message the text is trying to convey will be better understood, thus increasing the perceived effectiveness of the EL text.

Summary

The reciprocal and multiple relationships between spoken and written language make it appropriate for SLPs and ESOL professionals to play an integral role in helping children become literate. These roles are implemented in collaborative partnerships with other professionals (general education teachers, bilingual education teachers, special education teachers, reading teachers, literacy coaches) who have expertise in the development of reading and written language and vary with settings and the experience of those involved. The knowledge of how the fundamentals of literacy apply to the instruction of ELs and ELs with communication disorders is a sine-qua-non condition for SLPs and ESOL professionals who are contributing to their L2 literacy. Therefore, this chapter provided a definition of literacy and discussed the operations of the construct of literacy, placing a strong emphasis on L2 reading, L2 writing, and schema, as well as how these operations contribute to the literacy development of ELs and ELs with communication disorders. The following chapter comprehensively examines the assessment instruments and procedures that are in place for ELs, from the incipient stages of placement to the final stages of exiting or dismissal.

6

Assessing Language Proficiency Levels for Identification and Disability Determination

Introduction

The previous chapters set the stage for the framework that guides this chapter and the subsequent chapter (7). The discussion of our assessment, intervention, and monitoring (AIM) framework begins with assessment, the first component of AIM. We consider assessment from the perspective of identification practices for ELs in general, to the educational identification of a speech-language impairment and the procedures used to determine the need for special education, related services, and/or accommodations. Chapter 7 will expand on the two remaining components of AIM, intervention and monitoring.

Assessment, Intervention, and Monitoring (AIM) Framework

There are numerous approaches to identifying, providing services and instruction for, and monitoring the progress of students who may or may not have disabilities/disorders. These include response to intervention (RtI) model or multitiered system of support (MTSS) (Burns, Appleton, & Stehouwer, 2005; Ehren, 2005; Halls-Mills, 2018; Jimerson, Burns, & VanDerHeyden, 2016; VanDerHeyden, Witt, & Gilbertson, 2007) and/or dynamic assessment (DA) (Lidz, 1991; Lidz & Peña, 1996). Dynamic assessment measures learning potential and RtI gauges progress. DA (Peña, Gillam, & Bedore, 2014) and RtI/MTSS (Esparza Brown & Doolittle, 2008) have been recommended as viable assessment strategies for bilingual children who are in the process of learning English as an additional language. Each are used to assess EL students for determination of possible disorders and to make informed decisions about when children might best benefit from intervention or related services (Lidz & Peña, 2009).

The AIM framework incorporates second language acquisition research and theory, in tandem with information about the learner's first language use, so that the learner's first and second language proficiency is considered during assessment and instruction/intervention. As discussed in Chapter 4, ELs typically move along a continuum of second language development, which is affected by a set of factors that are both external and internal to the learner. Common external factors include the language(s) used, as well as the perceived value of each language in the learner's community of residence, the socioeconomic status of the learner's family and its impact on the learner's formal education, and the second language instructional model and quality of instruction the learner experiences in acquiring a second language. Typical internal factors include the learners' age, personality, and their language-learning aptitude and motivation.

Clinicians and educators who work with ELs need to understand how these factors affect learners' progress in acquiring a second language. One important reason is to be able to detect if other issues, such as a disability or disorder, could be altering the normal progression of L2 acquisition. Together with formal and alternative assessments of disabilities, constructing a composite portrait of each EL's internal and external L2 learning factors offers a more complete and comprehensive evaluation. This ongoing evaluation occurs during what we have defined as a three-part cycle of assessment, intervention, and monitoring, known as the AIM framework (Figure 6–1). The acronym AIM is fitting because this cycle points educators and clinicians toward the successful

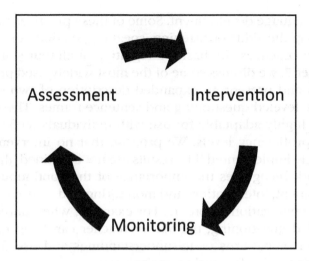

Figure 6–1. *AIM framework.*

progression across the second language development continuum through individualized and coordinated support.

The first step in the AIM framework is assessment. Assessment uses a variety of measures to identify ELs and potential disorders or disabilities. As we will discuss in this chapter, there are many standardized assessments of English proficiency that place ELs' listening, speaking, reading, and writing performance on a second language development continuum to determine their language and grade-level proficiency. In addition to English language proficiency assessments, a variety of assessment tools and strategies are used to establish whether a disorder or disability exists. For example, the Clinical Evaluation of Language Fundamentals (CELF) (e.g., CELF-4 and CELF-5; Semel, Wiig, & Secord, 2003; Wiig, Semel, & Secord, 2013) is a commonly used standardized test instrument for identifying and diagnosing disorders in language performance. Additionally, obtaining classroom-based language samples for analysis is a frequent type of alternative assessment (Heilmann, Nockerts, & Miller, 2010). Using an array of assessment information, in combination with a portrait of the individual student's internal and external factors, can lead to a substantiated identification of learning disorders/disabilities.

The second step in the AIM framework is intervention. Intervention uses research- and theory-based practices that promote second language development. Some of these practices focus on developing the skills or listening, speaking, reading, or writing, and other practices emphasize integration of all four skill areas. In Chapter 7, we discuss some of the most widely used practices with ELs and present an expanded description of two specific practices, leveled questioning and sentence frames. These practices are highly adaptable for use with individuals with varying English proficiency levels. We propose that no intervention is adequately implemented if its results are not examined; thus, our framework recognizes the importance of the continuous cycle of assessment, intervention, and monitoring and its use with ELs with communication disorders. For example, when implementing leveled questioning, the SLP or teacher can keep notes of student error patterns or misunderstandings and use these as language samples for further analysis.

The last step in the AIM framework is monitoring. Common language proficiency assessments can be used to assist clinicians and educators in determining if interventions are appropriate for ELs and, specifically, ELCDs. The continuous AIM cycle serves to inform assessment and intervention, as the learner's first and second language proficiency is documented and used as a foundation to make evidence-based decisions.

Assessment and Collaboration

Much has been discussed in the literature about the importance of collaboration and in the assessment and management of ELCDs (ASHA, 2010a, 2017a; Berninger, 2015; Caesar & Kohler, 2007; Gutiérrez-Clellen, Restrepo, Bedore, Peña, & Anderson, 2000; Hammer, Detwiler, Detwiler, Blood, & Qualls, 2004; Hillier, Civetta, & Pridham, 2010; Johnson, Prelock, & Apel, 2016; Ludwig & Kerins, 2019). If you ask any SLP or educator if they collaborate, often, the answer would be yes. However, collaboration does not just happen. It needs a roadmap and a starting point.

Several scholars and practitioners have provided many definitions of collaboration. For example, Friend and Cook (2009) define collaboration as "a style for direct interaction between at least two coequal parties voluntarily engaged in shared decision making as they work toward a common goal" (p. 6). ASHA (2016a), in its guide on interprofessional education and interprofessional practice for audiology and speech-language pathology, highlights the difference between collaboration and interprofessional practice (IPP). It emphasizes that in IPP, various professionals "learn from, with, and about each other in order to develop a collaborative practice" (ASHA, 2016a, p. 57). Schrage (1995) describes collaboration as a process of shared creation where two or more individuals with complementary skills work toward creating a shared understanding that none had previously possessed or could have come to on their own. Thus, an important step in collaboration is to understand the unique contributions of each professional and how each can complement and augment those made by other professionals who also have unique perspectives and skills in working with ELs and ELCDs (Briggs, 1991; Giess & Serianni, 2018; Peña & Quinn, 2003; Rosa-Lugo & Fradd, 2000; Spencer, 2005).

As accountability for both SLPs and ESOL professionals has increased with federal and state legislation, the focus on student performance requires that each professional share their knowledge and skills. ESOL professionals and SLPs each have expertise that can address the impact of language differences and second language acquisition on students learning to promote efficient and effective outcomes for ELCDs. To ensure that ELs are being accurately identified as having a communication disorder and subsequently receiving quality, culturally responsive services, it is essential that these two professionals work with each other and additional professional partners (e.g., administrators, teachers, support services personnel, parents/guardians) to ensure that assessment for identification and placement of K–12 ELCDs aligns with federal regulations, state regulations, and/or local requirements; research; and best practices (Ireland & Conrad, 2016; Muñoz, White, & Horton-Ikard, 2014).

ASHA's 2010 position paper outlines the roles and responsibilities of SLPs in schools in prevention, assessment, intervention, and program design. Applied to ELs, one role of the SLP is to reduce disproportionate referrals of ELs to special education by using preventive evidence-based practice (EBP) approaches.

In the absence of improvement by using EBP strategies, SLPs are responsible for identifying and implementing evidence-based assessment methodologies and approaches to accurately identify whether the performance of an EL is reflective of a true disorder. TESOL's 2007 position paper addresses the identification of ELs with special needs and the role of the ESOL professional and bilingual educator. The position paper highlights its expertise in applying culturally responsive and comprehensible instruction. Specifically, both position papers emphasize the importance of purposeful collaboration in identifying ELs with special needs, developing goals, and identifying appropriate services and instruction for ELs (ASHA, 2010a; TESOL, 2007b).

To address the interdisciplinary nature and appropriate assessment of ELs and ELCDs, this chapter provides information to SLPs about the assessment procedures and instruments used by ESOL professionals in the assessment for identification of EL students with different language proficiency levels. Delving deeper, we describe the most common standardized and informal procedures and instruments used by SLPs to identify the category of communication disorders. Taking these quantitative measures into account, we further discuss other means of initial assessment for identification and placement, including home language surveys, oral interviews, review of student records, and classroom-based assessment, among other options. We discuss the importance of assessing language proficiency and how the assessment of language proficiency impacts the identification, placement, and exit of ELs from special programs.

Identification Practices and Protocols for English Learners

Procedures for Identification and Placement of ELs

Before we discuss the identification and placement protocols for ELCDs, it is beneficial to look at the procedures that are in place for the identification and placement of the general EL population. The policies in Florida, California, and Minnesota to identify ELs will serve as examples.

Florida

In Florida, the identification and placement of ELs is based on the steps outlined in the Consent Decree (*League of United Latin American Citizens (LULAC) et al. v. State Board of Education Et al. Consent Decree*, 1990). The Consent Decree (also known as the META or ESOL Consent Decree) of 1990 is the state of Florida's framework for compliance with federal and state laws regarding the education of ELs. It addresses the civil rights of these students, with the primary right being that of equal access to comprehensible instruction (Florida Department of Education, 2001, 2011). This settlement agreement states how Florida is to address the needs of its EL students. According to the Consent Decree, when parents enroll their children in school, they are asked to complete a home language survey (HLS). The purpose of the HLS is to determine whether their children speak a language other than English at home. A series of questions are posed to obtain information on language acquisition and proficiency to guide educators to make an informed decision about whether a student needs EL services. An example of what a typical HLS might look like can be seen in Figure 6–2.

This survey (or a similar one) is the first protocol used to identify potential ELs in Florida. If the answers on the HLS reveal that the student speaks another language, then the school personnel responsible for testing ELs is informed that a potential EL student has registered to attend the school. After the notification, the student's English language proficiency must be assessed within 20 days of entry in the school using specific state-approved tests.

Students may also be referred to an English Language Learner (ELL) team or committee by a parent or teacher to determine if the student meets the criteria to be identified as an EL. The criteria to be identified as an EL are determined by results on an English language measure and at least two of the following criteria: proficiency test, previous educational and social experiences, student interview, written recommendation and observation by current and previous instructional and supportive services staff, level of mastery of basic competencies or skills in English and/or home language according to appropriate criterion-referenced standards, and previous or current grades and test results.

Home Language Survey

To be completed for all students enrolling in the district.

School:_____   Date:_____

Name of person completing this survey: (Please Print)

_____

Student's Name:_____

Date of Birth:_____   Grade:_____

1. Is a language other than English used in the home? Yes___ No___

2. Did the student have a first language other than English? Yes___ No___

3. Does the student most frequently speak a language other than English? Yes___ No___

4. What is the predominant language spoken in the home by the parent(s)/guardian(s)?

_____

5. What is the country of national origin of the student?

_____

Figure 6–2. *Generic example of a home language survey.* continues

6. If the student was born in another country, what is his/her date of entry in the United States?

_____

7. Number of years of school outside the U.S._____

8. Number of years of school inside the U.S._____

_____   _____

Signature of person completing this survey   Date

Relationship to student: (Circle One) Mother   Father   Guardian   Self

_____

Signature of translator (if necessary)

Figure 6–2. continued

California

California does not have a Consent Decree as we have seen in Florida's case, but the steps of identification and placement of ELs are somewhat like Florida. California state law (EC sections 313 and 60810) and federal law (ESEA; Title I and Title III of the Elementary and Secondary Education Act [ESEA]) require that local educational agencies (LEAs) administer a test of English language proficiency (e.g., listening, speaking, reading, and writing) to newly enrolled students whose primary language is not English (California Department of Education, n.d.). If the HLS indicates English as the primary/native language, the student is classified as English only (EO) and the process stops. If the HLS indicates a language other than English as the primary/

native language, the student must take the Initial English Language Proficiency Assessments for California (ELPAC) (California Department of Education, n.d.-a).

Minnesota

The identification and placement procedures for ELs in Minnesota are very similar to Florida and California. All students, regardless of perceived native language, require a home language questionnaire called Minnesota Language Survey (MNLS) upon initial registration in the district. Then, based on the answers provided through the MNLS, students complete an approved English Language Proficiency (ELP) screener. There are three approved ELP screeners in Minnesota: the WIDA Screener (either an online version or a paper version), the Kindergarten W-APT, and the Kindergarten MODEL service. The districts also have a process to determine if students who were not initially identified as ELs may in fact be eligible for EL instruction (Minnesota Department of Education, 2017).

As illustrated in the above examples, an HLS is used by each of these states to identify ELs and determine which students should be tested more thoroughly for special language programs (bilingual or ESL). Most HLSs have a series of questions that survey the language(s) spoken in the home and to identify the first language learned by the child. Although many states use HLSs to identify ELs, there is variation across states in the specific measures that are used to determine eligibility for identification and placement in an instructional program for ELs.

Instruments and Techniques Used for EL Identification and Placement

Common to Florida, California, and Minnesota is the use of home language surveys and language proficiency tests as a means of identifying and placing ELs in programs that will help them transition from limited English proficiency to full English proficiency. In the past, a variety of instruments and techniques were used by K–12 school districts to assess and identify ELs, including home language surveys, achievement tests, and criterion referenced tests (Table 6–1; Rhodes, Ochoa, & Ortiz, 2005). Currently, identifying ELs is generally a two-step process: First, students and parents/legal guardians are asked to fill out an HLS, which identifies students who may need English development services based on degree of English language exposure. If students speak a language other than English at home, an English language assessment, which assesses the student's language proficiency and confirms the student's language status, is administered (OELA, 2016).

We have discussed the HLS and noted its use in identifying ELs. Also, we have emphasized the importance of the language proficiency instruments designed to identify and place ELs in appropriate instructional programs.

Table 6–1. *Past EL Identification Instruments and Protocols Nationwide*

Identification Technique	Number of States
Home language survey	46
Language proficiency test	45
Student records	40
Teacher observations	40
Parent information	38
Achievement tests	36
Informal assessment	34
Referral	34
Student grades	34
Teacher interview	31
Criterion-referenced test	20
Other	13

Source: Adapted from *Assessing Culturally and Linguistically Diverse Students: A Practical Guide,* by R. L. Rhodes, S. H. Ochoa, & S. O. Ortiz, 2005, New York, NY: Guilford Press.

Before the ESSA, the NCLB required states to test the oral language, reading, and writing skills of ELs each year to determine their language proficiency in English. Title III of the NCLB was even more focused on language proficiency. First, it defined English language proficiency according to comprehension, listening, speaking, reading, and writing skills. Next, Title III required annual English language testing to assess the progress of ELs learning English and to determine their level of English proficiency. Starting with the NCLD and continuing with the ESSA, to monitor the progress of ELs and their growth in English proficiency, a variety of tests have been used. Their use by SLPs and ESOL and bilingual professionals is key in determining the communicative competence of an EL with communication disorders.

Assessing ELs' Language Proficiency for Identification and Placement

Traditionally, language proficiency has been measured using discrete-point assessment measures that yield a proficiency score in each language assessed. Often students are determined to be proficient in a language when they can understand and speak with a rudimentary level of conversational fluency. Many tests that measure language proficiency focus solely on listening and speaking skills and do not provide information about the child's functional use of language and their skill in using language across social demands. The absence of information about the child's language competence in reading and writing also provides a limited view of the student's language capabilities. Nonetheless, there are students that have no formal schooling or who have interrupted formal education that would perform poorly if they were required to read and/or write in their first language (Calderón, 2018). Professionals must remember that a student's level of proficiency will depend on the aspect of language that is being assessed. For this reason, professionals must recognize that formal language proficiency tests do not always provide a comprehensive view of a student's language capabilities (Albers, Kenyon, & Boals, 2009; Esquinca, Yaden, & Rueda, 2005; MacSwan & Rolstad, 2006; Ortiz & Yates, 2002).

Several tests have been commonly used to determine whether ELs need to be placed in an instructional program for ELs. These include the IDEA Language Proficiency Test (IPT) (2005), the Language Assessment Scales-Links (LAS Links) (Indiana Department of Education, 2006), and the Woodcock-Muñoz Language Survey–Revised Normative Update (WMLS-R NU) (Schrank, Wendling, Alvarado, & Woodcock, 2010), a revision of the 2005 Woodcock-Muñoz Language Survey–Revised (WMLS-R, 2005) (Woodcock, Muñoz-Sandoval, Ruef, & Alvarado, 2005), now revised to the Woodcock-Muñoz Language Survey®–Third Edition (WMLS™ III; Woodcock, Alvarado, Ruef, & Schrank, 2017) . The instruments noted above are often administered by a designated professional in the school system (e.g., ESOL professional, general education teacher, bilingual teacher), as designated by policies and procedures (Loop, 2002). In addition to these three tests, many states currently use the WIDA Screener and Kindergarten WIDA-APT (Assessing Comprehension and Communication in English State to-State for English Language Learners) Placement Test (W-APT) developed by the World-Class Instructional Design and Assessment (WIDA) consortium. To better understand these assessment measures, we provide a brief overview of each of the tests and their use and importance in determining language proficiency and identifying ELs.

IDEA Language Proficiency Tests (IPT)

The IPT (2016) is a nationally normed series of language proficiency assessments for ELs in grades preK–12. It is currently available for students in English and Spanish in a paper-based format and an online format. Many of the tests within the IPT family of tests were renormed for the 2017 to 2018 school year to make sure that the score interpretation norms are relevant to the current student population. This test is widely used in many districts and schools across the nation to determine if a student is a non-English speaker, a limited English speaker (LES), or a fluent English speaker (FES) or competent language learner. To determine an EL's oral, reading, and writing proficiency in English, the IPT is administered according to a student's age and grade level. The Pre-IPT is used for ELs aged 3, 4, and 5; the IPT I is used for ELs in Grades K to 6; and the IPT II is used for ELs in Grades 7 to 12. Two examples of an oral task from the IPT II for Level A (the levels range from A to F) are provided below:

Example 1. (Examiner points to a picture of a dog and a horse) Tell me what these animals are.

Example 2. Point to the astronaut at the bottom left corner of the picture.

The IPT also evaluates a student's oral, reading, and writing proficiency using specific tests organized by grade level. ELs in Grades K to 1 take the Early Literacy test, ELs in Grades 2 and 3 take the IPT I, ELs in Grades 4 through 6 take the IPT II, and ELs in Grades 7 through 12 take the IPT III. Reading tasks ranging from vocabulary in context to reading for life skills are found in the IPT II Reading test. An example of a *vocabulary in context* reading task is presented below. This measure is often used by an ESOL professional to identify and place an EL, monitor the progress of an EL, or redesignate a student's language proficiency.

Tom _____ to the store to buy bread.
   A. laughed
   B. added
   C. skated
   D. rested

Language Assessment Scales–Links (LAS Links)

The LAS Links test (Indiana Department of Education, 2006) is designed to place students upon initial entry into appropriate instructional programs. The LAS Links addresses the four language domains of speaking, listening, reading, and writing. The LAS Links consists of short placement tests, two summative test forms (Forms A and B) for each grade span, one Spanish form, and three parallel benchmark assessment forms. Instructional guidance binders are available for teacher use and to augment professional development/training. The LAS Links assessment is divided into five grade level spans: primary (K–1), early elementary (2–3), elementary (4–5), middle school (6–8), and high school (9–12). A rubric is used to grade students' responses. An example of the rubric is presented in Table 6–2.

A combination of the LAS Links test and results is used by ESOL and bilingual professionals (a) for English language development, (b) to monitor student progress, (c) to link results to teaching strategies, and (d) to create remedial instruction to ensure the successful academic achievement of ELs in all English academic settings.

Woodcock-Muñoz Language Survey III (WMLS-III)

The Woodcock-Muñoz Language Survey III (Woodcock, Alvarado, Ruef, & Schrank, 2017) is the third edition of the language survey and replaces the revised normative update (WMLS-R NU). This individually administered test provides a norm-referenced measure of listening, speaking, reading, and writing, for ages 2.5 to 21. The instrument features two English forms and one Spanish form and comprises eight individually administered tests that provide a broad sampling of proficiency in listening, oral language, language comprehension, reading, and writing in English and Spanish (Figures 6–3 and 6–4).

This test assesses basic and applied language skills and considers the influence of the child's language background and academic language exposure. This test situates students in one of six levels of language proficiency levels (Figure 6–5), provides the examiner with the general characteristics of each of the levels of language proficiency (Table 6–3), and uses language proficiency cutoff scores to identify or reclassify an EL as English proficient. The information generated from an assessment is entered into a software program that generates several online reports (e.g., teacher report; parent report; English/Spanish table of scores). These reports provide useful information about the linguistic status of the examinee and language proficiency, and they recommend intervention strategies for teachers. This test also provides home-based activities for parents with the goal of promoting family participation in language instruction (Duffy, Stephens-Pisecco, & Schultz, 2018).

Table 6–2. LAS Links Speaking Rubric

Score	Descriptor	Example
0	No response in English, response only in home language, or response does not relate to the prompt, including "I don't know."	**Student response to any task:** I don't know.
1	Response relates to the prompt but does not satisfy the task. Lack of sentence form, errors in grammar and vocabulary, and insufficient vocabulary interfere with communication. Response consists of at least one on-topic English word. If a text prompt is given, a single-word response may not be a repetition of the prompt.	**Grade:** 3 **Picture prompt:** A man who is sitting in a wheelchair is feeding a couple of birds. **Teacher prompt:** Tell me what is happening in the picture. **Student response:** A man in a wheelchair.
2	Response satisfies the task and is in sentence form (subject/predicate) with errors in grammar and/or vocabulary or insufficient vocabulary not typical of a native speaker.	**Grade:** 1 **Picture prompt:** A boy is eating vegetables. **Teacher prompt:** Tell me what is happening in the picture. **Student response:** That boy is eating with broccolis and carrots.
3	Response satisfies the task, is in sentence form, and is spoken with the vocabulary, grammar, and ease of expression of a native speaker.	**Grade:** 10 **Picture prompt:** A girl is at the doctor's office and the doctor is consulting her. **Teacher prompt:** Tell me what is happening in the picture. **Student response:** The doctor is checking the little girl's heart.

Source: Adapted from Academic Language Programs Department—LAS Links. Retrieved from http://www2.yisd.net/education/components/docmgr/default.php ?sectiondetailid=162164&catfilter=10502#showDoc

Figure 6–3. WMLS III: English Selective Table.

	Listening and Speaking					Reading and Writing						Cross-Domain Clusters		
	Listening	Speaking	Broad English Oral Language	Basic English Oral Language	Applied English Oral Language	Reading	Writing	Broad Reading and Writing	Basic Reading and Writing	Applied Reading and Writing	Comprehension	Broad English Language Ability	Basic English Language Ability	Applied English Language Ability
Test 1: Analogies	■		■		■							■		
Test 2: Oral Comprehension	■		■		■						■	■		
Test 3: Picture Vocabulary		■	■	■								■	■	
Test 4: Oral Language Expression		■	■	■								■		
Test 5: Letter-Word Identification						■		■	■			■	■	
Test 6: Passage Comprehension						■		■		■	■	■		
Test 7: Dictation							■	■	■			■	■	
Test 8: Written Language Expression							■	■		■		■		

■ Tests required to create the cluster listed.

Figure 6–3. WMLS III: English Selective Table. From Woodcock–Muñoz Language Survey (WMLS III) Copyright © 2017 by Riverside Assessments, LLC. All rights reserved. Used by permission of the publisher.

Figure 6–4. WMLS III: Spanish Selective Table. From Woodcock-Muñoz Language Survey (WMLS III) Copyright © 2017 by Riverside Assessments, LLC. All rights reserved. Used by permission of the publisher.

	Escuchar y hablar						Leer y escribir					Compuestos entre dominios		
	Escuchar	Hablar	Lenguaje oral amplio en español	Lenguaje oral básico en español	Lenguaje oral aplicado en español	Leer	Escribir	Lectura y escritura amplias en español	Lectura y escritura básicas en español	Lectura y escritura aplicadas en español	Comprensión	Habilidad amplia de lenguaje en español	Habilidad básica de lenguaje en español	Habilidad aplicada de lenguaje en español
Prueba 1: Analogías	■		■								■	■		
Prueba 2: Comprensión oral	■		■								■			■
Prueba 3: Vocabulario sobre dibujos		■	■	■							■	■		
Prueba 4: Expresión de lenguaje oral		■	■	■							■			
Prueba 5: Identificación de letras y palabras						■		■			■	■		
Prueba 6: Comprensión de textos					■	■		■			■			■
Prueba 7: Dictado							■		■		■	■		
Prueba 8: Expresión de lenguaje escrito					■		■		■		■			■

■ Tests required to create the cluster listed.

Figure 6–5. WMLS III language proficiency levels.

Table 6–3. WMLS Language Proficiency Level Descriptions

Initial Development	Receptive and expressive skills are very limited and he or she has minimal comprehension and speech. The individual is often at the preproduction or silent stage of academic language learning and typically struggles to understand simple conversations/discussions, even when topics are familiar and the speaker uses linguistic supports. Spoken language often consists of single words or familiar phrases. In reading and writing, an individual derives little or no meaning from grade-level text and has little or no ability to use reading or writing in the academic context. Participation in the classroom may be minimal unless substantial instructional scaffolding is provided for all language and academic content.
Early Development	Receptive and expressive skills are very limited but he or she is beginning to understand and speak high-frequency words and phrases.
Continuing Development	Sufficient conversational proficiency to interact with others in day-to-day situations and is beginning to grasp academic language. Moderate instructional scaffolding in the classroom environment is needed for effective learning. In oral language, the individual's receptive and expressive skills are at a level sufficient for most context-embedded conversations and discussions.
Emerging Proficiency	Demonstrates understanding of the specialized academic language required in the school setting but still requires some instructional scaffolding in the classroom environment for effective learning. The individual's oral receptive and expressive proficiency is near the level of average native-language peers. Understands the majority of elaborate classroom conversations. Spoken language consists of complete, and often complex, sentences. Grammatical and pronunciation errors are still evident, but his or her language is easily understandable.

Table 6–3. *continued*

Proficiency	Achieved language proficiency comparable to that of average native-language speakers. Able to communicate effectively and handle the demands of the mainstream classroom with no instructional support needed. Listening and oral speaking skills are comparable to those of average native-language speakers. On-level literacy skills comparable to those of average native-language speakers. Understands standard classroom interactions and instruction. Has a substantial vocabulary, rarely struggling finding words.
Advanced Proficient	Has achieved proficiency at a level above that of average native-language speakers. Communicates clearly in all domains of language and manages the demands of the classroom easily. In oral language, has an expansive vocabulary and advanced understanding of language, above the level of average native-language peers. Literacy is above the level of average native-language peers and the individual can perceive complex relationships and ideas in written language.

Source: From Woodcock-Muñoz Language Survey (WMLS III) Copyright © 2017 by Riverside Assessments, LLC. All rights reserved. Used by permission of the publisher.

The WMLS III is often used by the ESOL or bilingual professional to (a) determine English and/or Spanish language proficiency, (b) determine eligibility for bilingual education/ESL services, (c) assess readiness for English-only instruction, (d) monitor growth or change, and (e) assist in educational planning and evaluating programs.

WIDA Screener

The WIDA Screener Online is an English language proficiency assessment administered to new students in Grades 1 to 12 to help educators identify them as ELs. The test, developed by the WIDA consortium, is an individually administered test that addresses the academic English language proficiency (ELP) standards at the core of the WIDA consortium's approach to instructing and evaluating the progress of ELs.

The WIDA consortium was founded in 2002 with the purpose of meeting the requirements of the NCLB for ELs with standards and assessment instruments. This assessment provides information about the ELP level of ELs in kindergarten through Grade 12 in the skill areas of listening, speaking, reading, and writing and discriminates across the full proficiency range of the WIDA ELP scale. The WIDA framework recognizes the continuum of language development within the four domains, with six English language proficiency levels ranging from Level 1: Entering (reflecting only rudimentary knowledge of and skills in English) to Level 6: Reaching (the level at which students can succeed academically in English on par with their English-proficient peers in speaking, listening, reading, and writing) (Figure 6–6). Below is a more detailed description of WIDA levels.

At **Level 1: Entering**, ELs have little or no understanding of English, and most of the time they respond nonverbally to simple commands or questions. It is important to remember that ELs at Level 1 build meaning from text from nonprint elements such as illustrations, graphs, or tables. Therefore, for EL students at Level 1, teachers should select texts that are rich in illustrations or, if such texts are not available, make illustrations, graphs, or charts available to ELs as supplementary materials.

At **Level 2: Emerging**, ELs are beginning to understand phrases and short sentences. They can communicate limited information in routine situations by using memorized chunks of language. ELs at Level 2 begin to use general academic vocabulary and familiar expressions used in everyday communication.

At **Level 3: Developing**, ELs have a more developed vocabulary and start to understand more complex speech. They use English spontaneously, using simple sentences that are both comprehensible and appropriate but frequently marked by grammatical errors. They understand not only general academic vocabulary but also specialized vocabulary. However, they still have some problems understanding and producing complex structures and academic language.

Figure 6–6. WIDA English language proficiency levels.

At **Level 4: Expanding**, ELs have language skills that are adequate for everyday communication demands, but they still make occasional structural and lexical errors. At this level, ELs are proficient in communicating in new or unfamiliar settings but have some difficulty with complex language structures and abstract academic concepts.

ELs at **Level 5: Bridging** are not fully proficient in English but can express themselves fluently and accurately on a wide range of social and academic topics in a variety of contexts. ELs at this level of proficiency need very minimal language support to function in English-based instructional environments.

The WIDA Screener test adapts to the test taker's ability level and is considered fully adaptive. For example, if the test taker performs well on a test item of moderate difficulty, then the test taker is presented with a more difficult test item. Likewise, if the test taker performs poorly, they are presented with a simpler test item. The speaking subtest of the WIDA Screener requires up to 25 minutes to administer and is scored using a rubric (available at http://www.perryschools.org/ell/wp-content/uploads/sites/30/2017/06/Screener-Speaking-Scoring-Rubric.pdf). The listening and reading subtests take up to 15 minutes to administer and are scored using an answer key. The writing subtest takes up to 25 minutes to administer and is scored using a rubric. For example, for the writing section of WIDA Screener, test raters use a rubric organized around the six levels of language proficiency developed by WIDA. This rubric (available at http://www.perryschools.org/ell/wp-content/uploads/sites/30/2017/06/Screener-Writing-Scoring-Rubric.pdf) is used to measure three components of writing: linguistic complexity, vocabulary usage, and language control. The use of this rubric on an authentic student response is highlighted in an example provided in Figure 6–7. Here, the EL was required to generate a list of important details associated with an event and then use the information to generate a written narrative. The examiner, using the writing rubric, graded this response at Level 1: Entering because the text produced by the test taker did not demonstrate the ability to write full sentences and the syntactic errors contained in the text obstructed comprehensibility. A score of 2 could have been obtained if the test taker had written a full, syntactically correct sentence.

Event	lisen mexico musica
Who	six friends
When	monday 8:00 PM
Where	is my house
Other Information	my cousin is they Mexico

My cousin is they mexico
is you come to house my lisen musica
it will be this monday 8:00 PM

Figure 6-7. Example of student response for assessing writing.

Kindergarten WIDA ACCESS Placement Test (W-APT)

The Kindergarten WIDA-ACCESS Placement Test (Kindergarten W-APT) is an English language proficiency screener administered to incoming kindergarteners to identify ELs. The Kindergarten W-APT helps teachers and administrators make decisions about whether incoming kindergarteners would benefit from English language support services. The Kindergarten W-APT does not assign scores across the full range of WIDA English Language Proficiency Levels 1 (Beginning) to 6 (Reaching). Instead, scores for Speaking and Listening are marked as showing low, mid, high, or exceptional proficiency.

State-Developed Instruments for Assessing English Language Proficiency

Although some states have decided to use language proficiency instruments developed either by multistate consortia or by national test development companies, others continue to develop and administer their own assessment of EL language proficiency.

For example, two states fall into this category: Texas (with the Texas English Language Proficiency Assessment System [TEL-PAS] and Texas English Language Proficiency Assessment System [TELPAS] Alternate Assessment) and New York (with the New York State Identification Test for English Language Learners [NYSITELL]).

Texas English Language Proficiency Assessment System (TELPAS)

In general, the TELPAS assesses the English language proficiency of K–12 ELs in four language domains: listening, speaking, reading, and writing. English language proficiency assessments are federally required to be administered to students in Grades K–12 to evaluate the progress that ELs make in becoming proficient in the use of academic English. The TELPAS assesses the English language proficiency standards (ELPS), which districts are required to implement as an integral part of each foundation and enrichment subject of the Texas Essential Knowledge and Skills (TEKS) state-required curriculum.

The TELPAS Alternate is administered to ELs with the most significant cognitive disabilities who cannot participate in the general ELP assessment, even with allowable accommodations. The TELPAS Alternate uses the same language domains (listening, speaking, reading, and writing) as the TELPAS; however, the definitions of the TELPAS language domains are broader in the TELPAS Alternate to allow for alternate forms of expressive and receptive language (Texas Education Agency, 2019).

Similar to other English language proficiency tests, the TEL-PAS measures English learning based on identifiable stages of second language development. There are four proficiency levels assessed through TELPAS: beginning, intermediate, advanced, and advanced high (Texas Education Agency, 2019). The proficiency language descriptors measure how well ELs at the four proficiency levels can understand and use English in grade-level academic settings. The descriptors serve as a guide for teachers to modify instruction based on the language proficiency and needs of the student.

At the **Beginning** level, students are typically new to the English language. They have little or no ability to derive meaning from English text. They generally understand very little English and tend to read very slowly and word by word. In order to figure out the meaning of what they read, they rely heavily on previous knowledge of the topic, the small bank of English words and phrases they have learned, and information from pictures. Because their English is so limited, their comprehension quickly breaks down when they try to read English in authentic social and academic contexts. At the **Intermediate** level, students have a somewhat larger English vocabulary and a basic sense of simple English language structures. However, they tend to interpret English very literally and have difficulty following storylines that have a surprise twist or nonstandard format. They still rely heavily on what they already know about a topic to confirm meaning and increase comprehension, and pictures that illustrate meaning are still a needed support. Students at this level can read and understand short connected texts on familiar topics when high-frequency English is used. They have difficulty reading and understanding materials written for their grade level. **Advanced** students have an emerging grade-appropriate reading vocabulary and a grasp of the structure and grammatical features of the English language. They have the ability to read grade-level texts with some success, although second language acquisition support is still needed to help them understand language that is typically familiar to native English-speaking peers. With linguistic support, these students can often demonstrate comprehension of main and supporting ideas on topics they know little about. Additionally, they can often understand English beyond its literal meaning, and they have an emerging ability to think analytically to build conceptual understanding as they read grade-level materials in English. Finally, students who are **Advanced High** have the ability to read and understand, with minimal support related to second language acquisition, grade-appropriate English used in academic and social contexts, with some exceptions when low-frequency or specialized vocabulary is used. With minimal visual and textual support and at a level nearly comparable to their native English-speaking peers, they are able to understand both explicit and implicit ideas, think analytically, and build conceptual understanding as they read grade-level materials in English.

New York State Identification Test for English Language Learners (NYSITELL)

The NYSITELL serves as the state's formal English language proficiency assessment in the process for initially identifying English Language Learners/Multilingual Learners in New York State. This assessment tests students' English language skills and determines if the students need bilingual and/or English as a New Language (ENL) services. The test is administered to eligible students within 10 school days of their initial enrollment and assesses the English language proficiency of K–12 ELs across four modalities: speaking, listening, reading, and writing.

The NYSITELL is composed of eight distinct levels (I–VIII) and is aligned with the expectations for an English Language Learner/Multilingual Learner, depending on the grade and when in the school year the new student arrives. Comparable to other English language proficiency tests, the NYSITELL assesses language proficiency across five proficiency levels: Entering/Beginning, Emerging/Low Intermediate, Transitioning/Intermediate, Expanding/Advanced, and Commanding/Proficient. These levels are known as Performance Level Descriptions (PLDs) (New York State Education Department, 2018). For students with disabilities, testing accommodations must be provided in the administration of the NYSITELL based on the student's IEP or 504 Plan and consistent with state policy for the administration of this state assessment.

Exiting Procedures for ELs

When ELs are identified as not being fully proficient in English, they are placed in educational programs that, regardless of format, have as their main goal the improvement of their English language proficiency. As the student becomes more proficient in English, a decision must be made: Should the EL student remain in a program for ELs or exit the program? The procedures used in three states (i.e., Michigan, Florida, and Massachusetts) provide examples of exiting procedures for ELs.

In Michigan, once EL students have been placed in the EL/ limited English proficient (LEP) program, they are evaluated on an annual basis to determine how well they are learning English and if they are becoming more proficient in the areas of listening, speaking, reading, and writing of the English language. ELs are also tested in the academic content areas of reading/language arts, math, and other core academic subjects. The purpose of this evaluation is to determine whether their level of proficiency is adequate to meaningfully participate in regular educational programs. To exit the EL/LEP program, students need to receive a composite score of 4.5 or higher on the WIDA ACCESS for ELLs (a language proficiency test that will be discussed in the next chapter), obtain minimum scores of 4.0 in the reading and writing domains, and demonstrate grade-level proficiency in reading on the state-approved local reading assessment. Upon exit from the EL/LEP program, schools must monitor ELs for 4 years and continue to provide the necessary support to them in the domain (listening, speaking, reading, or writing) in which they scored less than 5.0, even if they meet the minimum criterion for exit.

In Florida, an EL student may be eligible for exit based upon teacher recommendation or observation. The student's name is provided to the ESOL teacher, who is responsible for the reevaluation process and procedures designed to determine exit eligibility. The ESOL teacher and the ELL Committee (which includes the ESOL teacher) can use other information to determine if the student should be exited from the ESOL program. Examples of the type of information that the ELL Committee considers include portfolio with student work, language proficiency scores, academic performance data (grade level), writing samples that demonstrate proficiency and performance in English, performance on norm-referenced standardized English test, and grades in a mainstream classroom.

In Massachusetts, an EL student exits the English language development program when it is determined, in consultation with the classroom teacher and/or a guidance counselor, that English language development instruction is no longer necessary.

In making this determination, the school district uses multiple means of assessment, which include student grades, reports of teacher observation, and WIDA ACCESS for ELLs' standardized test scores. Once a student has exited the program, the student is reclassified.

All reclassified students must be monitored for 4 years and be provided support if needed to progress. In addition, schools serving former ELs should consider:

- ◆ assigning reclassified students (students whose EL classification has been removed), at least initially, to Sheltered English Immersion endorsed teachers licensed in the appropriate content area to enhance the likelihood of continued growth in their English language proficiency and academic content learning;
- ◆ providing regular, structured times during the school day or week for sheltered content area and ESL teachers to plan instruction collaboratively for reclassified EL students;
- ◆ providing additional opportunities for the student to participate in small group instruction and learning throughout the school day, as well as after school and during the summer; and
- ◆ designing and providing additional individualized learning support and opportunities to check on academic progress.

If former EL students fail to make academic progress, as measured by their grades and content-area assessments, after their EL classification has been removed, and if a school-based team determines that this failure is due to the lack of English proficiency, then students are reclassified as ELs and the instructional programming for these students is redesigned. So far, we have examined assessment instruments that are used to identify and classify the general EL population and procedures used in EL programs to exit students. What are the policies that are put in place for ELs with disorders?

States often diverge on policies and procedures to identify ELs who need special services. They are challenged to a varying degree to determine whether a student's academic difficulties stem from learning a second language or from the presence of a communication disorder or from both. The framework in which states must identify, evaluate, and provide evidence-based intervention for ELs with communication disorders are couched in IDEA (2004), NCLB (2001), and ESSA (2015). The subsequent sections focus on the identification practices and protocols used by SLPs to identify ELs with a communication disorder and to determine eligibility for speech-language services and/ or programs.

Identification Practices and Protocols for ELs with a Communication Disorder: Disability Determination, Eligibility, and Intervention

Different states have developed their own criteria or relied on the skilled judgment of professionals responsible for conducting special education assessments to guide the assessment and identification process (Scott, Boynton Hauerwas, & Brown, 2014). According to parents and school personnel, variations in these criteria and how they are applied have contributed to confusion when children move within and across school districts (Ireland & Conrad, 2016). In addition, as school administrators and boards of education have examined state special education prevalence data, increasing attention has been given to discrepancies among districts in the numbers of children identified as having speech-language disabilities, particularly in ELs. In a study conducted by Klingner and Harry (2006), researchers examined the special education referral and decision-making process for ELs in an urban school district in a southern state. Specifically, the researchers focused on the Child Study Team (CST) meetings, placement conferences/multidisciplinary team meetings, and the process that was used to determine if ELs who were struggling had disabilities. The researchers posed the following questions: (1) How is it determined whether ELs who struggle academically have a disability? (2) What is the decision-making process? (3) To what extent do the professionals involved understand second language acquisition? and (4) What considerations are given to language issues?

The researchers found that professionals were confused about when to refer an EL, were not always able to differentiate between English language acquisition and a disability, depended on test scores, misinterpreted the child's lack of full language proficiency as having a disability, and did not fully consider other factors that might affect a student's performance (Rodriquez & Rodriguez, 2017). In general, the findings of this study revealed that in practice, only cursory attention was given to prereferral strategies and/or response to intervention (RtI) models with ELs. Most important, there was a great deal of variability across schools in how district policies were carried out, how assessments were conducted, and how decisions were made (Caesar & Kohler, 2007; Chu & Flores, 2011; Echevarria, Richards-Tutor, & Vogt, 2015; Linan-Thompson, 2010; Muñoz, White, & Horton-Ikard, 2014; Spaulding, Plante, & Farinella, 2006).

The steady increase in the number of students whose primary language spoken in the home is a language other than English has created a need for the development of consistent state policies and procedures to appropriately identify and provide educational interventions for ELs and bilingual students with disabilities. There is widespread anecdotal evidence suggesting that ELs may be either bypassed for consideration as a child with a disability because professionals assume the child is not achieving solely because of his or her language difference, *or* overrepresented on special education rosters due to inappropriate placement based on inaccurate measures and ill-conceived procedures (Bedore & Peña, 2018; Kangas, 2014; Paradis, Schneider, & Duncan, 2013).

Roseberry-McKibben (2018) outlines the procedure commonly used to determine a student's eligibility for special education and/or related services (Figure 6–8). The process routinely begins with a teacher referral. If an EL student is suspected of having a speech or language disorder, an interdisciplinary team (also often termed a "child study committee") convenes to review existing data and discuss possible interventions prior to referral for an evaluation. To reduce inappropriate identification and placement of ELs in special education, prereferral strategies are often implemented (Fuchs, Mock, Morgan, & Young, 2003; Sanford, Brown, & Turner, 2012). During this time, it is important that a team of professionals gather information about the stu-

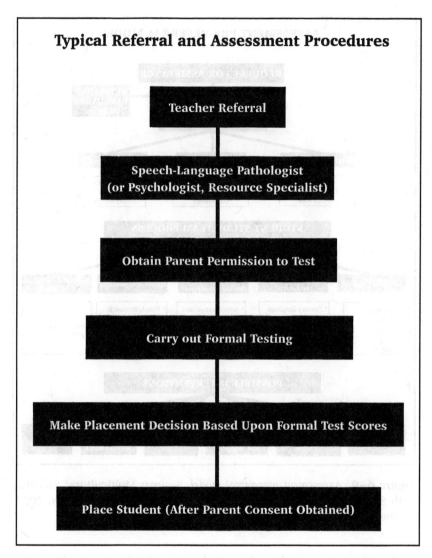

Figure 6–8. *Typical referral and assessment procedures.* Source: Multicultural Students with Special Language Needs *(3rd ed.), by C. Roseberry-McKibben, 2008, Oceanside, CA: Academic Communication Associates.*

dent using a variety of strategies to determine whether a formal evaluation is warranted. A model, such as the one shown in Figure 6–9, can be used to guide the process of data collection. The purpose of these strategies is to provide students with assistance

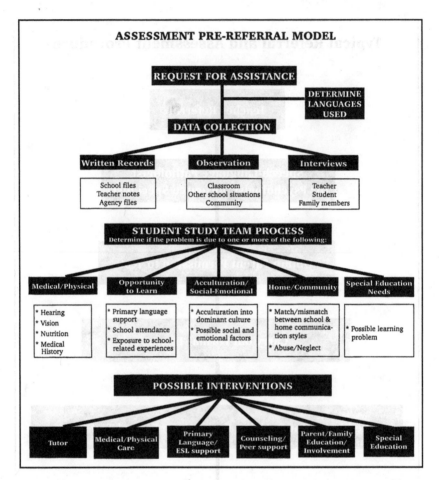

Figure 6–9. Assessment prereferral model. Source: Multicultural Students with Special Language Needs *(3rd ed.), by C. Roseberry-McKibben, 2008, Oceanside, CA: Academic Communication Associates.*

within the general education environment prior to conducting a formal evaluation to determine whether the student has a communication disorder.

With the reauthorization of IDEA (2004), RtI multitiered models have been established as a vehicle for supporting monolingual English students and ELs with meaningful prereferral strategies. RtI has been recognized as a promising alternative for use with ELs (Burns, Griffiths, Parson, Tilly, & VanDerHeyden, 2007; Collier, 2010; Echevarria & Vogt, 2011; Ehren, 2005; Esparza Brown & Sanford, 2011; Fuchs & Deshler, 2007; Klingner

& Edwards, 2006; Mellard & Johnson, 2007; Moore & Montgomery, 2008; Schraeder, 2008), and the SLP can collaborate with school professionals and specialized instructional support personnel in the implementation of RtI models.

Several RtI models, flowcharts, guiding questions, and recommendations have been offered to guide assessment professionals in the collection of critical student information. These resources can be used to facilitate decision making regarding the need for a more extensive formal evaluation of EL students (Batsche et al., 2005; Leung, 1993; Linan-Thompson & Ortiz, 2009; Rinaldi & Samson, 2008; Rosa-Lugo, Rivera, & Rierson, 2010). Specifically, RtI models that focus on the use of screening and progress-monitoring tools and effective, high-quality, and linguistically and culturally responsive core curricula as a precursor to the identification of ELs with communication disorders have been recommended (Figure 6–10) (Esparza Brown & Doolittle, 2008; Haas & Esparza Brown, 2019).

To determine the presence of a disability, the normal behaviors of dual code learners and users must be identified and differentiated from disabilities. Possible indicators of a language disorder have been described in the literature (Goldstein, 2004a, 2004b; Kayser, 1995; Kohnert, 2008; Ortiz, 1997; Paradis, 2005; Paradis, Genesee, & Crago, 2011; Roseberry-McKibben, 2018). These indicators offer assessment professionals a framework to establish if the child (a) meets the federal definition of a "child with a disability," (b) meets the criteria associated with one of the disability categories established in the law (e.g., speech-language impairment), and (c) if special education and/or related services are necessary to address the disability. For ELs, the disability determination of "language disorder" is appropriate only for students with disabilities affecting their underlying ability to learn any language (Paradis, 2018; Paradis, Schneider, & Duncan, 2013; Roseberry-McKibben, 2018). For example, the federal regulation at 34 CFR § 300.304 of IDEA (PL 108-146) (2004) requires that:

◆ assessments and other evaluation procedures are selected and administered to ensure that they measure the extent to which a child has a disability and needs special education, rather than measuring a child's English language skills;

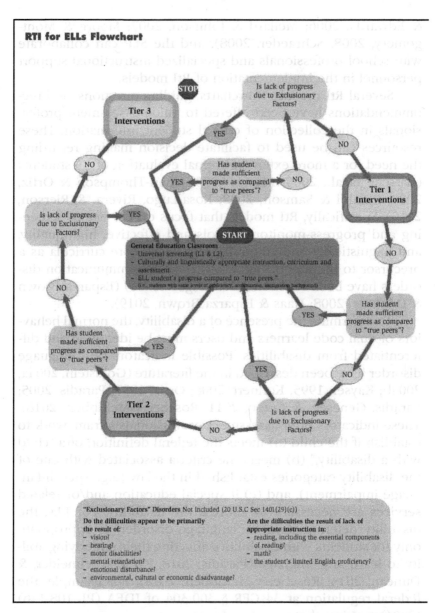

RTI for ELLs Flowchart

STOP

Tier 3 Interventions

Is lack of progress due to Exclusionary Factors?

YES

NO

NO

Has student made sufficient progress as compared to "true peers"?

YES

NO

Tier 1 Interventions

NO

Is lack of progress due to Exclusionary Factors?

YES

START

General Education Classroom
- Universal screening (L1 & L2).
- Culturally and linguistically appropriate instruction, curriculum and assessment.
- ELL student's progress compared to "true peers."
  (i.e., students with same levels of proficiency, acculturation, immigration background)

NO

Has student made sufficient progress as compared to "true peers"?

YES

NO

Has student made sufficient progress as compared to "true peers"?

YES

YES

Tier 2 Interventions

NO

Is lack of progress due to Exclusionary Factors?

"Exclusionary Factors" Disorders Not Included (20 U.S.C Sec 1401(29)(c))

Do the difficulties appear to be primarily the result of:
- vision?
- hearing?
- motor disabilities?
- mental retardation?
- emotional disturbance?
- environmental, cultural or economic disadvantage?

Are the difficulties the result of lack of appropriate instruction in:
- reading, including the essential components of reading?
- math?
- the student's limited English proficiency?

Figure 6–10. RtI for ELs flow chart. Source: Brown, J., & Doolittle, J. (2008). *A cultural, linguistic, and ecological framework for response to intervention with English Language Learners.* Teaching Exceptional Children, 40(5), 66–72. continues

Tier 1 Interventions
- Review of student's ecology (i.e., educational history, language proficiency in L1 and L2, family education and literacy, acculturation level, SES, etc.)
- Interventions are developmentally, culturally, linguistically and experientially appropriate for targeted students and may be the classroom curriculum but a "double dose" or extension of classroom curriculum
- Interventions provide by classroom teacher, instructional assistant or other specialist within the general education classroom in a small group

Tier 2 Interventions
- Small group in or outside of general education classroom
- Interventions are linguistically, culturally and experientially appropriate
- Interventions counter to address specific problem areas and progress is closely monitored

Tier 3 Interventions
- Small Group or 1:1 instruction with alternative curriculum in alternative setting
- Curriculum and instruction addresses the specific deficit(s)
- Interventions must continue to be culturally, linguistically and experientially appropriate
- Standardized assessment in both L1 and L2 could be considered at this tier to identify learning profiles

DECISION-MAKING POINT FOR SPECIAL EDUCATION CONSIDERATION
- If the student has not made sufficient progress, a psychoeducational evaluations may be considered that links to interventions.
- Parent rights and consent are required for standardized assessments.
- All information must be provided to parents in their native language, including parent rights.
- Using a discrepancy formula approach for learning disability is appropriate for ELL students.
- Interpretation of standardized test data must be done within the context of the student's language proficiency in L1 and L2 acculturation level.
- IEP goals must consider the student's developmental, cognitive, cultural, and linguistic abilities.

Figure 6–10. continued

- evaluators conduct assessments in the child's native/ dominant language;
- a variety of assessment tools and strategies are used to gather relevant functional and developmental information about the child;
- any standardized tests administered to a child are valid for the specific purpose for which they are used and are administered by trained and knowledgeable personnel in accordance with any instructions provided by the test publisher; and
- no single procedure is used as the sole criterion for determining whether an EL child or student has a disability.

When a speech-language disability is suspected in an EL, the SLP ideally must use a combination of assessment procedures and strategies that include:

- information obtained from the parents (medical, educational history; concerns regarding their child's communication);
- hearing screening;
- formal and informal assessment (e.g., standardized tests, language samples; alternative assessment strategies);
- review of classroom performance (e.g., work samples, journals, narratives, criterion-referenced tests);
- review of student record (e.g., performance on state or district assessments of prereading and reading abilities, attendance, discipline, health records, universal screening results);
- observation in the classroom, using checklists to quantify student behaviors, ideally during diverse instructional activities; and
- information obtained from teachers.

Roseberry-McKibben (2018) highlights a process that can be followed to determine if a language disorder is present (Figure 6–11). This assessment wheel highlights the various activities that SLPs use in the evaluation of ELs.

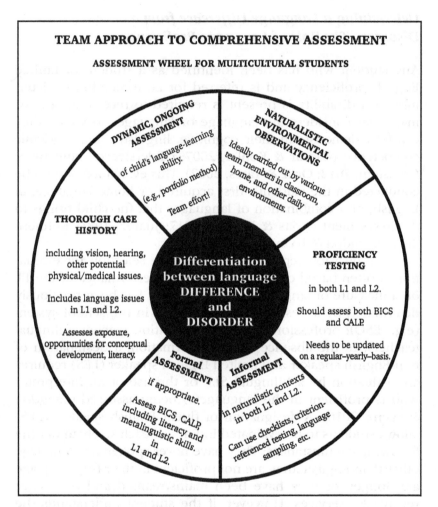

Figure 6–11. The assessment wheel. Source: Multicultural Students with Special Language Needs (3rd ed.), by C. Roseberry-McKibben, 2008, Oceanside, CA: Academic Communication Associates.

Practices Used by SLPs for EL Identification, Disability Determination, and Placement

Determining a Language Difference from a Disorder: The Role of Language Proficiency

Any student who has been identified as a student of limited English proficiency and is referred for an evaluation to determine if a disability is present is required to receive an assessment that considers the language or languages in which they can best demonstrate their cognitive, linguistic, and academic competence (Caesar & Kohler, 2007; Gildersleeve-Neumann & Goldstein, 2012; Ortiz & Yates, 2002). This evaluation should be conducted in the student's first acquired or home language, in English, or a combination of languages that the child brings to the assessment (Arias & Friberg, 2017; Juarez, 1983; Kohnert, 2010; Langdon & Irvine Saenz, 1996).

The decision regarding the language selection for evaluation is often based on the results of the performance of the EL on a measure of language proficiency that has been previously determined by a designated professional in the school system (e.g., ESOL professional, general education teacher, bilingual teacher). In the absence of this information, a designation of non-English speaker and limited English speaker (LES) requires an evaluation by a bilingual SLP or the use of an interpreter who is proficient in the language(s) being assessed (Langdon & Saenz, 2016). A designation of fluent English speaker (FES) allows students to be evaluated in English exclusively under the following circumstances: They have never spoken any language other than English, they are not proficient in their first language any longer, or they have been mainstreamed and no longer receive EL services. However, if the student understands the non-English language spoken in the home at a conversational level but speaks only a few basic words or phrases, the evaluation should be done bilingually to determine the extent of the low functioning in the both languages. Often students who come from code-switching communities must also be provided with the opportunity to demonstrate their language use to determine if the code-switching behaviors are appropriate or indicative of a communication disorder.

Instruments and Assessment Practices Used by SLPs for EL Identification, Disability Determination, and Placement

IDEA (1997) requires that ELs be assessed in their native language(s) (L1) and English (L2) using appropriate test instruments and assessment practices. Despite the persistent shortage of norm-referenced assessment procedures in languages other than English (Bedore & Peña, 2008; Kohnert, 2010; Langdon & Cheng, 2002; Peña, Iglesias, & Lidz, 2001; Solórzano, 2008), SLPs typically administer tests normed on monolingual English speakers and then use measures normed on a specific language group (e.g., monolingual Spanish speakers) to determine if the EL has a disorder (McLeod & International Expert Panel on Multilingual Children's Speech, 2017).

Prior to determining if the child has a language difference or a language disorder, the SLP must first obtain information about a child's language proficiency and functioning in L1 and L2. Similar to the ESOL professional, the SLP uses questionnaires and criterion-referenced and/or language proficiency tests to assess the level of English language proficiency (ELP) in ELs and to help them decide whether or not a bilingual speech-language assessment is warranted. This practice can be problematic because of the questionable psychometric properties and conceptual framework of language proficiency found in such measures (e.g., Larkin, Restrepo, & Morgan, 2007; Liu, Ward, Thurlow, & Christensen, 2017; MacSwan & Rolstad, 2006; Pray, 2005). For example, if the child obtains a low score in the primary language (e.g., Spanish) on a language proficiency measure (e.g., Woodcock-Muñoz Language Survey III, 2017) the SLP might assume that the child does not need to be assessed further in that language. It is possible that the child may receive a low score in Spanish on this measure and yet perform within normal limits on other measures of language tasks in Spanish. This is particularly likely to occur when the child is not being instructed in Spanish or has experienced interrupted formal education (MacGregor-Mendoza, 2000; Schiff-Myers, 1992; Zacrian & Haynes, 2012). Therefore, it is recommended that SLPs assess the child's academic, developmental, and functional language more holistically across languages and, as with all measures, careful interpretation of results is warranted (Arias & Friberg, 2017; Custodio & O'Loughlin, 2017; Duffy, Stephens-Pisecco, & Schultz, 2018).

Despite the limitations found with using static, standardized, quantitative, norm-referenced approaches to assess ELs, several standardized assessment instruments and practices are consistently used by bilingual and monolingual SLPs (with the assistance of a translator when warranted) to determine whether a student has a language delay, difference, or disorder (Betz, Eickhoff, & Sullivan, 2013; Caesar & Kohler, 2007; Fulcher-Rood, Castilla-Earls, & Higginbotham, 2019; Langdon, 1989; Langdon & Saenz, 2015). Of the norm-referenced measures, the Clinical Evaluation of Language Fundamentals–Fifth Edition (CELF-5 English; Semel, Wiig, & Secord, 2013) and the Clinical Evaluation of Language Fundamentals–Fourth Edition (CELF-4 Spanish; Wiig, Semel, & Secord, 2006) are one of the most frequently used standardized tests (Arias & Friberg, 2017; Senaga & Inglebret, 2003). This is often followed by the Expressive One-Word Picture Vocabulary Test 4: Spanish-Bilingual Edition (EOWPVT-4: SBE; Martin, 2011); the Receptive One-Word Picture Vocabulary Test-4: Spanish-Bilingual Editions (ROWPVT-4: SBE; Martin, 2011); the Preschool Language Scales–Fifth Edition (PLS–5 English; Zimmerman, Steiner, & Pond, 2011), or the Preschool Language Scales–Fifth Edition (PLS-5 Spanish; Zimmerman, Steiner, & Pond, 2012), as appropriate, and/or the Structured Photographic Expressive Language–Third Edition (SPELT-3) (Dawson, Stout, & Elyer, 2003) or the Spanish Structured Photographic Expressive Language Test 3 (Spanish SPELT-3; Langdon, 2012).

To better understand these assessment measures, we provide a brief overview of each of the measures that SLPs have used often to identify ELs, to make an appropriate diagnosis, and to determine eligibility for intervention and accommodations, as well as their importance in determining a language difference or disorder. In some instances, there have been revisions to some of the assessment instruments that have been used over time and/or the introduction of new tests, such as the Bilingual English-Spanish Assessment (BESA; Peña, Gutiérrez-Clellen, Iglesias, Goldstein, & Bedore, 2018).

Clinical Evaluation of Language Fundamentals–Fifth Edition (CELF-5 English; Semel, Wiig, & Secord, 2013)

The Clinical Evaluation of Language Fundamentals (CELF-5) (Semel, Wiig, & Secord, 2013), administered primarily by the speech-language pathologist, is used to determine whether a student has a language disorder or delay. This test assesses oral and written language as well as nonverbal communication skills of individual students, ages 5 to 21. The test is divided into five areas—Language Content, Language Structure, Oral-Written Language Connection, Pragmatics, and Language and Memory—and consists of 16 age-specific standalone tests. Twelve of the tests differentially combine to yield core (e.g., measure of overall language performance) and index (e.g., information about specific language skills) scores (Coret & McCrimmon, 2015).

A major revision of this test was its focus on assessing social language in authentic settings, such as in the classroom setting. An observational scale is available to obtain information about a student's language performance in the classroom and to plan for intervention or treatment. The CELF-5 is a comprehensive and flexible assessment that correlates with current educational practices by implementing common core standards that link assessment with instruction and intervention.

Clinical Evaluation of Language Fundamentals–Fourth Edition (CELF-4 Spanish; Semel, Wiig, & Secord, 2006)

The Spanish edition of the CELF-4 (Semel, Wiig, & Secord, 2006) is an individually administered clinical tool for the identification, diagnosis, and follow-up evaluation of language and communication disorders in Spanish-speaking students aged 5 to 21. The CELF-4 Spanish is a norm-referenced standardized assessment developed specifically for Spanish speakers living in the United States as a parallel test to the CELF-4. It is not a translation of the English edition of the CELF-4. The test is normed on a current sample of Spanish speakers in the United States, representing many countries of origin (25% from the Caribbean [Puerto Rico, Dominican Republic, and Cuba], 28% from Central and South America, and 46% from Mexico). This test evaluates interpersonal communication (BICS), assesses elements of more advanced academic language (CALP), and includes a Pragmatics Profile and an Observational Rating Scale. It consists of 16 subtests, exemplified in Table 6–4.

To date, this instrument remains one of the most commonly used standardized measures to assess and identify Spanish-speaking

Table 6–4. *CELF-4 Spanish Subtests*

Subtest	Subtest Task
Concepts and Following Directions (Conceptos y siguiendo direcciones)	The student points to pictured objects in response to oral directions
Word Structure (Estructura de palabras)	The student completes sentences using the targeted structure(s)
Recalling Sentences (Recordando oraciones)	Examiner presents sentence and student is required to imitate the sentence
Formulated Sentences (Formulación de oraciones)	The student formulates a sentence about visual stimuli using a targeted word or phrase
Word Classes—1 and 2 (Clases de palabras 1 y 2)	The student chooses two related words and describes their relationship
Sentence Structure (Estructura de oraciones)	The student points to a picture that illustrates the given sentence
Expressive Vocabulary (Vocabulario expresivo)	The student identifies a pictured object, person, or activity given a stimulus
Word Definitions (Definiciones de palabras)	The student defines a word that is presented and used in a sentence
Understanding Spoken Paragraphs (Entendiendo párrafos)	The student responds to questions about orally presented paragraphs; questions target main idea, details, sequence, inferential, and predictive information
Number Repetition 1 and 2 (Repetición de números 1 y 2)	The student repeats a series of numbers forward, then backward
Familiar Sequences 1 and 2 (Secuencias familiars 1 y 2)	The student names days of the week, counts backward, orders other information while being timed

Table 6–4. *continued*

Subtest	Subtest Task
Rapid Automatic Naming (Enumeración rápida y automática)	The student names colors, shapes, and color-shape combinations while being timed
Word Associations (Asociación de palabras)	The student names words in specific categories while being timed
Phonological Awareness (Conocimiento fonológico)	The student rhymes, segments, blends, identifies sounds and syllables in words and sentences
Pragmatics Profile (Clasificación pragmática)	The examiner elicits information from a parent or teacher about the student's social language skills.
Observational Rating Scales Escala de valoración del lenguaje)	Parent, teacher, and student each rate the student's classroom interaction and communication skills.

Source: Adapted from *The Clinical Evaluation of Language Fundamentals—Fourth Edition, Spanish Edition (CELF-4 Spanish)*, by E. Semel, E. H. Wiig, & W. A. Secord, 2006, San Antonio, TX: Pearson.

children with language disorders (Arias & Friberg, 2016). Since it is widely used to identify language disorders in ELs whose primary language is Spanish, it is critical that SLPs consult research on the use of this measure with Spanish-English ELs. For example, Barragan, Castilla-Earls, Martinez-Nieto, Restrepo, and Gray (2018) conducted a study to explore the performance of a group of Spanish-speaking, dual-language learners (DLLs) on this measure. Specifically, they wanted to examine if the CELF-4S accurately differentiates between children with and without LI in students from low-income and low-parental education backgrounds who attended English-only schools. In general, they found that this measure, when used alone, overidentifies low-income Spanish-English DLLs attending English-only schools as having a language disorder. They concluded that practitioners should use the results of the CELF-4 Spanish with this specific population with caution.

Receptive One-Word Picture Vocabulary Test and Expressive One-Word Picture Vocabulary Test, English and Spanish Editions

The Expressive One-Word Picture Vocabulary Test, Fourth Edition (EOWPVT4) (Brownell, 2010) and the Receptive One-Word Picture Vocabulary Test, Fourth Edition (ROWPVT4) (Brownell, 2010) are administered to children aged 2 to 18 years and 11 months. The EOWPVT is designed to assess expressive vocabulary, whereas the main purpose of the ROWPVT is to measure receptive vocabulary. Test administration for each is approximately 20 minutes. To administer the EOWPVT, the examiner presents a series of illustrations showing objects, actions, or concepts. The child is asked to name each illustration. The test begins with an illustration the child is expected to name successfully. The examiner then presents items that become progressively more difficult. When the examinee is unable to correctly name several consecutive illustrations, testing discontinues.

To administer the ROWPVT, the examiner presents a series of test plates that each shows four illustrations. The examiner orally presents a stimulus word, and the child is expected to identify the illustration that depicts the meaning of the word. Like the EOWPVT, the test begins with a word the child should be able to identify. The examiner then presents items that become progressively more difficult. When the examinee is unable to correctly identify the meaning of a specified number of items, testing is stopped. EOWPVT was co-normed with the ROWPVT, so accurate comparisons can be made between a student's receptive and expressive vocabulary skills.

Both the EOWPVT (Brownell, 2010) and the ROWPVT (Brownel, 2010) have bilingual versions assessing expressive and receptive vocabulary of individuals, ages 2 to 70+, who demonstrate varying levels of proficiency in Spanish and English: the Expressive One-Word Picture Vocabulary Test 4: Spanish-Bilingual Edition (EOWPVT-4: SBE; Martin, 2011) and the Receptive One-Word Picture Vocabulary Test-4: Spanish-Bilingual Editions (ROWPVT-4: SBE; Martin, 2011). These versions assess total acquired vocabulary by allowing examinees to respond in both languages. The record forms include acceptable responses and stimulus words in both languages. It is important to emphasize that these assessment tools are not measuring language proficiency but are measuring an individual's total acquired vocabulary.

Preschool Language Scale–Fifth Edition (PLS–5), English and Spanish Editions

The PLS-5, Fifth Edition, English edition (Zimmerman, Steiner, Pond, & Evatt, 2011), is designed to identify young children from birth to 7 years, 11 months old to determine the presence of a language delay and/or disorder. This test is also used to determine eligibility for early intervention or speech-language services and can be administered between 45 and 60 minutes in a play-based format requiring the child to interact appropriately with different toys and manipulatives. The PLS-5 consists of two subscales, Auditory Comprehension (AC) and Expressive Communication (EC). The Auditory Comprehension subscale measures a child's ability to understand spoken language; the Expressive Communication subscale measures the ability of a child to communicate with others. The test also provides three supplemental measures, which include an articulation screener, a language sample checklist, and a home communication questionnaire. The PLS-5 yields norm-referenced scores such as standard scores, percentile ranks, and age equivalents for the AC and EC scales as well as for Total Language (TL) (Zimmerman, Steiner, Pond, & Evatt, 2011).

Although current studies document that the PLS is a widely used measure for assessing child language (e.g., Arias & Friberg, 2017; Betz, Eickhoff, & Sullivan, 2012), practitioners have raised concerns about this instrument's psychometric properties, such as its reliability, validity, and diagnostic accuracy, particularly with children from diverse backgrounds (Denman et al., 2017; Leaders, 2013; Smith, 2014).

The Preschool Language Scales–Fifth Edition, Spanish edition (PLS-5 Spanish; Zimmerman, Steiner, & Pond, 2012) was normed on 1,150 monolingual and bilingual Spanish-speaking children in the United States and Puerto Rico. The goal of this assessment instrument is to determine if a monolingual or bilingual Spanish-speaking child, from birth to 7 years, 11 months old, demonstrates age-appropriate communication skills. The SLP initially administers the Auditory Comprehension (AC) and Expressive Communication (EC) subscales in Spanish and English, and the child may respond to the examiner in either language. Only those items missed by the child in Spanish are readministered in English. The PLS-5 Spanish has supplemental measures that include a questionnaire (Cuestionario de Comunicación en el Hogar), an Articulation Screener, and a Language Sample checklist; however, these are optional and not incorporated in the AC, EC, or Total Language scores.

Thus, a major feature of this test is that the child's responses in both English and Spanish are accepted and scored using a dual-language scoring system. The use of a dual-language assessment approach instead of a single-language scoring system has been discussed in the literature as a way to adequately capture a child's vocabulary knowledge across languages (Anaya, Peña, & Bedore, 2018; Bedore, Peña, Garcia, & Cortez, 2005; Core, Hoff, Rurniche, & Senor, 2013). While scholars agree that the use of conceptual scoring appears to show promise in identifying bilingual children at risk for language delay, others have pointed out that single-language measures may still be useful to practitioners when they want to know about a child's English proficiency or academic performance relative to monolingual peers (Paradis, 2005; Pearson et al., 1993; Thordardottir et al., 2006).

Structured Photographic Expressive Language–Third Edition (SPELT-3) (Dawson, Stout, & Elyer, 2003)

The Structured Photographic Expressive Language Test–Third Edition (SPELT-3) (Dawson, Stout, & Elyer, 2003) assesses morphosyntactic skills in children aged 4 years to 9 years and 11 months. It requires the child to look at color photographs of everyday situations and familiar objects and answer simple questions about each one. These questions, presented orally by the examiner, elicit specific morphological syntactic structures and are used nationally to assess children who experience language problems. The SPELT-3 is a revision of the SPELT-2 (Werner & Kresheck,1983), and it not intended to diagnose language impairment in ELs; however, this tool has been shown in the past to have high levels of discriminant accuracy in identifying preschoolers with language impairment (Perona, Plante, & Vance, 2005). Using 54 (4 by 6 inches) stimulus pictures, the examiner elicits simple verbal questions and statements to elicit specific morphological and syntactic structures. This assessment tool allows for analysis of specific language structures that may not occur in spontaneous language samples. The manual includes explicit scoring guidelines, listing expected responses, and typical errors. A separate chapter addresses African American vernacular response variations, but the authors note that appropriate cautions and care should be applied with using this measure to assess ELs.

Spanish Structured Photographic Expressive Language Test 3 (Spanish SPELT-3; Langdon, 2012)

The importance of measuring language proficiency in the development of a second language resulted in the development of the Spanish SPELT-Preschool-Spanish and the Spanish SPELT-2 (Werner & Krescheck, 1983, 1989). The Spanish SPELT-3 (Langdon, 2012) assesses the expressive language of Spanish-speaking children. Although this test is not a direct translation of the English SPELT-3, it also assesses morphology and syntax skills in monolingual or bilingual children aged 4 years to 9 years and 6 months. It also samples the child's ability to use pragmatically appropriate language for various purposes.

The primary purpose of the Spanish SPELT-3 is to (1) aid in identifying children who may need language intervention and (2) assist in targeting intervention that considers the child's strengths and weaknesses. This test utilizes actual photographs of children in contexts that are conducive to specific utilization of linguistic markers, particularly those related to noun, adjective, and verb morphology. This test allows analysis of a child's ability to express common grammatical form, as well as to perform rule-governed changes in sentence structure.

In a study conducted by Arias and Friberg (2017) to identify current bilingual assessment practices of school-based SLPs, they disseminated a national survey yielding results from 34 different states in the United States. The Structured Photographic Expressive Language Test (SPELT) was one of the 20 most frequently administered instruments with bilingual students.

BESA: Bilingual English Spanish Assessment (Peña, Gutierrez-Clellen, Iglesias, Goldstein, & Bedore, 2018)

The Bilingual English-Spanish Assessment (BESA) was developed to identify phonological and/or language impairment in Spanish-English bilingual students ages 4 years through 6 years and 11 months old. The test is also used with ELs to differentiate between a delay in English language acquisition and a true language disorder. Norming of the BESA consisted of bilingual children who varied in their Spanish-English language proficiency and geographic region of the United States.

The BESA consists of two questionnaires, one criterion-referenced activity, and three standardized norm-referenced subtests in English and Spanish that address morphosyntax, semantics, and phonology. The two questionnaires, the Bilingual Input-Output Survey (BIOS) and the Inventory to Assess Language Knowledge (ITALK), are used to elicit information from parents and/or teachers about the child's language environment. These tools can be used to provide much-needed information and context to determine language(s) of testing, guide the assessment, and contextualize test results (Peña, Gutierrez-Clellen, Iglesias, Goldstein, & Bedore, 2018). The criterion-referenced activity is designed to observe the child's language use. Each component may be used independently or combined as part of an assessment battery. Depending on whether both languages are tested, and which subtests are included, administration of all BESA components may take between 1 hour (for one language) and 2 hours (for both languages) (Peña et al., 2018).

Several studies have been published that have included the use of the BESA in the assessment of bilingual children (e.g., Kapantzoglou, Fergadiotis, & Restrepo, 2017; Rodriguez, Bustamante, Wood, & Sundeman, 2017). The study by Lazewnik et al. (2019) indicated that the two BESA subtests (Morphosyntax and Semantics) were effective in identifying a language disorder in bilingual children. They noted that the use of this measure, combined with a language sample assessment, increases the likelihood of differentiating a language difference from a language disorder. Continued research to determine the diagnostic accuracy of this measure will be useful to practitioners in assessing ELCDs.

Important Considerations Regarding Language Assessment Instruments for ELs with Communication Disorders

SLPs have become increasingly aware of the inappropriateness of many standardized tests used with ELs; however, they continue to rely primarily on the use of norm-referenced tests to determine if an EL has a disorder (Arias & Friberg, 2017; Crowley, 2003; Kriticos, 2003; Roseberry-McKibben, 2018). Reliance on these instruments often occurs because SLPs and other professionals believe that federal law (i.e., IDEA) requires their use to determine a disability and subsequently eligibility for special education intervention. According to federal law, however, standardized tests are not required. Yet, they are often used because they provide scores (i.e., percentile ranks, standard scores) that are used as guidelines to determine if a student is eligible for special education services. Furthermore, they are often used because they are perceived as more expedient and convenient to administer. Given the paucity of standardized tests for ELs in most languages and the continued use of standardized tests to assess the language development of ELs, several important considerations regarding their use are provided.

Standardized Testing and Bias

Selecting an appropriate standardized test is a challenging task. It is often recommended that professionals examine test items and consult test manuals to review the adequacy, reliability, and validity of tests used with ELs with different language profiles (Betz, Eickhoff, & Sullivan, 2013; Caesar & Kohler, 2007; Dollaghan & Horner, 2011; Hutchinson, 1996). While evidence-based practice encourages practitioners to select standardized measures based on their psychometric properties, this is often not the case (Betz, Eickhoff, & Sullivan, 2013).

Many standardized tests, designed from a middle-class, literate Western framework, contain many potential sources of bias (Goldstein, 2000; Kayser, 1998; Roseberry-McKibben, 2018). These may include content bias (use of activities and items that are not familiar to the child), value bias (use of a test item that is inconsistent with the child's value system), format bias (using test procedures and/or materials that are unfamiliar to the child), and/or examiner bias (examiner may be unfamiliar with the cultural and/or linguistic characteristics of the child and/or have low expectations of the child and interpret results based on these assumptions). These tests are also designed with the assumption that a child will have the experiential background to perform optimally in a testing situation with test tasks that are administered by an unfamiliar adult using a language that the child might not yet have mastered.

Test Administration and Interpretation

Modifying how a test is administered, scored, and interpreted has been discussed as one way to minimize test bias (Bedore et al., 2005; Denman et al., 2017; Greenfield, 1997; Hamayan & Damico, 1991; Kayser, 1995, 1998; Saenz & Huer, 2003). Although a variety of recommendations to modify standardized tests for ELs have been offered, these have not always resulted in eliminating test bias. Some of the modifications have included:

- Providing instructions to the child in L1 and English.
- Rephrasing of instructions.
- Providing the student with extra time.
- Asking the child to clarify an "incorrect" response and score the response within the context of the child's cultural and linguistic background.
- Using a dual scoring system.
- Completing the assessment over a period of time.

Some recommendations to reduce bias in test *interpretation* have included:

- Consulting the literature to determine if the errors demonstrated by the child are typical of other ELs from similar backgrounds.
- Incorporating cautionary statements and disclaimers regarding deviations from standardized assessment procedures.

◆ Avoiding the use of only standardized test results to determine disability and eligibility for special education services.

Translated Tests

Determining which tests are most appropriate for a given purpose requires that the SLP be familiar with the theoretical framework of the test and the possible limitations of the test (Caesar & Kohler, 2007; Goldstein, 2000; McCauley & Swisher, 1984; Plante & Vance, 1994). Often, translated versions of speech-language tests have been used with ELs without considering the inherent problems in their use. For example, many translations provide word-for-word translations that do not account for a lack of equivalent linguistic form in the second language. Additionally, translated tests do not consider the effects of second language acquisition on a student's performance. As a precaution, scores from these translated versions should not be used to diagnose a communication disorder.

Tests in the Primary Language

To counteract the practice of using translated versions of English assessment instruments, many professionals use tests specifically developed for bilingual children, some of which were discussed above. These tests have been specifically developed in the primary language to assess the language skills of ELs. Although many tests have proven to be useful in the identification and diagnosis of language and communication disorders in children (i.e., Semel, Wiig, & Secord, 2006), the use of tests in the primary language has also been problematic (Peña & Kester, 2004; Perona, Plante, & Vance, 2005; Restrepo & Silverman, 2001). For example, several assessment instruments developed to accommodate a child's various proficiency levels in Spanish and English do not represent all the existing dialects of Spanish. Therefore, the SLP will need to be familiar with different dialects and what is acceptable across dialects to determine acceptable and unacceptable responses.

Another challenge is the availability of reliable phonological and language development norms. Although developmental norms have been developed for Spanish (e.g., Acevedo, 1993; Anderson, 1995; Fantini, 1985; Goldstein & Iglesias, 1996; Jimenez, 1987; Merino, 1992), developmental data on languages other than English continue to be limited.

Alternatives to Standardized Assessment

A critical question often asked by SLPs is: if standardized testing has such limitations and challenges, then what should we use to identify ELs with possible disabilities and to determine appropriate services? We have previously discussed that IDEA (2004) requires that ELs be assessed in their native language(s) (L1) and English (L2) using appropriate test instruments and assessment practices. We also noted that although IDEA allows for the use of norm-referenced standardized tests, it also allows for the use of subjective and qualitative measures. One option often recommended to SLPs is to use alternative assessment procedures (Gorman, 2015; IDEA, 2004; Kohnert, 2008; Roseberry-McKibben, 2008; Saenz & Huer, 2003). Several alternative assessment procedures have been recommended. These include (a) criterion-referenced testing, (b) language sampling, (c) dynamic assessment, (d) observation, and (e) use of interpreters. Each of these is briefly described.

Criterion-Referenced Testing

Criterion-referenced testing differs from norm-referenced testing. Criterion-referenced tests are administered to primarily gauge a child's skill level or capability, as opposed to determining a child's overall level as compared to others who are given the same test. The SLP often uses criterion-referenced measures to obtain a profile of a child's strengths and weaknesses. Criterion-referenced measures allow for reporting results using percentage of items passed, instead of normative standard scores (Battle, 2002; Laing & Kamhi, 2003).

Criterion-referenced tests are often used when norms that might be used to provide a norm-referenced interpretation of test performance are unavailable or inappropriate, or when information concerning specific skills or behaviors of a test taker is required by the clinical question being posed (McCauley, 1996). One drawback for using criterion-referenced measures is that their use still presumes a developmental framework that might not be appropriate or available for ELs (Goldstein, 2000).

Language Samples

Another alternative assessment technique used by SLPs is language sampling (Beck, 1995; Caesar & Kohler, 2007; Hux, 1993). Often referred to as the "gold standard" in assessing bilingual children, many experts (Gutierrez-Clellen, Restrepo, Bedore, Peña, & Anderson, 2000; Heilmann et al., 2008; Kayser & Restrepo, 1995) suggest that this approach allows the SLP to obtain language information about the conversational skills, syntactic structures, grammatical competency, and language use of ELs. They also note that language samples are useful in differentiating between a language disorder and a language difference.

Gathering a language sample in all languages used by the EL requires that the SLP have language proficiency in the child's language. If the child's primary language is not English, then the SLP should enlist the services of a bilingual SLP or use a properly trained interpreter to assist in the collection and analysis of the language sample. Additionally, the SLP should be familiar with a variety of elicitation techniques and analysis protocols and use these appropriately in analyzing the obtained sample (Retherford, 2000).

Although conversation followed by narration (i.e., giving a child a book to read) has been identified as the technique most often used by SLPs to elicit language samples, several alternative techniques have been recommended (Cornejo, Weinstein, & Najar, 1983; Hux, Morris-Friehe, & Sanger, 1993; Kayser, 1995, 1998; Langdon, 1992). These include having a child describe an object, engage in a game or problem-solving activity to verbalize an answer to a problem, and narrate or describe a sequence of events. When storytelling is used in the context of a spontaneous language sample, the SLP should use procedures to analyze story structures in a narrative (see Bloome, Champion, Katz, Morton, & Muldrow, 2001; Champion & Mainess, 2003; Champion & Seymour, 1995; Gutierrez-Clellen & Quinn, 1993; Hester, 2010; Rollins, McCabe, & Bliss, 2000). It is also recommended that SLPs obtain language samples as the child engages in activities across settings (e.g., home and school) with a variety of conversational partners to yield a more representative and reliable measure of the child's language abilities.

A variety of strategies are available to analyze language samples (see Bliss, 2002; Gutierrez-Clellen et al., 2004; Linares, 1981; Long & Channell, 2001; Owens, 2004; Roseberry-McKibben, 2007). The main areas of language sample analysis are form (morphology, syntax, discourse structure), content (objects, actions), and use (semantics) (Swisher, 1994). Although many of these procedures require time, training, and skill in their application, they are effective in assessing the language skills of ELs and capturing their strengths and weaknesses (Kemp & Klee, 1997; MacWhinney, 1996, 2000a, 2000b). The following are examples of analysis techniques used by SLPs to describe the child's language.

Mean Length of Response (MLR)

One of the frequently reported measures of linguistic skill in young children has been the mean length of response (MLR). MLR is a measure of expressive language development and has been defined as the average number of words used in 50 consecutive verbal utterances. Normative data are available and MLR measurement is known to be reliable (Webster & Shelton, 1964). MLR has also been recommended for languages that are highly inflected (i.e., Spanish) (Schnell de Acedo, 1994).

Mean Length of Utterance (MLU)

Mean length of utterance (MLU) is a measure of linguistic productivity in children. MLU is the average length of morphemes in the child's utterances and is traditionally calculated by collecting 100 utterances spoken by a child and dividing the number of morphemes by the number of utterances (MLU = number of morphemes/number of utterances). A higher MLU is taken to indicate a higher level of language proficiency (Owens, 2004). To measure morphological production in Spanish-speaking children, Linares (1981) recommended a procedure to calculate the mean length of utterance-morphemes (MLU-m) in Spanish.

The use of MLU has been challenged, specifically for counting verb inflections, and the use of mean length of utterance words (MLU-w) has been offered as an alternative (Gutierrez-Clellen, Restrepo, Bedore, Peña, & Anderson, 2000; Rojas & Iglesias, 2013; Schnell de Acedo, 1994).

MLU-w is calculated by summing the number of words for each utterance and dividing by the number of utterances. This measure of analysis focuses on syntactic complexity, and its use has been suggested for identifying developmental differences in young Spanish speakers with limited or no English proficiency. Caution in using MLU as the only diagnostic measure of language proficiency in children is recommended.

Type-Token Ratio (TTR)

Language samples can also be analyzed using the Type-Token Ratio (TTR). TTR is a measure of vocabulary variation that a child uses expressively and measures the proportion of different words (types) to total words (tokens). The TTR is calculated by the ratio TTR = number of different words in a sample/total number of words in a sample and reflects the diversity of words used by the client during a language sample.

Terminal Units (T-Units)

Another measure of analysis used in language sampling is the T-unit (minimal terminal unit). T-unit analysis, developed by Hunt (1965), has been used extensively to measure overall syntactic complexity, especially in older children. T-units are defined as any clause and its subordinate clauses that are attached to or embedded in the main clause. The application of this analysis technique to measure the syntactic language skills of school-age children (Klecan-Aker & Hedrick, 1985) and specifically bilingual Spanish children is offered as one way to quantify and analyze the language assessment of ELs with different levels of English proficiency (Gutiérrez-Clellen, Restrepo, Bedore, Peña, & Anderson, 2000; Kayser & Restrepo, 1995).

Computer-Aided Language Sample

Recent advances in computer technology have made analysis of language samples a realistic option (Long & Channell, 2001). Wider availability of software and hardware technologies has increased an SLP's potential for using Computer-Aided Language Sample Analysis protocols (Pavelko, Owens, Ireland, & Hahs-Vaughn, 2016). Despite their availability, many SLPs continue to analyze their language samples based on nonstandardized, self-designed procedures (Hux, Morris-Friehe, & Sanger, 1993). Programs such as the CLAN program (Child Language Analysis) used in the CHILDES project (MacWhinney, 1996, 2000), the SALT (Systematic Analysis of Language Transcripts) software (Miller, Andriacchi, & Nockerts, 2015; Miller & Iglesias, 2016), the PAL (Pye Analysis of Language; Pye, 1987), and the CP (Computerized Profiling) program (Long, Fey, & Channel, 2000) are some of the computer-aided language sample analysis protocols that are available to SLPs. Although some programs now include separate databases to compare Spanish-English bilinguals and African American English (AAE)–speaking children, overall tools or established protocols remain limited for other languages (Hammett Price, Hendricks, & Cook, 2010; Hux et al., 1993; Kemp & Klee, 1997; Kohnert, 2008; Miller & Iglesias, 2006; Miller, Freiberg, Rolland, & Reeves, 1992).

There are many ways the SLP can analyze language samples. In general, the use of this alternative assessment can provide the SLP with information on the language proficiency of the EL. Observation of the child with different language partners, across settings, using all languages, and including code-switching or use of dialects assists the SLP to obtain a more comprehensive view of the EL.

Dynamic Assessments

Static procedures to assess ELs are often used by SLPs to make disability determinations. One challenge with this practice is that judgments about the language proficiency of ELs are made using the results of testing that measure the student's skills at one point in time and do not consider the child's ability to learn. In recent years, dynamic assessment has been recommended as an alternative means of assessing ELs who are suspected of having language disabilities (Hux, 1993; Laing & Kamhi, 2003; Lidz & Peña, 1996; Peña, Quinn, & Iglesias, 1992; Petersen, Chantthongthip, Ukrainetz, & Steeve, 2017). Initially described by Vygotsky (1986) as part of his model of cognitive development, dynamic assessment refers to approaches that evaluate a student's ability to learn when provided with instruction, such as the test-teach-retest paradigm. Studies (Butler, 1997; Gutierrez Clellen, 2000; Lidz & Peña, 1996; Peña, Iglesias, & Lidz, 2001) have addressed the use and effectiveness of dynamic assessment with ELs and note its promise for distinguishing language differences from language learning disabilities (Gorman, 2015; Gutierrez-Clellen & Peña, 2001; Hasson, Camilleri, Jones, Smith, & Dodd, 2013).

Response to intervention (RtI), discussed earlier in this chapter, uses the principles of dynamic assessment. The focus in RtI is on measuring the students' response to effective instruction. As appropriate and comprehensible instructional support is provided to ELs, a variety of informal assessment tools and observational protocols can be used to assess how ELs use language in the classroom and across social contexts (Collier, 2010). Their performance can be compared to their similar classmates rather than using national norms (Mattes & Saldana-Illingworth, 2009). Portfolio methods of assessment can also be used to evaluate samples of student work over time. It has been suggested that RtI, used as a form of dynamic assessment, can be helpful in discriminating language differences from language disorders in ELs (Rosa-Lugo, Rivera, & Rierson, 2010).

Observations

SLPs are often required to obtain information on the student's use of language in various academic and social contexts. By observing and examining the language strategies used by students to communicate with their peers and others, the SLP can obtain information about the child's language performance and identify observed behaviors that are characteristic of children in the normal process of acquiring a second language and children with a communication disorder.

The use of observation as an alternative assessment is highly recommended by many researchers (Caesar & Kohler, 2007; Collier, 2011; Kayser, 2008; Waxman, Padron, Franco-Fuenmayor, & Huang, 2009). Observation is a quantitative method of measuring specific behaviors observed in children and teachers as they interact in the classroom setting. Rating scales, interviews, and observational techniques and protocols have traditionally been used by SLPs to gather information about the child's language capabilities over multiple contexts with a variety of communication partners. Most observations require that the observer use a coding system to record what students and teachers do during learning activities within the classroom and often include the following (Stallings & Mohlman, 1988):

- ◆ A purpose for the observation.
- ◆ Operational definitions of all the observed behaviors.
- ◆ Training procedures for observers.
- ◆ A specific observational focus.
- ◆ A unit of time.
- ◆ An observation schedule.
- ◆ A method to record the data.
- ◆ A method to process and analyze data.

To determine whether a communication disorder exists in an EL, it is important that all data obtained through rating scales, interviews, and observational techniques and protocols support the diagnosis of a language disorder. Observation protocols that have been used to observe teachers and EL students as they work in classrooms are the Sheltered Instruction Observation Protocol (SIOP; Short & Echevarria, 1999), used to observe and rate teachers in the classroom, and the Transitional Bilingual Pedagogical (TBP) Observation Protocol (Bruce et al., 1997), used to observe instructional practices in transitional bilingual classrooms. The Bilingual Classroom Communication Profile (BCCP; Roseberry-McKibben, 1993) is another protocol that is used in conjunction with other alternative measures to provide a comprehensive picture of the student's use of language. Mattes and Saldana-Illingworth (2008) have compiled a few observational communication protocols and interview questionnaires that are useful for assessing the speech and language of ELs.

Use of Interpreters

As a supplement to the alternative assessments described above, the use of interpreters plays a critical role in assessing ELs. Interpreters convey information from one language to the other and facilitate communication between individuals who do not speak the same language, whereas translators translate written documents from one language to another (Kayser, 1995; Langdon & Cheng, 2002; Langdon & Saenz, 2016; Roseberry-McKibben, 2018). During a student evaluation, the interpreter usually takes a leading role. Langdon and Cheng (2002) and Matsuda and O'Connor (1993) have discussed the role and responsibilities of an interpreter/translator and the criteria that should be used in their selection (Hegde & Maul, 2006; Pretto, 2012). Specifically, the SLP and the interpreter must work together to assess ELs in the absence of a bilingual SLP who speaks the client's language and adheres to legal requirements and professional ethics (Rosa-Lugo & Abreu, 2017). The interpreter must have excellent communication skills in the language of the child and must be trained in the role of interpreter (Langdon & Saenz, 2016).

Langdon and Cheng (2002) outline a three-step process that can be used by the SLP as they work with interpreters. The three steps of the process are (1) briefing, (2) interaction, and (3) debriefing (BID). During the *briefing* step, the SLP and the interpreter review the client's background information and outline the purpose of the assessment. The use and review of materials, seating arrangements, and type of interpreting is planned. During the *interaction* step, the interpreter and the SLP work as a team in test administration or use of alternate assessments. In this task, the interpreter acts as a bridge between the SLP and the client and attempts to engage and elicit responses from the student. The third step, *debriefing*, consists of reviewing the process as well as the outcome of the assessment process. The SLP and interpreter discuss the student's performance during tests, the interpreter's observations, test scoring, and the challenges encountered during the testing session. If the interpreter has been appropriately trained, he or she can provide the SLP with valuable information that will shed light on the linguistic functioning of the child.

Final Thoughts Regarding Assessment

Alternative assessments are promising tools that should be included as part of an assessment battery. The use of these tools and strategies can contribute to the accurate identification of ELs with communication disorders. These measures can also be used by the SLP to plan intervention programs, document treatment effectiveness, and determine when services are no longer necessary.

The assessment process is incomplete without a final written report outlining the findings of the evaluation. Report formats vary from school district to school district; however, certain information should consistently be included in the diagnostic report. Information obtained through the case history should be included (i.e., client's language history, schooling history, and language proficiency) as well as all testing results (to include standardized and alternative assessments), modifications, and use of interpreters.

Ultimately, the written report should serve as a document that presents an accurate representation of the student written in a language understood by all professionals that will work with the student and the families of the child. SLPs are responsible for supporting the diagnosis of a communication disorder. Because this report is used to determine eligibility for speech and language services or programs, document progress, or determine if a child no longer needs services, it is extremely important that this report be detailed and precise (Burrus & Haynes, 2009; Goldfarb & Serpanos, 2009; Shipley & McAfee, 2016; Stein-Rubin & Fabus, 2011).

Eligibility and Dismissal Decisions

Eligibility Decisions

Determining whether a child has a communication disorder is a significant decision because of its educational consequences. The SLP is responsible for gathering all the critical information, obtained through formal testing and informal procedures, to determine whether the EL is experiencing challenges due to a true communication disorder or to something else, such as a communication difference. To determine the presence or absence of language impairment and if the student meets the eligibility criteria for speech-language services or programs in the schools, the SLP must address three questions:

1. Does the student have a communication difference or disorder? In other words, is there a disability that is manifested across all languages spoken by the child?
2. If so, does the disability have an adverse effect on educational performance resulting from the disability?
3. Are specially designed instruction and/or related services and supports needed to help the student make progress in the general education curriculum?

If it is determined, after supporting the student with meaningful RtI strategies, that the student demonstrates a language disorder in L1 and L2, then best practice is for the student to receive specially designed instruction and support for students with disabilities (Linan-Thompson & Ortiz, 2009; Restrepo & Gutierrez-Clellan, 2004). It is important to note that a child cannot be determined to have a disability if one of the determinant factors is limited English proficiency (IDEA, 2004). Assessment results should support that the disorder is having an adverse impact on performance in the general education classroom. It is critical that the SLP and other professionals remember that if the EL has a communication problem, it must be present across languages (Goldstein, 2004b; Kayser, 2002; Kohnert, 2008; Restrepo, 1997; Roseberry-McKibben, 2018).

Determining if a student has a disability is not the sole responsibility of the SLP. It is critical that *all* school professionals share information on the student with each other and that parents serve as active partners to help determine eligibility and appropriate educational services (Garcia, 2002). If the student is found to be eligible to receive services from the SLP, then an Individual Education Plan (IEP) must be developed. The IEP should contain clear goals and objectives that will consider the student's strengths in L1 and L2. Information about each student's language proficiency should be clearly documented in the IEP so that SLPs can work with school professionals (e.g., ESOL professionals) and the parents to plan an appropriate and culturally responsive instructional program that addresses which language will be primary in instruction. It is important that SLPs know the eligibility criteria for their state.

Dismissal Decisions

Parents, teachers, SLPs, and professionals from other disciplines are encouraged to play a role in all aspects of decision making and problem solving related to the eligibility, placement, intervention, and dismissal of ELs with a communication disorder. Usually, the decision to dismiss a student from speech-language services begins with the SLP. According to ASHA's best practices, students with communication disorders may be dismissed from receiving services only when they are no longer identified as having speech-language impairments and are no longer in need of special education services (ASHA, 2004a). The SLP determines if the student met IEP annual goals, conducts an assessment, and reviews all evaluation data to consider if the student no longer needs the services of the SLP. Dismissal from services may occur if the EL with a communication disorder meets the following criteria:

A. no longer has speech-language impairment;
B. has a speech-language impairment, but it no longer affects his or her educational performance;
C. has received speech-language services as special education and still has a speech-language impairment that affects his or her educational performance, but the child study team determines that he or she does not need special education; or

D. has received speech-language services as special education and still has a speech-language impairment that affects his or her educational performance, but the child study team determines that he or she does not need related services to benefit from special education.

When making decisions regarding dismissal, SLPs should work with the appropriate professionals to determine whether the child is not eligible to receive services in schools under IDEA and follow the procedures established by their state and districts (Ireland & Conrad, 2016). Although all states adhere to IDEA requirements regarding dismissal, it is possible that various state laws and regulations may create additional requirements. For example, in Florida, the dismissal policies and procedures are often found in the Special Programs and Procedures document of each respective school district as well as in technical assistance papers that provide guidance regarding state board rules (Florida Department of Education, 2015).

Steppling, Quattlebaum, and Brady (2007) have looked at the guidelines for dismissal as they are stated in IDEA and ASHA and identified several issues that the SLP needs to consider during the dismissal process. The IDEA guidelines for dismissal focus on measuring disabilities that affect educational performance, whereas the ASHA guidelines include educational goals and items that are linked to health status. The IDEA dismissal guidelines give the appearance that they are a broad outline that relates to educational performance and that there are just a few questions that need to be answered for an EL with a communication disorder to be dismissed from SLP programs. On the other hand, the ASHA guidelines offer a more detailed list of considerations for dismissal. This important difference between the two sets of guidelines might create a situation with important educational consequences for ELs with communication disorders if a child meets the criteria for dismissal under IDEA but still displays a disorder according to the ASHA criteria. For example, the IEP team might determine that the communication disorder of an EL with a communication disorder does not affect educational performance any longer, but still has a negative influence on social interaction. From an IDEA point of view, the student can be dismissed from the program, but from an ASHA perspective, the student needs to continue to be in the program.

Summary

In this chapter, we examined the first element of our assessment/intervention/monitoring (AIM) model. We looked at a variety of instruments and procedures ESOL professionals and SLPs can use for assessing ELs and ELs with communication disorders. Although ESOL or bilingual professionals are knowledgeable about the identification practices and assessments used to identify and place ELs in accordance to their language proficiency, it is the SLP, a key member of an interdisciplinary team, who determines if an EL has a communication disorder by making use of the information provided by the selected measures of language proficiency. In Chapter 3, we emphasized the importance of collaboration between these two categories of professionals. In this chapter, we continued to highlight how critical the relationship between SLPs and ESOL professionals is in the assessment of ELs and specifically ELs with communication disorders.

Since collaboration is the recurring theme of this text, we wanted to provide a comprehensive description of what each professional is doing at the identification stage, during the ongoing language proficiency assessment, and at the exiting/dismissal phase. When team members are familiar with the context in which their colleagues function, they can complement each other and collaborate to facilitate language and literacy development in ELs. The next chapter will discuss approaches and strategies and address the next component of the AIM framework: intervention.

7

Intervention and Monitoring—Approaches and Practical Strategies to Facilitate and Monitor Language and Literacy Development in English Learners

Introduction

Language and literacy development in ELs shares many commonalities with language and literacy development in native speakers of English. Yet there are several critical variables unique to ELs that affect the process and outcomes of literacy development. For example, depending on age and educational background, ELs may have varying degrees of oral proficiency in English and literacy skills in their native language. Often, typically developing ELs require additional language support than typically developing native speakers of English (Francis, Rivera, Lesaux, Kieffer, & Rivera, 2006; Petersen & Spencer, 2014). In particular, the language and literacy development of EL students with communication disorders often requires necessary supports, modifications, and accommodations to facilitate their academic success (Hoffman & Ireland, 2018). Understanding the needs of ELs and ELs with communication disorders can be difficult for all literacy professionals, given their complex profiles.

School-based SLPs are increasingly being asked to show that their intervention efforts result in positive educational outcomes for students in school-based settings (ASHA, 2010a). Likewise, ESOL professionals are required to monitor the progress of all ELs in achieving English language proficiency (ELP) and gain content knowledge. Regularly monitoring ELs' progress in ELP and content knowledge allows SLPs and other professionals to determine how well students are mastering academic content standards, meeting benchmarks, and responding to instruction and intervention (Brown & Sanford, 2011; Ehren, Montgomery, Rudebusch, & Whitmire, 2009; Power-de Fur, 2016; Selin, Rice, Girolamo, & Wang, 2019).

In this chapter, we address the second and third components of the AIM framework: intervention and monitoring. First, we discuss findings from major reports on reading research, including the Institute of Education Sciences (IES) (2010, 2016, 2018), National Early Literacy Panel (NELP) (2008), and National Reading Panel (NRP) (2000). Following the discussion of research findings, we survey several widely used instructional practices for developing reading, oral language, and writing skills in English. Specifically, we offer guidance on using two interventions that are highly adaptable by EL proficiency level, leveled questioning and sentence frames. We highlight how the SLP and the ESOL professional can partner to implement high-quality approaches and practical strategies to facilitate and monitor language and literacy development in ELs and ELCDs using some of the strategies that are discussed in this chapter. The last section of this chapter addresses the use of formal assessment to monitor English language development, as well as acquisition of academic content.

Knowledge and Skills Necessary for Learning to Read

Learning to read for the first time involves developing the same knowledge and skills, regardless of whether the learner speaks one or two languages. According to the NELP (Lonigan,

Christopher, & Shanahan, 2009), research shows that preschool-age children must master six precursor skills to begin reading successfully.

The first skill, alphabet knowledge, pertains to knowing the names and sounds of printed letters. The second skill, phonological awareness, includes detecting, manipulating, or analyzing the sounds of spoken language. This involves separating or segmenting words, syllables, or phonemes, which are the smallest distinctions in sound that differentiate meaning (i.e., such as /p/ in pit; /b/ in bit versus [ph] in pat and [p'] in spat). Phonological awareness is independent of meaning. The third skill is rapid automatic naming of letters or digits. Similarly, the fourth skill involves the rapid automatic naming of common objects, such as a car or tree. The fifth skill is writing letters in isolation or writing one's name. Last, the sixth skill is phonological memory, which is the ability to remember what someone said for a brief time period. Table 7–1 summarizes the six skill areas.

In addition to these six necessary skills, the NELP (2008) found an additional five skills that are potentially important in developing the ability to read. These include (1) concepts of print—print conventions such as left to right, front to back, and print concepts such as book cover, author; (2) print knowledge—concepts of print, alphabet knowledge, and early decoding of sounds/symbols; (3) reading readiness—a combination of concepts of print, alphabet knowledge, vocabulary, memory,

Table 7–1. *Knowledge and Skills Necessary for Learning to Read*

Language knowledge and skills learners must develop from birth to age 5	Alphabet knowledge
	Phonological awareness
	Rapid automatic naming of letters
	Rapid automatic naming of colors
	Writing name
	Phonological memory

Source: From *Developing Early Literacy: Report of the National Early Literacy Panel,* by National Early Literacy Panel, 2008, Washington, DC: National Institute for Literacy. Retrieved from http://www.nifl.gov/earlychildhood/NELP/NELPreport.html

and phonological awareness; (4) oral language, including using vocabulary and grammar; and (5) visual processing, which involves matching or discriminating visual symbols.

Once the precursor reading skills are mastered, students in kindergarten through third grade develop more complex reading skills. The Center for Improvement of Early Reading Achievement (CIERA) reviewed more than 100,000 research studies on teaching reading in K–3 (Adler, 2001). From these studies, a clear picture of five necessary skills for successful reading emerged: (1) phonemic awareness, (2) phonics instruction, (3) fluency, (4) vocabulary, and (5) text comprehension.

The first necessary skill, *phonemic awareness*, is the ability to distinguish, identify, and manipulate phonemes. This is a skill that can be taught. Within the category of phonemic awareness, there are eight subskills, which we now examine in more detail.

The first subskill, isolating phonemes, is commonly taught by asking students to identify the first (or last) sound in a word. Phoneme identity involves asking learners to find the same sound in different words. Phoneme categorization requires learners to find the word that doesn't fit, such as in tip, cap, tap, and top. Blending phonemes requires learners to combine phonemes into a word, such as when a teacher pronounces the three phonemes /r/ /ə/ /g/ and asks children, "What words do those sounds make?" Segmentation of phonemes involves breaking words into separate phonemes. The teacher asks how many sounds are in the word "flat," and the students articulate each sound while clapping—/f/ clap /l/ clap /æ/ clap /t/ clap. In phoneme deletion, learners determine what remains when a phoneme is omitted, such as, "What is plate without the /p/?" The opposite of phoneme deletion, phoneme addition, involves adding a sound to an existing word, such as, "What is the word if you add /s/ to the word "top"? Last, phoneme substitution switches one phoneme for another, as in the case of, "What happens if you change the /l/ in the word 'look' to /b/?" Although there are eight subskills, research shows that it is important for teachers to focus on only one or two different phonemic awareness activities.

Phonics instruction teaches how to use the relationships between letters and sounds to read and write. Explicit and systematic phonics instruction involves direct teaching of sound-letter correspondences in a determined sequence. Research shows that explicit, systematic phonics instruction leads to better reading outcomes. Systematic phonics instruction should begin in kindergarten and continue through first grade for the greatest impact on children's reading achievement. Other findings regarding phonics instruction indicate that it improves reading comprehension and is effective for children from different social and economic statuses. In addition, it is beneficial for struggling and at-risk readers, and it is most effective when begun in kindergarten. It is important to note that phonics instruction is only one part of reading instruction during the K–3 continuum and is not sufficient for developing all the requisite skills.

Fluency is the rate and comprehension of reading. If a reader is fluent, then he or she can read text at his or her level accurately and quickly. When reading aloud, a fluent reader expresses the written text effortlessly and naturally. Fluent readers attend to meaning because they can decode the sounds of the letters with automaticity. Their main focus is on comprehension. Fluency is dependent on the subject and difficulty of the text, the reader's familiarity with the topic of the text, and the reader's amount of practice in reading the text. *The Nation's Report Card: Reading 2009* (National Center for Education Statistics, 2009) reported a close relationship between fluency and comprehension. Research shows that regular guided oral reading improves fluency and reading achievement. This can be accomplished by having students read a text multiple times (up to four times) until a particular fluency level is attained or by using instructional technology or peer tutoring. When selecting a text for building fluency, teachers should choose materials that are at the reader's independent reading level. The independent level text contains no more than 5% difficult words for the reader. Instructional-level texts contain approximately 10% difficult words, and frustration-level texts include more than 10% difficult words. Techniques such as taking turns reading a text with students (student-adult reading), choral reading, recorded reading, and peer reading help build fluency.

Vocabulary is one of the most important aspects of reading and involves both oral and print representation of words. Vocabulary comprehension consists of four modalities of language comprehension and expression: listening vocabulary (words comprehended by hearing others' speech), speaking vocabulary (words we use when speaking), reading vocabulary (words we understand when reading), and writing vocabulary (words we use in writing). Vocabulary is learned both informally and formally. Informal or indirect vocabulary learning comes from conversations with adults, listening to adults read, and independent reading.

Direct instruction of vocabulary is important and includes teaching specific words as well as strategies for learning new words. Specific word instruction techniques support learners' comprehension and use of new vocabulary and include (1) pre-teaching words prior to encountering them in a reading passage, (2) multiple exposure to new terms, and (3) access to the same terms in different contexts. In selecting words to teach, three considerations can be helpful: the importance of the word, the usefulness of the word, and the difficulty of the word. Difficulty encompasses words with multiple meanings and idiomatic expressions. In learning new words, students move through becoming acquainted with the term to establishing meaning. There are four types of word learning: (1) learning a new meaning of a known word, (2) learning the meaning of a new word whose concept the learner knows, (3) learning the meaning of a new word whose concept the learner does not know, and (4) clarifying and enhancing the meaning of a word the learner knows. Developing strategies for learning new words include using dictionaries; learning about word parts, such as prefixes, word roots, and suffixes; and using context clues to understand word meaning.

The last skill, *text comprehension*, is the purpose of reading. According to the National Reading Panel (2000) report, good readers have a purpose for reading and think actively as they read. Research shows that specific comprehension strategy instruction improves text comprehension. The report identifies six strategies that improve text comprehension.

The first strategy, monitoring comprehension, indicates that readers are aware of what they understand and do not understand and use strategies to repair comprehension problems. Examples of monitoring comprehension strategies include identifying where and what the difficulty is, restating the difficult passage in the reader's own words, and reviewing previous and upcoming parts of the text.

The second strategy, using graphic and semantic organizers, enables learners to comprehend concepts and relationships among the concepts in a text. These tools help students see the text structure, examine relationships, and summarize the content of a text. Answering questions, the third area, gives a purpose for reading, focuses attention on key elements, promotes active thought while reading, supports monitoring comprehension, and connects content of the reading to learners' background knowledge of the topic.

Similar to answering questions, the fourth area involves having students generate questions. This strategy promotes active processing of the text and monitoring of comprehension.

The fifth area, recognizing story structure, involves identifying the setting, events, reactions, and so forth and how they are pulled together in a plot. Story maps are an effective means of depicting story structure.

Lastly, summarizing the important ideas in a text helps students identify and connect main ideas, omit unnecessary information, and remember what they read. Table 7–2 summarizes the National Reading Panel Report's (NRP, 2000) findings.

Adapting Literacy Activities for English Learners

As stated previously, developing ELs' reading skills has much in common with developing the reading skills of native speakers of English. Chapter 5 offered a detailed description of how teaching reading to ELs differs from native speakers. We will highlight several effective reading development activities that work for ELs as well as native speakers; however, we will first present simple guidelines developed and used with preservice and in-service general education teachers (Nutta, Mokhtari, & Strebel, 2012; Nutta, Strebel, Mihai, Crevecoeur-Bryant, & Mokhtari, 2018).

Teaching Reading

Unlike teaching subject matter content such as science or social studies to English learners, teaching language arts focuses primarily on language development. When teaching subject matter

Table 7-2. The National Reading Panel Report's (2000) Findings

Language knowledge and skills learners must develop, K–3	Phonemic awareness—Phoneme isolation, identity, categorization, blending, segmentation, deletion, addition, and substitution
	Phonics—Graphophonemic (combined letter and sound representation) relationships, letter-sound associations, letter-sound correspondences, sound-symbol correspondences, sound-spelling correspondences
	Fluency—Read a text accurately and quickly, focusing on comprehension
	Vocabulary—Listening, speaking, reading, and writing
	Text comprehension—Use strategies such as comprehension monitoring, graphic and semantic organizers, answering questions about the reading, generating questions about the reading, recognizing story structure, and summarizing.

Source: From *Teaching Children to Read: An Evidence-Based Assessment of the Scientific Research Literature on Reading and Its Implications for Reading Instruction—Reports of the Subgroups,* by National Reading Panel, April 2000. Retrieved from http://www.nationalreadingpanel.org/Publications/subgroups.htm

content, the point is for ELs to learn the concepts and skills of the discipline—language growth occurs as a collateral effect of comprehending those concepts and skills in the second language. However, when teaching language arts, including listening, speaking, reading, and writing in English, the point is to learn about the language and how to use it—in other words, the aim is language growth.

Teachers of native speakers of English may assume that common techniques for teaching reading and writing are similarly appropriate for ELs and native speakers. This assumption is partly fueled by the use of the same terminology in both fields.

For example, the emergent literacy development technique for native speakers, known as the Language Experience Approach (LEA), is also used for ELs in sheltered environments (i.e., classes with ELs only) (Dixon & Nessel, 2008). However, the *way* the technique is used differently with ELs than with native speakers who possess oral proficiency in English is the focus here.

The goal of this approach is to use the students' own experiences and descriptions as reading material, ensuring that the content is familiar to all. During the initial phase of the LEA, the steps are the same for ELs and non-ELs: Students participate in a shared experience and then recount their experience while the teacher transcribes their description. However, during the recounting of the experience, the teacher of ELs needs to scaffold his or her oral description of the experience by eliciting and elaborating on the input of the ELs and focusing attention on linguistic errors as appropriate. Although the outcome, having all students recite the finished product as the teacher leads them in choral reading of their class-generated text, is the same, the intermittent step of generating the oral description of the dictated text is very different. In addition, the complexity of the oral description that is transcribed will differ based on the students' level of English proficiency.

As a rule of thumb, Nutta et al. (2018) categorize the difference between the way a language arts (including reading) activity is used with ELs versus native speakers of English in four areas: *pitch*, *pace*, *portion*, and *perspective*.

Pitch refers to targeting the language used to the students' level of English proficiency. This is similar to using the appropriate reading materials for a particular grade level; however, age and grade do not determine English proficiency. An EL in first grade may be at a near-native level in English proficiency, and an EL in fifth grade may be at a beginning level of English proficiency. If the two students attempted to read a first-grade text, everything else being equal, the first grader would perform better than the fifth grader. If the fifth-grade EL were in a sheltered reading class, the teacher would attempt to match the reading materials to the student's vocabulary and grammar knowledge and skills in English. In addition to the pitch of the reading text, the pitch of the teacher's oral language use (giving definitions, explanations, directions, etc.) needs to be adjusted to the level of the EL. In addition to matching reading materials and instructional discourse to the EL's level of English proficiency, the content of the reading activity needs to be scaffolded to facilitate comprehension. Scaffolding takes place through controlling the **pace** of the lesson and the portion of the materials. The lower the EL's level of English proficiency, the slower the pace to unpack and scaffold the content. Providing ample time for frequent comprehension checks, repetition and rephrasing, giving definitions (which can often include acting out, drawing, etc.), and explaining new grammar is important. In a mixed classroom with ELs and native speakers, taking this extra time may not be practical, so coteaching or follow-up may be necessary.

Similar to the time constraints of pacing, the **portion** or amount of reading material in an activity must be adjusted for ELs. Native speakers may read four pages during a class and then answer comprehension questions, but ELs at low levels of proficiency may only be able to fully comprehend four sentences during the lesson. If the reading lesson focuses on understanding details, then the teacher may limit the material to four sentences from the text. If the reading lesson focuses on getting the main idea, then the teacher may choose to extract four key points and organize them in an outline. Because ELs need to understand new vocabulary, grammar, and often cultural references, they can be overwhelmed with too much content and will come away from the lesson without making gains.

Perspective pertains to the focus of the instruction. For a native speaker, a lesson using LEA may focus primarily on properly spelling and sounding out words the students dictate. For an EL, a lesson using LEA may focus on syntactic errors, such as stating an adjective after a noun. Because ELs do not have the same oral proficiency and cultural background as the native English-speaking students, the issues that arise during reading instruction may be very different for ELs.

As we look at the following literacy development activities, we need to consider the English proficiency of ELs and how this will affect the pitch, pace, portion, and perspective of the lesson.

Developing Reading Skills

The U.S. Department of Education Institute of Education Sciences, through its What Works Clearinghouse (see https://ies
.ed.gov/ncee/wwc/), has reviewed high-quality research on a variety of educational issues, compiling the findings in IES Practice Guides. Building on the research-based recommendations of the National Early Reading Panel and National Reading Panel, IES provides recommendations for teaching reading through two Practice Guides, *Foundational Skills to Support Reading for Understanding in Kindergarten Through Third Grade* (IES, 2016) and *Improving Reading Comprehension in Kindergarten Through Third Grade* (IES, 2010).

One key recommendation is to teach academic language skills (IES, 2016), which includes inferential and narrative language skills and academic vocabulary and grammar. IES suggests including conversations before, during, and after read-alouds, using open-ended questions that ask about connections to students' lives, relationships among concepts or themes, and solving problems. They also recommend teaching narrative structures as well as corresponding complex grammatical structures. For example, they recommend engaging students with descriptions and examples of compound sentence (e.g., I like to read, and my favorite book is *Charlotte's Web*), subordinate clause (e.g., The ping pong ball will float **because it is full of air**), adverbial clause (e.g., I'm speaking **as quietly as I can**), and prepositional phrase structures (e.g., Our flag is **above the whiteboard**). Elements of linguistic structure, such as connectives (e.g., because, later), noun phrases (e.g., my dog's squeeze toy), verb phrases (e.g., I **might be** late tomorrow), and pronoun references (**Jelitza** is my friend. **She** lives next door) should also be taught.

Another emphasis of the IES Practice Guides is to teach students how to use reading comprehension strategies (IES, 2010). This includes activating prior knowledge related to and predicting upcoming elements of the text, questioning ideas in the text, visualizing what is described in the text, monitoring/clarifying/fixing up parts of the text that are unclear to the reader, drawing inferences about what is not explicitly stated in the text, and summarizing/retelling the text's main points. They refer to the Reading Framework from the National Assessment of Educational Progress (2008) and suggest that teachers lead discussions of the text's meaning, including questions that guide students to locate and recall (e.g., What is the main idea of Chapter 3?), integrate and interpret (How did Charlotte feel when she heard what would happen to Wilbur?), and critique and evaluate (What is the most important point in this section?) (IES, 2010).

The Center for Applied Linguistics (CAL) (n.d.) offers a variety of excellent activities for reading development. For example, some ideas for developing phonemic awareness (CAL, 2007, pp. 144–145) include:

- ◆ Rhyme hunt—Have students identify objects in the classroom and school that rhyme with words the teacher supplies. For example, students are told to find something that rhymes with "hat" and identify "mat." ELs may intersperse words from their native language or may mispronounce words in a way that makes them rhyme (spot and hat could rhyme if the EL pronounces /æ/ as /ɑ/).
- ◆ Find and say—Paste clip art or magazine pictures of at least two objects that begin with the same sound on card stock, putting together a set of different pictures depicting a variety of beginning sounds. Ask the student to pick a card, say the word and its beginning sound, and find another picture card of an object that begins with the same sound.
- ◆ Ball toss—Using a beach or NERF ball, state a word and toss the ball to a student, who then says another word that begins with the same sound. Keep tossing the ball until no one can think of another word for the sound. The game can be changed to say words that use the same vowel sound in a one-syllable word, such as hat and nap.

In the area of phonics, CAL (2007, p. 147) provides some examples of activities:

- ◆ Sorting alphabet cereal—Give each child a cup full of alphabet letter cereal and a paper plate. Each student (or pairs of students) should sort the letters and count the multiples. The teacher then makes a graph with each letter across the bottom and asks students to raise their fingers to show how many of the letters they have, plotting the total number of each letter on the graph.

◆ Letter formation—Have pairs or small groups use their bodies to form different letters and have the class state the letters.

To develop reading fluency, CAL (2007, p. 166) recommends Adler's (2001) activities. These include:

◆ Choral reading—Fluent reader reads the passage aloud while students listen, then class reads along in chorus with the fluent reader. Repeat the process four or five times to prepare students to read the passage independently.

◆ Reading in pairs—Pair students up, pairing one student who reads fairly well with another student who does not read as well. Have the better reader read the text while the other reader listens and follows the text silently. Switch readers and have the stronger reader assist the other with word recognition as needed. For ELs, the pairs can consist of an EL and a native speaker or an EL at one level of English proficiency and an EL at a higher level of English proficiency.

Vocabulary development, the fourth area of the National Reading Panel's research review, is especially critical for ELs. Peregoy and Boyle (2017, pp. 269–281) offer several suggestions for EL vocabulary development that can be used for ELs at the beginning, or intermediate levels, for example:

◆ Word wheels—Make a circle in the center of a poster board and write a common word in the middle, for example, the word "good." Draw six lines like spokes outward from the circle, leaving enough space to write synonyms for good between each pair of lines.

◆ Teaching affixes—Show students a prefix in a common word and define it; for example, in "un-happy," "un" means "not." Ask students to think of other examples using this prefix. Make index cards with adjectives that can serve as base words with the prefix "un-" and have students work in pairs to match, define, and illustrate them.

The last area of the NRP (2000) findings focuses on text comprehension and teaching strategies for comprehension. CAL (2007, pp. 77–78) suggests Stauffer's (1975) sequence, the Directed Reading-Thinking Activity (DRTA). This sequence of five steps involves:

1. Previewing the content of the reading—vocabulary, structures, background knowledge—and introducing them to students
2. Predicting: The teacher prepares questions that guide students to scan passage headings and graphics.
3. Reading: Students read alone, in pairs, or while someone else reads aloud and they note where predictions are confirmed or disproven.
4. Checking: Students report prediction results and where the answers are found in the text.
5. Summarizing: Students read the main points in the text and write them in their own words.

Developing Oral Proficiency in ELs

Depending on the learning context and age of the learner, specific activities for developing oral proficiency are helpful. These activities may take place in the mainstream classroom, in self-contained ESOL classes, or in consultation with the SLP. In general, ELs and English-speaking students in the lower grades are immersed in activities that build their oral proficiency, such as show and tell, picture books, and more. As they move to upper grades, students have fewer nonverbal cues to connect with new terms and phrases; therefore, working on specific speaking activities can help mitigate this shift. In addition, older students are more likely to have literacy skills in at least one language, so these can be used to foster oral proficiency as well (e.g., in a dialogue memorized for a skit). Last, some students in the upper grades may benefit from specific pronunciation exercises to help them distinguish phonemes that may not be the same in their native language.

Information Gap

An information gap is a second language learning activity intended to promote real communication in the language being acquired. In contrast with language learning approaches such as the audiolingual approach of the 1960s, which focused on learning contrived dialogues to facilitate conversational skills (Richards & Rodgers, 1986), information gap activities set up communication situations that are real.

For example, using a dialogue in an audiolingual approach, a person may ask where the library is, and the other person responds that it is two blocks down the street on the right. Both speakers know that this is not a real dialogue; therefore, they do not use language spontaneously or for their own immediate communication needs. In contrast, an information gap activity creates a reason for one person to gather information from the other, thus prompting each person to use language purposefully. An example of an information gap activity follows:

> A teacher brings in a variety of clothing that she hangs up for the class to see. She calls upon two volunteers to role-play the information gap situation. Person 1 is given a card with a picture of a piece of clothing, such as a corduroy jacket with elbow patches. She must describe the jacket to Person 2, who takes the role of the salesperson, and ask if she has anything in the store that is similar. Person 2 finds the corresponding jacket from the clothes hung in the classroom and offers to let Person 1 try it on. They then improvise from there until completing the transaction.

Information gaps promote the use of vocabulary and phrases specific to a situation, and they spontaneously emulate real communication. They are used to allow ELs to practice any type of vocabulary or discourse. Examples of information gap activities can be found at http://bogglesworldesl.com/information_gap.htm

Jazz Chants

Invented by Carolyn Graham, an ESOL teacher with a jazz background, jazz chants (Graham, 1978) are similar to raps and choral activities. They focus on particular topics, vocabulary, and phrases to give ELs practice in pronouncing new words and sentences. Because they are chanted chorally, the intonation is exaggerated, which helps with prosody. There are a number of prepared jazz chant books with accompanying audio files; however, they are easy to create. Graham (1978, 2000) recommends identifying vocabulary and phrases for a topic of focus, then isolating a small sample for a jazz chant. She recommends selecting words that are one, two, or three syllables. For example, in a lesson on moon phases, some of the words might be "moon," "full," "new," "phases," "waxing," "waning," "gibbous," "crescent," "quarter," and "full."

> Full moon, waxing gibbous
>
> New moon, waning crescent
>
> First quarter, last quarter
>
> Phases of the moon

Jazz chants can also be used to help students learn language functions and the proper intonation for expressing them. For example, in asking and giving permission:

> Is this seat taken? May I sit here?
>
> Is this seat taken? May I sit here?
>
> Is this seat taken? May I sit here?
>
> No, it's free. Have a seat! It's yours!

Each of the chants would be accompanied by rhythmic clapping and exaggerated intonation, and stress on the stressed syllables and music can also be added.

Minimal Pairs

Minimal pairs focus on phonemes of contrast to help students whose native languages do not have the same distinctions. For example, Arabic-speaking ELs do not have a /p/ sound in their native language. This often leads to confusion, because the Arabic language does have the /b/, which is a similar sound. This can result in misunderstandings of both languages and often leads to errors stemming from not hearing the difference between the /p/ and /b/ sounds (e.g., pat and bat). If the EL were told, "Give him a pat," he or she may understand, "Give him a bat." Similarly, not having the phoneme /p/ in Arabic results in substituting the phoneme /b/ when attempting to pronounce a word in English, such as "Bark the car."

Minimal pair exercises often involve the selection of two words that differ in one phoneme. The first step is to have the learner identify which word has the targeted phoneme. For instance, the teacher would say, "park, bark" and would ask the learner to raise her hand when she heard the /p/ sound. After "park, bark," the teacher would say "bin, pin," and so forth. The /p/ phoneme could then be used in the medial position, such as "cable, maple," and also in the final position, "cap, cab." After the student develops a high success rate of identifying the /p/ phoneme, the teacher can then move to having the student pronounce each pair, ensuring that the /p/ sound is included in words that use it. It then becomes a type of pronunciation drill. Although minimal pairs is primarily a listening and speaking activity, it has implications for reading and writing. An EL who could not distinguish the sounds would then have trouble spelling the word "park" in writing and might confuse the word "pole" for the word "bowl" in the sentence, "She was carrying a pole." Helping students to differentiate between sounds has far-reaching implications.

Cooperative Learning

The cooperative learning strategy is not specific to ELs, although it has many features that promote the development of oral language skills. Students work in teams and must interact to complete a given task. The interaction involves conversation and discussion, and it often occurs between pairs or small groups of up to four people. This allows for multiple opportunities for negotiating meaning, which facilitates second language development. According to Kagan (1994), a leading proponent of cooperative learning, a group activity must include four elements: positive interdependence, individual accountability, equal participation, and simultaneous interaction. In other words, everyone in the group is dependent on each other for the outcome, each member is evaluated for his or her contributions, everyone contributes and is on task, and everyone has a concurrent task. An example of a cooperative learning activity for pairs is the think-pair-share strategy. The first step is for individuals in each pair to think about a question or problem that the teacher poses. Step 2 requires two students to share their thoughts with each other. The final step involves grouping the pairs with another pair to report their conclusions or share the pairs' conclusions with the entire class. The amount of time that each student spends speaking is greatly increased by participating in pair and small group activities rather than whole-class instruction.

Developing Writing Skills

Writing skill development spans emergent writing stages—including letter formation, invented spelling, and approximated spelling—all the way to advanced composition skills, such as writing a research paper. The IES Practice Guide *Teaching Elementary School Students to Be Effective Writers* (2018) offers guidance in best practices. The first suggestion is to teach strategies for the elements of the writing process. This involves planning, drafting, sharing, evaluating, and revising and editing. They also recommend teaching writing for different purpose, including description, narration, information, persuasion, and analysis. They suggest using examples of good writing for students to emulate, unpacking the features and using them to elicit variations on the language patterns and style. Techniques for developing sentence-level fluency, accuracy, clarity, and style include sentence framing (discussed in detail in the following section), sentence expanding (e.g., The bird chirped. → The red bird chirped on the oak tree branch.), and sentence combining (e.g., Our school is new. Our school is big. → Our new school is big.).

In the following section, we highlight a sampling of writing activities. Peregoy and Boyle (2008, 2017) offer a wealth of resources that promote writing skill development at K–12 levels.

Language Experience Approach

The Language Experience Approach (Peregoy & Boyle, 2017, pp. 356–359), described above as a reading skill development activity, can also be used as an early writing skill development activity. Using this approach, students participate in a shared experience that serves as the basis for subsequent storytelling. For example, the teacher and students may use a blender to grind peanuts into peanut butter. Following the experience, the teacher leads the students to retell what happened and then writes the students' dictation sentence-by-sentence on chart paper. The teacher then leads the class in a choral reading of the descriptive paragraph. Depending on the children's age, they may copy the paragraph or write and/or draw their own version of the story. If they have difficulty writing their own version, they can dictate the story to the teacher or an aide, who helps reinforce the narrative structure of a descriptive paragraph and grammar and usage conventions.

Dialogue Journals

Peregoy and Boyle (2017) point out that emergent writers need to develop fluency and automaticity in writing. The development of fluent writing skills requires practice in purposeful writing that is engaging and interesting to the student. Dialogue journals are like personal journals. Students share their personal thoughts and the teacher responds to the student by sharing his or her own personal thoughts. There is a regular exchange of journaling between the teacher and students. The role of the teacher is not to correct grammar or any other aspect of form but to reply to the content of the entry. Students should be reminded that the teacher cannot necessarily respond to every issue raised in the dialogue journals, but if they would like a response on a specific point, they can underline it or write it in a different color.

It is also important to set parameters for dialogue journals, as students may address inappropriate topics or reveal issues that the teacher must report.

Clustering and Mapping

Peregoy and Boyle (2017) suggest two types of graphic organizers to help plan for writing: clustering and mapping. Clustering helps writers identify vocabulary for their composition. The subject of the composition is placed at the center of the cluster. Students then begin to draw spokes from the center circle with words that relate to the topic. Words on the spokes can be added to the cluster as necessary (Figure 7–1).

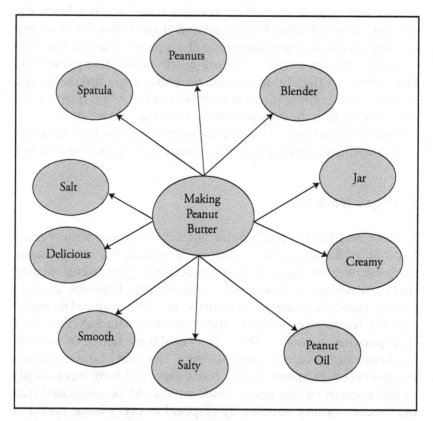

Figure 7–1. Cluster about making peanut butter.

Mapping is more detailed and organized than clustering and can be used by writers at all levels. It uses more than single words in the graphic and moves the writer into the next stages of composition. If students were to take the composition of making peanut butter to the next step, they could first make a cluster and then categorize the content. Maps assist students to write about a topic in a logical and descriptive way (Figure 7–2).

Sentence Combining and Shortening

More advanced ELs, especially at the secondary level, can benefit from writing exercises that emphasize varied sentence construction. Peregoy and Boyle (2017) suggest sentence combining and

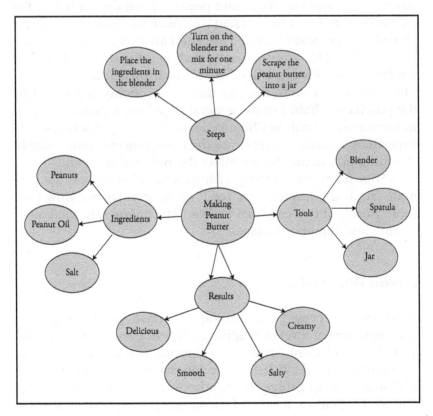

Figure 7–2. *Map of making peanut butter.*

sentence shortening as a way to help students write with more sophistication. In sentence combining, writers are given two or more sentences that present information on the same topic. Students are then required to find the best way to combine the sentences into one sentence, using relative phrases, subordinate clauses, and so on. For example: (1) Mary ate her lunch, (2) Mary's lunch was delicious and nutritious, (3) Mary was in a hurry, and (4) Mary only had a 15-minute lunch break. The combined sentence might look like this: Mary ate her delicious and nutritious lunch in a hurry because she only had a 15-minute lunch break.

Sentence shortening addresses verbose sentences, challenging students to revise them into the shortest sentence possible without losing meaning. Sometimes this involves dividing a run-on sentence into two sentences, and sometimes it simply requires omitting extraneous words and phrases from the sentence. For example, in the sentence, "I had ice cream for dessert and it was chocolate chip, and I liked it a lot, and I ate every bite," the writer could revise it to two sentences, such as, "I had chocolate chip ice cream for dessert. I liked it so much that I ate every bite." The sentence, "Due to the fact that the economy is affected by the purchasing habits of the general population, people have an influence on the nation's financial health," can omit a number of superfluous words and rephrase the main concepts more simply, "People's purchasing habits affect the national economy."

After featuring a variety of instructional practices that promote language development for English learners, we now look more closely at two essential tools and techniques, leveled questioning and sentence frames.

Leveled Questioning

Teachers use leveled questioning to phrase questions at each student's current level of English proficiency and to elicit, recast, and expand students' responses through communicative interaction (Nutta et al., 2018). These interchanges between teacher and student help bridge the gap between the student's current English proficiency level and the language demands of instruction. The language of the question is adjusted to the English proficiency of the student, and images, objects, and actions are used to support comprehension and responses when the language is necessarily a bit more complex than the student's current level of English proficiency.

You can plan to ask leveled questions before, during, or after a lesson to gauge students' prior knowledge of the topic, to check for comprehension of instruction, and to assess their learning. In addition, you can ask questions as part of a whole-class activity, during small group and pair work, and while consulting one-on-one with your EL students.

The first step in employing leveled questioning with English learners is creating the questions. When writing questions for your English learners, especially those who are at beginning and intermediate levels of English proficiency, be sure to find, organize, and provide images and objects that are related to the instructional topic. These will be helpful to indicate details that the students may not be able to comprehend or describe completely through language.

While English proficiency is divided into different numbers of levels, such as WIDA, which has six levels (e.g., entering, emerging, developing, expanding, bridging, and reaching), we have found that it is practical to differentiate questions by three levels: beginning, intermediate, and advanced. Beginning-level questions tend to be short, with simple grammar focusing on the here and now and frequent vocabulary. Intermediate-level questions are longer and use more specialized vocabulary and more complex grammar, such as simple past, present, and future tenses. Advanced-level questions use complex phrasing, a wide variety of vocabulary, and grammatical tenses and moods that sequence events in past or future and address hypothetical and conditional circumstances. In Table 7–3, sample question types and examples are organized by three levels of proficiency.

Sentence Frames

Sentence frames provide academic language phrasing that English learners cannot yet produce without support (Nutta et al.,

Table 7–3. *Sample Question Types Organized by Three Levels of Proficiency*

Beginning Question Phrasing	
Short, simply phrased questions that use frequent vocabulary and verb tenses that focus on the here and now (simple present tense).	
Question Type	**Example**
Questions that elicit nonverbal responses	Where is the equator? Answer: points to globe
Yes/No	Is this a triangle?
Either/Or	Is this a triangle or a square?
Wh questions that elicit one-word answers	What is this? Answer: a triangle Who is this (point to drawing)? Answer: Galileo What is your name? Answer: student's name
Wh questions that elicit two- or three-word phrase answers	Where is the cup? Answer: on the table When is lunch? Answer 11:30 or at 11:30
Frequently used, formulaic questions How much or how many	How much does this cost? How many pencils are there?
Intermediate Question Phrasing	
Longer, more complexly phrased questions that use less frequent vocabulary and verb tenses that focus on the present, past, and future.	
Question Type	**Example**
Wh questions that elicit description	What does a metamorphic rock look like?
How and why questions that elicit explanation	How is sedimentary rock formed? Why is erosion bad for the environment?

Table 7–3. *continued*

Intermediate Question Phrasing *continued*	
Question Type	**Example**
Questions using simple verb tenses	
Present progressive	What **is** the water **doing?**
Simple past	What **caused** the levees to break?
Past progressive	What **was** the geologist **doing** when the rock cracked?
Simple future	How **will** she solve the problem?
Present perfect	Why **has** pollution **increased** so much this century?
Negative questions	When **isn't** water a liquid?

Advanced Question Phrasing	
Complexly phrased questions that use a wide range of vocabulary and verb tenses that discuss sequences of events in the past or future or are hypothetical or conditional.	
Question Type	**Example**
Hypothetical/conditional Past perfect	What **would have happened** if the Allies had lost the Battle of Midway?
Future perfect	**Will** scientists **have completed** exploration of Mars by the next century? Why or why not?

Source: Nutta, J., Strebel, C., Mihai, F., Crevecoeur-Bryant, E., & Mokhtari, K. (2018). *Show, tell, build. Twenty key instructional tools and techniques for educating English learners*, p. 6. Cambridge, MA: Harvard Education Press. Used with permission from Harvard Education Publishing Group.

2018). English learners at a given English proficiency level cannot yet independently and spontaneously phrase sentences with the sentence frame's grammatical complexity and density because the ELs' process of acquiring English morphology and syntax is still in development. Sentence frames provide both explicit instruction on more complex and dense grammatical phrasing than the EL is currently capable of producing as well as support for ELs to express different language functions during academic discussions and in academic writing. Sentence frames also model common phrasing of different language functions, such as describing, comparing, disagreeing, and so on.

Let's take a look at a sentence frame that would be appropriate for an English learner at WIDA Level 2. At this level, English learners can **comprehend** as follows (from the WIDA Performance Definitions Listening and Reading, Grades K–12, p. 8):

◆ General content words and expressions, including cognates.
◆ Social and instructional words and expressions across content areas.
◆ Compound grammatical constructions.
◆ Repetitive phrasal and sentence patterns across content areas.
◆ Multiple related simple sentences.
◆ An idea with details.

The same student at Level 2 in Speaking and Writing can **produce** as follows (from the WIDA Performance Definitions Listening and Reading, Grades K–12, p. 9):

◆ General content words and expressions.
◆ Social and instructional words and expressions across content areas.
◆ Formulaic grammatical structures and variable use of conventions.
◆ Repetitive phrasal and sentence patterns across content areas.
◆ Phrases or short sentences.
◆ Emerging expression of ideas.

These Performance Definitions describe what an English learner at WIDA Level 2 can comprehend and produce without support. For example, a Level 2 EL could independently and spontaneously produce "I like ice cream" and "We like science," and after learning the discipline-specific words "seismologist" and "earthquake," they could produce "Seismologists study earthquakes." They could also produce compound sentences with the same patterns, such as, "Seismologists study earthquakes, and botanists study plants." All of these examples are formulaic, repetitive sentence patterns. A student at Level 2 would probably not need a sentence frame to express those ideas (a sentence starter could be provided, such as Seismologists _____).

To get a sense of what types of sentences they would need sentence frame support for, we can look to Level 3 Performance Definitions at WIDA Level 2. At this level, English learners can **comprehend** as follows (from the WIDA Performance Definitions Listening and Reading, Grades K–12, p. 8—differences from Level 2 are **bolded**):

- **Specific content language**, including expressions.
- Words and expressions with **common collocations and idioms** across content areas.
- Compound and **some complex** (e.g., noun phrase, verb phrase, prepositional phrase) **grammatical. constructions**.
- Sentence patterns across content areas.
- Discourse with a **series of extended sentences**.
- **Related ideas**.

At Level 3 in Speaking and Writing, English learners can **produce** as follows (from the WIDA Performance Definitions Listening and Reading, Grades K–12, p. 9):

- **Specific content language**, including **cognates** and expressions.
- Words or expressions with **multiple meanings** used across content areas.
- Repetitive grammatical structures with **occasional variation** and **emerging use of conventions**.
- **Sentence patterns** across content areas.
- Short and **some expanded sentences with emerging complexity**.
- **Expanded expression of one idea** or emerging expression of **multiple related ideas**.

If a Level 2 English learner were given an assignment to write a persuasive paragraph about a global problem, the sentence frames should provide collocations and idioms across content areas, some complex grammatical constructions, and extended sentences with related ideas. For example, in response to the prompt, "What is the biggest problem of the world today?"

_____ is the biggest problem that the world is facing today

        name the problem that you identified (Noun—N)

because _____.

       state the reason why the problem is important
                      (Noun Phrase—NP)

Despite some anecdotal evidence, research shows that
_____.

       describe the results of research about the problem (NP)

One example of the effect of this phenomenon is _____
_____.

       provide an example of the effect of the problem (N or NP)

When _____, _____
_____.

       state the previous example in present tense (NP)
      state its effect in present tense (NP)—*what happens?*

Climate change is the biggest problem that the world is facing today

because it affects every continent and every person.

Despite some anecdotal evidence, research shows that temperatures are increasing.

One example of the effect of this phenomenon is polar icecaps are melting.

When polar icecaps melt, sea levels rise.

    The process of understanding the elements of, filling in, reflecting upon feedback, and supporting independent writing based on the sentence frames is similar regardless of the level of proficiency.

1. SLP introduces sentence templates (i.e., sample sentences for specific language functions) as well as their corresponding sentence frames, each of which use structural complexity and density just above the ELs' level as models (consult WIDA Performance Definitions for guidance in selecting or adapting appropriate sentence frames).
2. SLP reviews the grammar of the sentence frames— their formal (e.g., word endings), structural (e.g., word order), and functional (e.g., purpose of statement) aspects—with the EL students.
3. EL students independently use sentence frames for writing a description of something learned in a previous lesson or for writing a response to a prompt.
4. SLP reviews ELs' sentences/paragraph and provides corrective feedback. For the example above, an EL student might write something like, "it affect every continent and every person," leaving the "s" off the word "affect." In this case, the teacher could point out the missing "s" and link it to the subject, "it," which requires an *s* ending verb in the simple present tense.
5. EL students are given a writing task using similar functions and requiring similar structures but without sentence frames. EL students can refer to previous materials, notes, and writing samples to support their efforts. For instance, the prompt might be "What is the best way to stay healthy?"
6. SLP provides feedback for the completed paragraph, focusing on the structural and formal accuracy of elements from the previous sentence frames used.

This cycle would be repeated with new language functions (e.g., evaluating an idea) and once the EL student can independently and consistently construct sentences using the form and structure correctly from the sentence frames, new sentence frames with increased density and structural complexity of the sentence patterns can be introduced. In addition, if the student struggles with writing in response to a prompt that is similar to previous ones, sentence starters (e.g., I disagree with _____) can be used to "prime the pump."

To create your own sentence frames, determine the main language functions of the sentences you want to focus on for your EL students and look at common phrasing for that language function (e.g., describing). For example, if you want your EL students to describe the three types of rocks (igneous, metamorphic, and sedimentary), you can start with writing your own descriptive sentences using academic language and then omit elements of the sentences with a blank.

> *Three major types of rocks have been identified by geologists. Rock classification is determined by, among other factors, texture, streak, and means of formation. **Igneous rocks**, such as basalt and obsidian, are formed as hot magma cools. **Sedimentary rocks**, for example sandstone, are found on the earth's crust, appear grainy, and are formed by time and pressure. **Metamorphic rocks** like gneiss have been changed by heat or pressure and were previously igneous or sedimentary rocks. Although these three rock types differ in appearance, they are all a result of the rock cycle, which forms them.*

This paragraph uses academic language to describe the three types of rocks. Some characteristics of this academic language are discipline-specific vocabulary and dense and complex grammatical construction (e.g., passive voice, relative clauses, etc.). Making sentence frames by omitting segments from each of these complex sentences would be appropriate for English learners at WIDA Level 4. For example, the first sentence, "Three major types of rocks have been identified by geologists," could be converted to a sentence starter such as, "Three major types of rocks _____." This would require the EL to use sentence patterns characteristic of particular content areas (in the case, science, which uses the passive voice).

If the sentence frames were to be used with a WIDA Level 2 English learner, the sentences could be rewritten to use the active voice, which is a more common and less complex/dense sentence pattern. For example, "Geologists identify three major types of rocks." The sentence frame could be "_____ three major types of rocks." A correct answer might be "There are" or "Scientists categorize" or any number of variations on this simple active voice phrasing.

In summary, leveled questioning and sentence frames are level-adjustable teaching techniques that can be incorporated into instruction focusing on EL oral language or literacy skills.

Roseberry-McKibben (2014) discusses specific strategies for developing language and literacy skills of ELs with language impairment through the use of a holistic strategies approach to intervention. Within this framework, she advocates the importance of working collaboratively to used research-based approaches to develop language and literacy skills within meaningful contexts. Emphasis is placed on the importance of structuring the environment and presenting information that is comprehensible for the EL learner. In particular, Roseberry-McKibben (2014) highlights the importance of incorporating the principles of Universal Design for Learning (Meyer, Rose, & Gordon, 2014; Ralabate & Nelson, 2017) and using recent technological developments (e.g., iPad apps) to support the attainment of standards in EL students. She outlines six compensatory strategies that can be used by ELs to learn and remember information. These include:

◆ Writing down important information in a notebook or technological device (e.g., iPad)
◆ Writing down key words
◆ Use of visualization to form mental pictures of information
◆ Use of metacognitive strategies
◆ Use of reauditorization/silent rehearsal
◆ Attend to the speaker

While there are many different evidence-based strategies that support EL students' development of reading, listening/speaking (oral proficiency), and writing skills (e.g., teaching high-frequency vocabulary; dialogic reading), further research continues to be necessary to determine which strategies and approaches are successful across proficiency levels, grade levels, and disability with EL students.

The last section of this chapter focuses on the third element of our assessment, intervention, and monitoring (AIM) model: monitoring. We have explored several educational strategies that

SLPs and ESOL professionals may consider using when working with ELs with communication disorders. In order to monitor the progress of ELs when it comes to not only their English language acquisition but also their academic language development, we need to explore how formal assessment can provide vital information in those two key areas. Therefore, we look at formal assessment as a means of monitoring school progress of ELs with communication disorders. Special attention will be paid to test accommodations and their effectiveness to ensure that large-scale assessment results are a valid measure of language and academic development of ELs with CDs.

Monitoring Through Large-Scale Assessments

We have discussed several intervention strategies that facilitate literacy acquisition for ELs and ELCDs (the intervention component of our AIM model). Given the importance of monitoring ELCDs' progress in language and literacy acquisition, we consider two types of large-scale assessment, one for language proficiency and another for content-area assessment.

Monitoring Language Proficiency Development Through Large-Scale Assessments

Consortium (Multistate) Instruments for Assessing English Language Proficiency

For accountability purposes, many states have developed English language proficiency standards (i.e., the WIDA consortium) and designed instruments based on these new language proficiency standards.

WIDA's ACCESS for ELLs Test

After completing the English language proficiency standards in 2004 (revised in 2007), WIDA developed several assessment instruments for ELs based on the WIDA/TESOL language proficiency standards. In the previous chapter, we discussed the WIDA Screener and WIDA ACCESS Placement Test (W-APT). WIDA has also developed another instrument called WIDA Assessing Comprehension and Communication in English State-to-State for English Language Learners for ELLs (ACCESS for ELLs). These three instruments allow teachers and administrators to separate the purpose of language proficiency assessment from placement and monitoring progress. The placement of ELs is addressed by using the WIDA Access Placement Test (W-APT) and WIDA Screener, two tests previously discussed in detail, whereas the question of ongoing language proficiency assessment is addressed by ACCESS for ELLs.

ACCESS for ELLs is a large-scale assessment. Summative in nature, it is used to measure the annual language proficiency development of ELs. ACCESS for ELLs consists of the following grade level clusters: 1, 2 to 3, 4 to 5, 6 to 8, and 9 to 12. Each cluster addresses the five WIDA/TESOL standards: social and instructional language, English language arts, math, science, and social studies. For each grade level, the standards further specify one or more performance indicators for each of the four language domains: listening, speaking, reading, and writing. ACCESS for ELLs has three tiers (A, B, and C) that correspond to the proficiency level of each EL taking the test. The tiers overlap in an effort to have a test designed for ELs within a particular grade-level cluster and range of proficiency level.

◆ Tier A covers Level 1 (WIDA Entering/TESOL Starting)
  to Level 3 (WIDA/TESOL Developing)
◆ Tier B covers Level 2 (WIDA Beginning/TESOL
  Emerging) to Level 4 (WIDA/TESOL Expanding)
◆ Tier C covers Level 3 (WIDA/TESOL Developing) to
  Level 5 (WIDA/TESOL Bridging)

As research in second language acquisition suggests, ELs are rarely fully at one level or the other. Quite often, they are in the process of moving from one level (tier) to the next. Attaining a certain level of English proficiency is not similar to leaving a room, closing the door, and never looking back. Rather, it is more like being in constant transition, at times fully comfortable at one level with certain skills but not with others. For example, an EL can be at Level 3 in speaking but at Level 1 or 2 in reading. The decision as to which tier version of the test ELs should take is made by their teachers based on information generated by other language tests, for example, the W-APT.

An example of an ACCESS for ELLs test item for the reading domain in Tier B of the grade cluster 1 addressing social and instructional language (WIDA/TESOL Standard 3) is provided in Figure 7–3. Given a picture of a bulletin board, the EL is required to extract information from environmental print (such as signs, bulletin boards, or menus). The EL then reads a scenario and responds to corresponding questions. In the example provided in Figure 7–3, three test items associated with this particular scenario are provided below.

The first test item covers Level 2, which has the following model performance indicator (MPI), very similar to TESOL's sample performance indicators previously discussed.

Figure 7–3. *ACCESS for ELLs test sample for the reading domain (bulletin board). Source: ACCESS for ELLs®. Listening, Reading, Writing, and Speaking sample items, Grades 1–12, by World-Class Instructional Design and Assessment (WIDA), 2008. Retrieved from http://www.wida.us/assessment/ACCESS/ ACCESS_Sample_Items.pdf. Reprinted with permission.*

When did the class visit the aquarium?
A. March
B. May
C. September

The second test item listed below measures the following MPI, associated with Level 3 of language proficiency: "Restate information found in visually supported print such as school schedules, field trips, or celebrations."

What was everybody's favorite animal?
A. Octopus
B. Shark
C. Seal

The third test item, designed for ELs at Level 4, is based on the following MPI: "Summarize information found in visually supported print on classroom or school activities."

What kind of animals are in the aquarium?
A. Animals that live on land
B. Animals that live in water
C. Animals that live in the air

Participation Requirements for ACCESS for ELLs for ELs with Communication Disorders

State and federal laws require that all ELLs participate in annual ELP assessments (http://www2. ed.gov/policy/speced/ guid/idea/memosdcltrs/q-and-a-on-elp-swd.pdf). These annual tests are designed to measure ELs' proficiency and progress in learning English in the language domains of listening, reading, speaking, and writing. All ELs are required to take these tests, including students with disabilities. However, the Individuals with Disabilities Education Act (IDEA) requires that states provide appropriate accommodations where needed, in accordance with a student's Individualized Education Program (IEP). Also eligible are students who have a 504 Plan or who are covered under Title II of the ADA.

The Every Student Succeeds Act (ESSA, 2015), however, requires that a state provide appropriate accommodations for ELs with disabilities. Moreover, ELs should not be assessed if there are not appropriate accommodations for one or more domains of the English language proficiency (ELP) assessment. ELs should be assessed based on the remaining domains in which it is possible to assess the student because appropriate accommodations are provided (34 CFR § 200.6(h)(4)). Determinations for a student to not participate in a specific domain must be carefully considered for each EL and for each specific domain.

For ELs identified as deaf or hard of hearing (DHH), including those for whom American Sign Language (ASL) is their primary mode of communication, the recommendation is that they can generally participate in the reading and writing domains of the assessment with few or no accommodations. Students who use speech reading as part of their communication system may use the Human Reader of Items accommodation to access the listening domain. IEP teams should determine on a case-by-case basis how an EL student who has a hearing loss will participate in ACCESS for ELLs. Individual state policy may allow for some form(s) of manually coded English to provide access to the listening and speaking domains for ELs who are DHH and use other communication modalities or systems. ELs identified as DHH are not required to participate in paper-based testing, but it is strongly recommended for several reasons, including the following.

- ◆ Ease of providing manually coded test directions.
- ◆ Eliminating the need to force submit a domain.
- ◆ Eliminating the need to override tier placement.

The list of allowed ACCESS for ELLs accommodations includes:

- ◆ Braille (BR) interpreter signs test directions in ASL (SD).
- ◆ Extended testing of a test domain over multiple days (EM).
- ◆ Large print (LP).
- ◆ Extended speaking test response time (ES) manual control of item audio (MC).
- ◆ Extended testing time within the school day (ET) repeat item audio (RA).

- Human reader for items (HI) scribe (SR).
- Human reader for response options (HR).
- Student responds using a recording device, which is played back and transcribed by the student (RD).
- Human reader for repeat of items (RI).
- Test may be administered in a nonschool setting (NS).
- Human reader for repeat of response options (RR).
- Word processor or similar keyboarding device to respond to test items (WD).

The following accommodations are not allowed for ACCESS for ELLs or any other WIDA test:

- Reading aloud test items or passages on the reading test.
- Translating test items into a language other than English.
- Reading test items in a language other than English.
- Using a bilingual word-to-word dictionary.
- Responding to test questions in a language other than English.

State-Developed Instruments for Monitoring English Language Proficiency Development

As discussed in the previous chapter, some states use language proficiency instruments developed either by multistate consortia or by national test development companies, while others develop and use their own assessment of EL language proficiency. The state of Texas is one example that falls into this category: This state uses the TELPAS test.

Texas English Language Proficiency Assessment System (TELPAS)

Just like many of the other tests discussed in the previous chapter, the Texas English Language Proficiency Assessment System (TELPAS) was developed in response to the NCLB Act's requirement of assessing ELs' progress in learning English (TELPAS,

2011). Structurally, the TELPAS is organized in two major sections. For ELs in Grades K and 1, TELPAS is composed of listening, speaking, reading, and writing assessments rated holistically. For ELs in Grades 2 to 12, TELPAS consists of multiple-choice reading tests, holistically rated student writing collections, and speaking and listening assessment.

Similar to other English language proficiency tests, the TELPAS measures English learning based on identifiable stages of second language development. There are four proficiency levels assessed through TELPAS: beginning, intermediate, advanced, and advanced high (TELPAS, 2011). For example, for reading, descriptors are provided for each proficiency level, as seen in Table 7–4.

The majority of the test items in the TELPAS reading section of the test are organized under three TELPAS reading assessment objectives: (1) understanding of words and language structures, (2) basic understanding of a variety of texts, and (3) analyzing and evaluating information and ideas in a variety of texts. One example for understanding words and language structures is as follows.

Miguel uses a ruler to _____ the length of a pencil.

A. line
B. ask
C. measure
D. add

Table 7–4. *TELPAS Proficiency Levels*

Beginning:

Students at this level are typically new to the English language. They have little or no ability to derive meaning from English text. They generally understand very little English and tend to read very slowly and word by word. In order to figure out the meaning of what they read, they rely heavily on previous knowledge of the topic, the small bank of English words and phrases they have learned, and information from pictures. Because their English is so limited, their comprehension quickly breaks down when they try to read English in authentic social and academic contexts.

Table 7–4. continued

Intermediate:

Students at this level have a somewhat larger English vocabulary and a basic sense of simple English language structures. However, they tend to interpret English very literally and have difficulty following story lines that have a surprise twist or nonstandard format. They still rely heavily on what they already know about a topic to confirm meaning and increase comprehension, and pictures that illustrate meaning are still a needed support. Students at this level can read and understand short connected texts on familiar topics when high-frequency English is used. They have difficulty reading and understanding materials written for their grade level.

Advanced:

Students at this level have an emerging grade appropriate reading vocabulary and a grasp of the structure and grammatical features of the English language. They have the ability to read grade-level texts with some success, although second language acquisition support is still needed to help them understand language that is typically familiar to native English-speaking peers. With linguistic support these students can often demonstrate comprehension of main and supporting ideas on topics they know little about. Additionally, they can often understand English beyond its literal meaning, and they have an emerging ability to think analytically to build conceptual understanding as they read grade-level materials in English.

Advanced High:

Students at this level have the ability to read and understand, with minimal support related to second language acquisition, grade appropriate English used in academic and social contexts, with some exceptions when low-frequency or specialized vocabulary is used. With minimal visual and textual support and at a level nearly comparable to their native English-speaking peers, they are able to understand both explicit and implicit ideas, think analytically, and build conceptual understanding as they read grade-level materials in English.

Source: Adapted from *Educator Guide to TELPAS. Grades K–12*, by TELPAS, 2011. Retrieved from http://www.tea.state.tx.us/WorkArea/linkit.aspx ?LinkIdentifier = id&ItemID = 2147501849&libID = 2147501843

The TELPAS also assesses advanced and advanced high levels of language proficiency using cloze procedures. Content-area cloze selections require students to fill in blanks with words that appropriately complete the surrounding academic context. This test format provides evidence of the extent to which ELs are developing the academic literacy in English necessary for understanding language and constructing meaning in subject area instructional materials. This type of test item is designed to assess general comprehension of content-based instructional materials, not mastery of the subject area academic content, skills, or terminology. For example, the student reads a paragraph that has several sentences with missing words:

Matteo was very happy. His math teacher showed the students many different _____ of maps.

A. types
B. places
C. students
D. teachers

This test item is a possible example of a mathematics cloze selection designed to assess understanding of words and language structures for Grade 2.

In terms of accommodations for ELCDs, the allowed TELPAS accommodations include:

♦ Basic transcribing.
♦ Individualized structured reminders.
♦ Large print.
♦ Manipulating test materials.
♦ Extra day.

The following accommodations are not permitted:

♦ Students may not receive reading assistance.
♦ Students may not use English language or foreign language reference materials.
♦ Test questions, reading selections, and listening passages may not be translated.
♦ Test questions, answer choices, and selections may not be rephrased, clarified, or read to students.

Monitoring Literacy Development and Academic Knowledge through Large-Scale Assessments

Large-Scale Assessment Accommodations for ELs: Defining the Issues

Under Title III of the NCLB Act (2001), states were required to measure whether or not ELs were making progress in attaining full English language proficiency. The same requirement applied to measuring academic knowledge. Currently, as a direct consequence of the NCLB and ESSA, all public school districts must include ELs when reporting student progress in academic achievement goals. Title I of the NCLB Act strengthened the idea of accountability by requiring that all states had to develop annual assessments for Grades 3 through 8 and one assessment in high school that were aligned with state standards.

This increased level of accountability is bringing an increased focus on the academic needs of ELs from educators and school administrators. There have been many concerns regarding the quality of standardized assessments applied to ELs, especially whether the results from such large-scale tests are valid and reliable (Abella, Urritia, & Shneyderman, 2005). To address these critical issues, all states have developed and implemented accommodation policies for ELs when taking standardized large-scale tests that focus on content areas, such as language arts, math, science, or social studies.

Test accommodation for ELs can be defined as the support provided to ELs to access the English content of the assessment in order to demonstrate what they know academically. Accommodations can be either modifications of the test itself or modifications of the test procedure (Butler & Stevens, 1997). In the category of modifications of the test, the following may be included: bilingual translations and glossaries (either in English or the student's native language). Accommodations such as flexible time limits, flexible setting, and/or the reading and explanation of directions belong to the category of modifications of the test procedures.

Abedi, Hofstetter, and Lord (2004) focus their attention on the effectiveness of EL accommodations. Effective accommodations should level the playing field for the ELs, and test modifications should help ELs overcome the language barrier. If the language barrier is reduced, the test becomes a measure of ELs' academic content knowledge and not of their language proficiency.

An example of this would be using a specialized glossary (defined as a list of definitions for selected words, terms, or phrases in a text) as opposed to a standard dictionary. For example, in English, there are several definitions for the word "view."

Let us suppose that a test prompt asks students to "give their own view." If ELs look in the regular dictionary, they will note that the word "view" is defined as a noun and has at least six separate definitions for the word. Non-ELs would probably identify the correct meaning of the word without any linguistic support. However, ELs may be easily confused and overwhelmed by the number of possibilities. This might potentially affect test validity because it measures language proficiency and not content knowledge.

To address this potential validity concern, a specialized glossary that supplies only the definition appropriate to that context should be used instead of a general dictionary. Using a glossary can help ELs understand what the test questions require and will not give them an unfair advantage over their non-EL peers.

Modifications and Accommodations for ELs: Examples and Effectiveness

Testing accommodations have been separated into test modifications and modifications of test procedures. This two-category structure is very broad; therefore, it is more useful to further separate EL accommodation in order to eliminate ambiguity. Mihai (2017) proposed a six-category system to include

1. Accommodation related to time/scheduling (schedule changes, additional time, etc.).
2. Location (preferential seating, private setting, etc.).
3. Directions (in native language, read aloud).
4. Presentation (bilingual version, audio/video recorded).
5. Support (dictionaries, computers, etc.).
6. Response format (in native language, point to responses in English).

Table 7–5 lists the top five most allowed EL test modifications. Most of the elements comprising Mihai's (2017) six-category system are represented; these most popular accommodations also require the least administrative costs. Unquestionably, they are very practical, but are they effective?

Research in the area of accommodations has compared scores of ELs from accommodated and nonaccommodated test administrations in an effort to make sure the validity of the test has been preserved. According to Sireci, Li, and Scarpati (2003), more studies are needed on the effects of accommodations on the actual test performance of nonnative English speakers. For example, many studies have analyzed the adequacy of translation of tests in the native language of the ELs or whether the constructs that needed to be tested in accommodated tests are similar to the ones found in no accommodated versions of the tests.

There have been several studies that looked at the effectiveness of ELs using accommodations in large-scale assessments. For example, in one study investigating the extra time modification, Abedi, Courtney, and Leon (2003) found that ELs who received extra time had significantly higher scores than the students who were not given this accommodation. However, findings from a different study revealed that gains in scores

Table 7–5. *The Top Five EL accommodations*

Accommodation	Category	Number of States
Additional Time	Time/Scheduling	39
Use of Dictionaries	Support	38
Individual/Small-Group Administration	Location	34
Flexible Scheduling	Time/Scheduling	28
Read Aloud of Test in English	Presentation	25

Source: From *Assessing English Language Learners in the Content Areas: A Research-into-Practice Guide for Educators,* by F. Mihai, 2010, p. 72, Table 12, Ann Arbor: University of Michigan Press. Copyright 2010 by University of Michigan Press. Reprinted with permission.

were very small (Abedi, Hofstetter, Baker, & Lord, 2001). Hafner (2000) conducted another study that looked at the effectiveness of additional time for ELs in combination with another modification, extended oral presentations. The findings showed that giving students more time did increase ELs' and non-ELs' scores significantly, compared to the scores of the students who received only extended oral presentation of directions and test items.

Abedi, Courtney, and Leon (2003) looked at the effectiveness of several accommodations, such as a customized English dictionary, a computer test with pop-up glossaries (an option to pop up the glossary definition in a new window when the user clicks on a glossary term), additional time, and small-group administration with ELs in the fourth and eighth grades. Their findings revealed that the ELs in the fourth grade who had access to the computer test and additional time received significantly higher scores than the ELs who took the nonaccommodated version of the math test. ELs in the eighth grade who took the computer test with pop-up glosses scored significantly higher than the EL students who were provided with the customized dictionary or the ELs who took the test under standard conditions. One other important finding of the study revealed that at both grade levels, native English speakers did not perform significantly better when provided with any of the four accommodations. This is very strong evidence for the validity of such accommodations, which are supposed to level the playing field for ELs and not give them an unfair advantage over their non-EL peers.

In a study exploring the effectiveness of using an English glossary containing definitions of nontechnical words, Kiplinger, Haug, and Abedi (2000) administered items selected from the National Assessment of Educational Progress (NAEP) to fourth graders in Colorado. The study found that, after using this accommodation, the scores of ELs did not improve significantly compared to non-ELs. In fact, all students scored better when they took the test under accommodated conditions. The glossary accommodation generated the most gain in scores for ELs, although insignificant from a statistical point of view.

The research on EL accommodations for large-scale literacy assessment is still in beginning stages, and more examination is needed to ensure that the existing accommodations do level the playing field for ELs. Anderson, Liu, Swierzbin, Thurlow, and Bielinski (2000) looked at whether bilingual accommodations provided to ELs during a reading test had an effect on student scores. The bilingual accommodations for the experimental group focused on providing ELs with the questions for the reading test in both English and Spanish. The experimental group ELs had access to test directions and test questions read aloud in Spanish, as well as test questions presented in both languages in writing side by side. The findings revealed that the accommodated EL group had a higher mean score than the unaccommodated group, but the mean scores of the two groups were not significantly different from a statistical point of view. The data from the study also revealed that the accommodations in focus did not give ELs a significant advantage over the native English speakers who participated in the study.

Albus, Bielinski, Thurlow, and Liu (2001) studied whether using a monolingual English dictionary with ELs taking a reading test improved their test performance. The results of their study indicated that there were no significant differences in scores between ELs who received the accommodation and ELs who did not. However, there was a slight gain between the ELs who used the dictionary accommodation and the ELs who were part of the control group and had no access to a dictionary while taking the reading test.

The research on the effectiveness of accommodations for ELs brings to light several important points. First, research findings are mixed and present conflicting results. For some accommodations, some studies found significant gains in scores for ELs taking standardized math assessments, whereas others identified gains in EL scores but without registering a statistical significance. A second point is that accommodations need to be studied in isolation and not combined in clusters of accommodation. One example is additional time, where the effects on EL scores (not only for math but for other content areas as well) are not very clear, mostly because this accommodation was clustered with other accommodations. Finally, one accommodation does not fit all. The research of Abedi, Courtney, Mirocha, Leon, and Goldberg (2005) has revealed that an accommodation that resulted in significant score gains for ELs at one grade level did not work for ELs at a different grade level.

Undoubtedly, there is a need for more research not only on the accommodations that have been previously researched but also on the entire range of available and state-sanctioned EL accommodations. Educators and researchers need to identify what works best for ELs. One example where research has informed the practice of EL accommodations is the language support provided to ELs. Dictionaries and glossaries seem to have a much more positive impact on EL student scores compared to when the test is translated, and research shows there is very little evidence for the effectiveness of dual-language test booklets.

Modifications and Accommodations for ELs with Special Needs: Examples and Effectiveness

There has been an increased need to ensure academic achievement for all students due to current legislation. The NCLB Act required that at least 95% of every subgroup of students (for example, ELs and special education students) must participate in statewide assessment for a district to demonstrate that enrolled students make adequate yearly progress. Consequently, many special education students, ELs with communication disorders included, have access to testing accommodations so they can participate in large-scale tests designed to measure and monitor student progress. Therefore, effective accommodations for ELs with communication disorders are very important in documenting student proficiency in core content areas.

Similar to accommodations for ELs, accommodations for students with disabilities permit changes in the administration of the assessments, allowing students to show what they know academically without negatively affecting the validity of the assessment. Many special education students have difficulty with the nonaccommodated format of standardized assessment. Access to accommodations can potentially improve the test participation and accuracy of students with disabilities (McDonnell, McLaughlin, & Morison, 1997).

Specific accommodations for students with special needs have been recommended. For example, Thurlow, Lazarus, Thompson, and Robey (2002) have proposed a five-category accommodation system, which consists of the following: presentation (large print, Braille, etc.), scheduling/timing (extended time, breaks, etc.), response (proctor/scribe, tape recorder, etc.), equipment/ materials (calculator, abacus, etc.), and setting (carrel, separate room, etc.). Table 7–6 specifies in more detail this five-category accommodation system for students with disabilities.

However, what are some specific accommodations for ELs with special needs? Previously, we analyzed one test that measured English language and literacy proficiency for ELs: the ACCESS for ELLs. We also listed what accommodations are allowed for students with special needs and specifically ELs who are DHH and belong to the larger category of ELs with communication disorders. We noted that these students can participate in the reading and writing sections of the test with few or no accommodations necessary. For the listening and speaking parts of the test, speech-reading with spoken responses for those students who possess these abilities is allowed. This accommodation is determined on a case-by-case basis as determined by the Individual Education Program (IEP) team. Because translating the listening and speaking prompts into sign language is viewed as similar to translating into another spoken language, this accommodation is prohibited, as it changes the construct and has a negative impact on the validity of the test.

Table 7–6. *State-Sanctioned Accommodations for Students with Special Needs*

Category	Accommodations
Presentation	Large Print
	Braille
	Read Aloud
	Sign Interpretation
	Read/Reread/Clarify
	Visual Cues
	Administration by Other
	Additional Examples

continues

Table 7–6. *continued*

Category	Accommodations
Scheduling/Timing	Extended Time
	With Breaks
	Multiple Sessions
	Time Beneficial to Student
	Over Multiple Days
Response	Proctor/Scribe
	Computer or Machine
	Write in Test Booklets
	Tape Recorder
	Communication Device
	Spell Checker/Assistance
	Braille
	Pointing
Equipment/Materials	Amplification Equipment
	Light/Acoustics
	Calculator
	Templates/Graph Paper
	Audio/Video Cassette
	Noise Buffer
	Adaptive or Special Furniture
	Abacus
Setting	Individual
	Small Group
	Carrel
	Separate Room
	Seat Location/Proximity
	Minimize Distractions/Reduced Noise
	Student's Home
	Special Education Classroom

Source: Adapted from *2001 State Policies on Assessment Participation and Accommodations* (Synthesis Report 46), by M. L. Thurlow, S. Lazarus, S. Thompson, & J. Robey, 2002, Minneapolis: University of Minnesota, National Center for Educational Outcomes.

A brief overview of the types of accommodations for ELs with special needs has been discussed. However, these accommodations raise a critical question: Are these accommodations successful in leveling the playing field for ELs with special needs?

To address this question, we look to the research on the accommodations for ELs and non-ELs with special needs. Bolt and Thurlow (2004) surveyed the most allowed large-scale test accommodations for special education students, as well as their effectiveness. Table 7–7 lists the top five most frequent special needs accommodations.

In their analysis of accommodation effectiveness, Bolt and Thurlow (2004) focused on three accommodations: (1) dictated response to scribe, (2) access to large-print test materials, and (3) usage of Braille. These three accommodations have generated a lot controversy in terms of effectiveness (Thurlow, House, Boys, Scott, & Ysseldyke, 2000). The results of their meta-analysis are summarized in Table 7–8.

There has been very limited research done on the effectiveness of large-scale test accommodations for ELs with communication disorders. In general, studies focus on either EL accommodations for students who have no disabilities or on special education accommodations for students who are not ELs. Table 7–9 briefly summarizes the research done on assessing literacy for students with special needs, with an emphasis on students with communication disorders.

Table 7–7. *Most Frequent Special Education Student Accommodations*

Accommodation	Category	Number of States
Individual Administration	Setting	44
Dictated Response to Scribe	Response	43
Small Group Administration	Setting	41
Large Print	Presentation	40
Braille	Presentation	38

Source: Adapted from "Five of the Most Frequently Allowed Testing Accommodations in State Policy," by S. E. Bolt & M. L. Thurlow, 2004, *Remedial and Special Education, 25*(3), 141–152.

Table 7–8. *Research on the Effectiveness of Commonly Allowed Special Needs*

Type of Accommodation	Studies
Dictated Response to Scribe	*Fuchs, Fuchs, Eaton, Hamlett, and Karns (2000):* On math problem-solving items, students with learning disabilities benefited from this accommodation more than the students without disabilities.
	Johnson, Kimball, Brown, and Anderson (2001): Students with disabilities who received this accommodation received significantly higher scores.
	Schulte, Elliott, and Kratochwill (2001): On math assessments, students with disabilities found significant differences between their scores and the scores of students without disabilities on several accommodation clusters that included dictated response.
	De La Paz and Graham (1997): Only small differences between dictated response and written essays.
	Graham (1990): When using a scribe, students with learning disabilities produced longer and higher quality essays.
Large Print	*Fuchs (2000):* No significant difference in scores for students with disabilities.
	Fuchs, Fuchs, Eaton, Hamlett, Binkley, and Crouch (2000): No significant difference in scores for students with disabilities.
	Burk (1999): No significant increase in the scores of students with or without disabilities when using this accommodation on computerized assessments.
	Brown (1998): Significant gains for third grade students with learning disabilities.

Table 7–8. *continued*

Type of Accommodation	Studies
Braille	*Bennett, Rock, and Novatkoski (1989)*: Certain math items, such as the ones that depict certain figures or graphs or the ones that require knowledge of the tally system might be more difficult for students taking the Braille edition of the SAT.
	Bennett, Rock, and Kaplan (1987): Some items on the math portion of the SAT were significantly difficult for visually impaired students taking the Braille edition of the test.

Source: Adapted from *State Participation and Accommodation Policies for Students with Disabilities: 1999 Update* (Synthesis Report 33), by M. L. Thurlow, A. House, C. Boys, D. Scott, & J. Ysseldyke, 2000, Minneapolis: University of Minnesota, National Center for Educational Outcomes.

One important study conducted by Steinberg, Cline, Ling, Cook, and Tognatta (2009) does not directly address the issue of accommodations for ELs but emphasizes the achievement gap of ELs with communication disorders. The researchers looked at the validity and fairness of a state English language arts assessment for students who were DHH and analyzed score performance of four categories of students: nondisabled/non-EL, nondisabled/ELs, DHH/non-ELs, and DHH/ELs. Their analysis considered for consistency across the above-mentioned nondisabled and disabled groups for the fourth- and eighth-grade students. The findings revealed that the performance of students with disabilities was significantly below that of nondisabled students, with a difference of nearly one standard deviation between the mean performances of the two groups. On average, nondisabled ELs had scores slightly below those of non-EL DHH students but significantly below nondisabled non-EL students. A very important finding of the study showed that DHH ELs performed more than 1.5 standard deviations below nondisabled, non-EL students and significantly below the non-EL DHH students. Clearly, there is a very urgent need to reduce this critical achievement gap between ELs with communication disorders and non-ELs.

Table 7–9. Literacy Assessment for Students with Special Needs

Study	Summary
Lollis and LaSasso (2008)	The study analyzed the appropriateness of the North Carolina state-mandated Reading Competency Test when administered to students who are DHH. Eight reviewers, of which four were DHH, rated the reading passages of the exam for difficulty, appropriateness, interest, and structure. Their analysis took into account factors that might influence test performance due to the student's hearing loss, such as cultural bias or disability related stereotyping, content that would be less familiar to students who are DHH.
	50% of the reviewers rated six of the ten passages as being difficult for DHH students. Moreover, five items from the content passages and two items from the literary passages received negative comments from half the reviewers. The conclusion of the study was that a valid test for DHH students requires proactive input on test construction from teachers of DHH students.
Martin (2005)	The study examined the appropriateness of the New York State (NYS) English Language Arts Grade 8 Test for DHH students. For the first part of the study, eight experts (three of whom were deaf), who were teachers of DHH students evaluated the appropriateness of the ELA Grade 8 Test passages. In the second part of the study, the researcher analyzed the test responses of the 44 DHH student participants on the 2004 ELA Grade 8 Test. More than 60% of the reviewers rated the overall difficulty of the eight passages as being hard for students who are DHH and found that 18% of the multiple choice items and 28% of the constructed response ones did not pass the item quality indicators. Specifically, the reviewers identified three skills as not being taught to students prior to test administration: literary device, author point of view and author technique. The test results of 44 DHH students who had taken the exam revealed congruence between the expert opinions on the test items and the students' performances on the test. Only 6 of 25 multiple choice items were correctly answered by 50% of students.

Table 7–9. *continued*

Study	Summary
Cahalan-Laitusis, Cook, and Aicher (2004)	The study investigated test results on third and seventh grade assessments of English/language arts. The analysis employed differential item functioning (DIF), which identifies items that are much harder or easier for group if test takers when compare to a reference group of test takers of the same ability. The researchers compared students with learning disabilities that received a read-aloud accommodation or extra time to two separate reference groups: students with and without disabilities who received no accommodations. The research results indicated that 7–12% of the test items functioned differently for students with learning disabilities that received read-aloud accommodations when compared to either of the reference groups. However, providing the students with learning disabilities with extra time resulted in only 0–1% of the items showing DIF.
LaSasso (1999)	The study looked at the limitations of tests and other assessment instruments that are administered to students during or after reading to measure reading comprehension. The author stated that conclusions about what deaf students learned were based on standardized tests, informal tests, and portfolios The study reviewed documented differences in test-taking abilities of deaf and hearing students, and listed specific compensatory test-taking strategies used by deaf readers. The author suggested instruction needed to include specific test-taking abilities in order to demonstrate mastery of subject matter. Therefore, the author recommended that deaf students needed to be exposed to instruction in multipurpose reading and to different test formats.

A step in the right direction is to provide ELs with communication disorders with appropriate and effective accommodations that can have a positive impact on their academic performance. Based on available research done on EL accommodations, Abedi

(2009) outlines a set of recommendations that should be used in the classification, instruction, and assessment of ELs with special needs in general and ELs with communication disorders in particular:

1. Assessment instruments for ELs with communication disorders should be made as accessible as possible to control for cultural, linguistic, etc. biases. It is important to remember that instruments constructed for the general English-speaking population might not be valid for ELs with communication disorders.
2. Accommodations should level the playing field. For example, for ELs with communication disorders, selected accommodations should directly address either their communication disorder or their language needs.
3. Accommodations should not affect the construct being tested negatively. The validity of accommodations must be established so that the results obtained can be aggregated with the results of non-ELs.
4. Accommodations should be practical and easy to implement.
5. Accommodations should be used in the classroom before large-scale assessments are administered so students become fluent in using them.

The following section discusses how SLP and ESOL professionals can partner to further English learners' language and literacy development.

SLPs and ESOL Professionals—Partners in Language and Literacy Development

The ASHA 2001 position statement *Roles and Responsibilities of SLPs with Respect to Reading and Writing in Children and Adolescents* set the stage for the involvement of the SLP in reading and writing. Specifically, SLPs were challenged to address reading and writing for struggling students and those with communication disorders. The established connections between spoken and written language and the reciprocal relationship between language and literacy competence make the SLP a unique contributor in the implementation of evidence-based literacy strategies and interventions. Since the publication of this position statement, many scholars have discussed, debated, and affirmed the critical role of the SLP in the prevention, assessment, and intervention of reading disabilities (ASHA, 2016a; Catts & Kamhi, 2005; Ehren & Ehren, 2001; Kamhi, Allen, & Catts, 2001; Nelson, 2010; Power deFur, 2018; Ritter, 2009; Schuele, 2017; Schuele & Larrivee, 2004; Spracher, 2000; Zygouris-Coe & Goodwiler, 2013). ASHA's practice documents on written language disorders and spoken language disorders reiterates the relationship between spoken and written language, reading, and writing and highlights the importance of SLPs working collaboratively to develop culturally responsive and linguistically appropriate treatment plans (ASHA, n.d.-a, n.d.-b; Blood, Mamett, Gordon, & Blood, 2010).

A requirement of IDEA (1997) is that intervention must be relevant to the expectations of the general education curriculum. Although SLPs traditionally have been trained in the language base of curriculum, including reading and writing, they have not always been familiar with or involved in incorporating the curriculum in their intervention (Ehren, 2006; Justice, 2006). With the increased emphasis on high-performance standards brought on by educational reform and more emphasis in university training programs on the role of the SLP in language and literacy (Koutsoftas, Maffucci, & Dayalu, 2018; Rosa-Lugo, Mihai, & Nutta, 2017; Waller, 2012), many SLPs have become familiar with approaches and practical strategies that parallel the curriculum and facilitate language and literacy development. Specifically, SLPs work in partnership with other school-based professionals to help students meet the performance standards of a particular school district and state (Rosa-Lugo, Mihai, & Nutta, 2012; Roseberry-McKibben, 2013, 2015; Schraeder, 2012).

The No Child Left Behind Act of 2001 stressed that accountability for all students was the responsibility of all school-based professionals (e.g., mainstream, content area, ESL, bilingual education teachers, and SLPs) who worked with ELs. Specifically, several TESOL position and policy papers and documents

(TESOL, 2003a, 2005a, 2007a, 2010a, 2016) have focused on the preparation and roles of the ESOL professional in the development of language and literacy in ELs. Similar to the SLP, they are charged with implementing evidence-based instructional practices and making instruction comprehensible (Brisk, 2008; Menyuk & Brisk, 2005; Power deFur, 2016; Valdés, Kibler, & Walqui, 2014). However, unlike the SLP, the responsibilities of the ESOL professional primarily focuses on achievement in core subjects using standards-based instruction (TESOL, 2001a, 2001b, 2006, 2009b). What makes this challenging is that ELs must achieve the standards in a language other than their native language and often before the EL is literate in that language.

A significant amount of research has been conducted during the past decades on literacy development in ELs. However, research on effective practices for ELs with a communication disorder is limited. In many instances, research that has been conducted on ELs has been generalized and applied to ELs with language disorders. For example, models to address literacy in ELs that involve native and second languages have been proposed (Gorman & Gillam, 2003; Gutierrez-Clellan, 1994; Klingner, Artiles, & Barletta, 2006; Lesaux & Siegel, 2003; Proctor, August, Carlo, & Snow, 2006; Restrepo & Towle-Harmon, 2008; USDOE/Office of English Language Acquisition, 2017), as well as strategies for ELs in the beginning, intermediate, and advanced stages of literacy (Cloud, Genesee, & Hamayan, 2009). Systematic reviews have been conducted on ELs and literacy development. The goal of these reviews is to identify programs or interventions that can potentially have positive effects on reading achievement and English language development (Institute of Education Science, 2006, 2007a, 2007b; Richards-Tutor, Baker, Gersten, Baker, & Smith, 2016; Thomason & Gorman, 2008).

This chapter does not provide an exhaustive list of strategies and approaches that have been used with ELs or ELs with communication disorders. For example, underlying general principles for effective bilingual service delivery and literacy intervention and resources on clinical and professional are provided in the ASHA Practice Portal (see https://www.asha.org/practice-portal/). Readers are directed to more specific sources for that purpose (i.e., Calderon, 2007; Diaz-Rico, 2004; Cloud, Genesee, & Hamayan, 2009; Peregoy & Boyle, 2017; Pieretti &

Roseberry-McKibben, 2015; Roseberry-McKibben, 2018; Schatz, 2010). However, this chapter does serve as a starting point for the SLP and ESOL professional to consider *purposeful collaboration* in the planning and implementation of intervention services, specific treatment techniques, and programs for students exhibiting a communication disorder.

Summary

This chapter first provided several approaches and practical strategies to facilitate language and literacy development in ELs and ELCDs. Evidence-based approaches and strategies that will facilitate literacy skills in ELs continue to be needed. Research that informs practice suggests that ELs learn best when explicit instruction, modeling, and a multitude of effective strategies are used daily that involve students as active and engaged listeners. Additionally, we presented the third element of our assessment, intervention, and monitoring (AIM) framework (monitoring) and discussed how the effects of intervention or progress in developing English proficiency and literacy are measured through formal assessment. The involvement of all professionals in the development of language and literacy skills for ELs and ELs with communication disorders is necessary. The next chapter will detail concrete steps to be taken for an effective interprofessional collaborative practice (IPP) between SLPs and ESOL professionals, with the assistance and support of school staff and administrators.

8

Directions for an Effective Interprofessional Collaborative Practice (IPP) Between SLPs and ESOL Professionals: The Power of Two +

Introduction

Interprofessional collaboration among various categories of education professionals are key elements in working with ELs with communication disorders. The team-based approach in identifying and educating students with special needs has been mandated since 1975, when Congress passed Public Law 94-142 (Education for All Handicapped Children Act), now known as IDEA (Individuals with Disabilities Education Act) (2004). One of the key provisions of IDEA was the creation of an Individualized Education Program (IEP) for children with special needs, a concept that has at its core a group problem-solving approach to the identification and education of students with special needs. For this reason and many others, all categories of special education have strongly advocated interprofessional collaboration with other educational entities, parents, and school administrators.

Clearly, interprofessional collaboration among SLPs and ESOL professionals can potentially affect the instruction of ELs

315

with communication disorders in a very positive manner. However, in order to occur, interprofessional collaboration needs to be systematic and constant. It is not enough for SLPs, educators, and other decision makers to meet once a year to review IEPs. Meetings should occur regularly and in a very well-defined context. These meetings should not be driven exclusively by compliance issues to avoid litigations. Instead, meetings should be a supportive group process where teachers, SLPs, related service professionals, parents, and administrators work collaboratively as key decision makers in this process.

According to Rosa-Lugo, Mihai, and Nutta (2017), interprofessional collaborative practice or IPP requires providers from different professional backgrounds to work together to deliver culturally responsive, evidence-based services across settings by working with ELs and their families or caregivers to improve educational outcomes (Self, Coufal, & Francois, 2011; WHO, 2010; Zraick, Harten, & Hagstrom, 2014). Table 8–1 is an example of a competency framework, with a core set of descriptors, often used to formulate learning objectives and learning activities to develop and promote interprofessionalism and collaborative practice (D'Amour & Oandasan, 2005; Interprofessional Education Collaborative Expert Panel, 2011; Thistlethwaite, Moran, & World Health Organization Study Group on Interprofessional Education and Collaborative Practice, 2010; WHO, 2010).

Do SLPs and ESOL professionals feel encouraged to foster IPP when working with ELs with communication disorders? What are some of the perceptions, practices, and needs of educational professionals who work with ELs with special needs? A survey of 125 educational professionals working with ELs with special needs in the Washington, DC, area attempted to answer these significant questions (Roache, Shore, Gouleta, & Butkevich, 2003). Most of the participants' responses indicated that they had the training and skills to work with EL students with special needs but were unclear about the roles, responsibilities, and practices of other school professionals who worked with ELs with special needs. Additionally, they noted that they had not received appropriate training on establishing effective frameworks for collaboration.

Notably, another finding revealed that administration often did not provide adequate support to foster collaboration with other school professionals in serving EL students with special

Table 8–1. *Interprofessional Collaborative Practice (IPP) Competencies*

Competency	Examples of Behaviors
Values and Ethics for Interprofessional Practice	• Acknowledges the views and ideas of other professionals • Demonstrates high standard of ethical conduct and acts with integrity with team members • Accepts diversity and individual differences, and respects misunderstandings and shortcomings in other professionals
Roles and Responsibilities for Collaborative Practice	• Knowledge and understanding of the different roles, responsibilities, and expertise of diverse professionals • Recognizes similarities and differences relating to roles, attitudes, and skills • Understanding of role/professional boundaries
Interprofessional Communication	• Communicates effectively with other professionals • Listens to others/team members • Engages in shared decision making
Interprofessional Teams and Teamwork	• Knowledge of, skills for, and positive attitudes toward collaboration with other professionals • Integrates the knowledge and experience of other professionals • Cooperation and accountability

needs. To achieve a successful collaboration, the roles and responsibilities of each professional need to be well defined. Then, collaboration needs to be structured and modeled after successful research-based examples of SLP-ESOL partnerships that generated tangible results for ELs with communication disorders. Last, it is important to have visible support from administration for a successful collaboration effort (Roache et al., 2003).

The Roles of SLPs and ESOL Professionals in Working with ELs with Communication Disorders

A first step to establish an effective interprofessional collaborative practice between SLPs and ESOL professionals is to ensure that both disciplines know exactly what their respective roles and responsibilities are when working with ELs (Honigsfeld & Dove, 2019; Rosa-Lugo & Fradd, 2000). For this reason, let us first examine how the role of the ESOL professional is defined and how they perceive their role. Then, we will look at the role of the SLPs in working with ESOL instructors in school settings, using out our assessment, intervention, and monitoring (AIM) model.

ESOL Professionals: Roles and Perceptions

In accordance with state and federal laws, ESOL programs across the United States must make every effort to implement policies and procedures to meet the educational needs of students whose primary language is not English. A primary goal of all ESOL programs is to increase the proficiency levels of ELs in the areas of listening, speaking, reading, and writing. To achieve this goal, ESOL professionals assist in the identification of EL students, using appropriate and approved assessment tools. They create and maintain instructional classes that have a positive impact on students' learning the English language so that ELs can function independently and fully in general education classrooms upon passing English language proficiency assessments. To facilitate the academic success of ELs, the ESOL professional works with other instructional team members to (a) plan culturally responsive instruction, (b) use appropriate accommodations and modifications, and (c) implement evidence-based strategies and techniques to make instruction comprehensible for ELs while promoting academic language development.

In addition to addressing the language needs of ELs, ESOL professionals have other roles. They are not simply teaching language; they are also assisting their students with the sometimes-difficult transition to a new culture and set of expectations. As a resource teacher, they work with ELs to understand American culture and encourage students in regular education and work with school faculty and staff to understand other cultures. ESOL professionals also provide social and emotional support for ELs. While developing the language proficiency of their ELs, ESOL professionals promote academic achievement, social growth and acceptance, and self-confidence and self-worth. Many ELs arrive from countries and cultures that are different from the mainstream United States. ESOL professionals are expected to provide support not only for their ELs but also for students' families while they adjust to life in America. Providing opportunities for acculturation and socialization are important aspects of the ESOL professional's role.

ESOL professionals also act as student advocates in the school community. Many times, the parents of ELs do not have the language skills to participate in the decision-making processes involving their children. ESOL professionals often take on the roles and responsibilities of parents and act as a critical liaison between the student and other teachers and staff members. Consequently, ESOL professionals are an essential link between the school and the student's family. This connection can be vital when ELs or their families are isolated as a result of cultural differences or language barriers.

This description of ESOL professionals' roles is applicable to the expectations of ESOL professionals in many programs and schools across the United States. However, it is important to know what ESOL professionals think of their roles and how they view themselves in the educational context in which they function. Are these self-constructed roles congruent with the roles they are expected to perform in accordance with state and federal mandates?

DeGuerrero and Villamil (2000) explored ESL professionals' roles through metaphor analysis. In their study of 22 participants who were ESOL professionals in Puerto Rico, they looked at the metaphors ESOL professionals associated with their roles and identified no less than nine roles, listed in Table 8–2.

It is very important to note that most of the roles listed in Table 8–2 are exclusively addressing the language needs of ELs and do not focus on the other roles of ESOL professionals, such as advocating for their students or collaborating with other teachers and professionals who are teaching ELs. This reiterates

Table 8–2. *ESOL Professionals' Roles*

Role	Definition	Metaphor
Cooperative Leader	The ESOL professional guides and directs students, and establishes an atmosphere of trust in the classroom.	Coach
Challenger/Agent of Change	The ESOL professional creates challenges, brings about change, and procures opportunities for learning.	Gateway to the future
Knowledge Provider	The ESOL professional is the source of language.	Sun
Nurturer	The ESOL professional facilitates language growth and development and mediates language learning by giving constant feedback and support.	Gardener
Innovator	The ESOL professional keeps up with new methods and evidence-based research in the field for classroom implementation	Explorer
Provider of Tools	The ESOL professional makes language available to students as a tool to construct meaning.	Tool carrier
Artist	The ESOL professional approaches teaching as an aesthetic experience and molds learners into works of art.	Potter
Repairer	The ESOL professional corrects students' language, strategies, and attitudes.	Mechanic of the mind
Gym Instructor	The ESOL professional treats students' minds as muscles that need to be trained and exercised.	Aerobics instructor

Source: Adapted from "Exploring ESL Teachers' Roles through Metaphor Analysis," by M. de Guerrero & O. Villamil, 2000, *TESOL Quarterly, 34*(2), 341–351.

the idea that collaboration occurs only when there is administrative commitment and solid and well-established mechanisms in schools and districts.

Role of the Speech-Language Pathologists in ESOL Instruction

What is the role of SLPs in ESOL instruction? Because of SLPs' professional preparation, are they allowed to provide *direct ESOL instruction* to ELs? Briefly said, "no." SLPs do not necessarily have the specialized competencies and the required education necessary to provide ESOL instruction to ELs. ESOL instruction requires academic preparation and experience in areas such as second language acquisition, linguistics, language teaching methodologies, assessment, and practicum, which may or may not be covered in SLPs' preparation programs. Therefore, SLPs without the mandatory training should not provide direct ESOL instruction to ELs. Instead, SLPs should collaborate and consult with ESOL instructors (ASHA, 1998a, 2010a).

SLPs providing services to school-age ELs with communication disorders should know school district policy, state and federal laws, first and second language acquisition, culturally appropriate assessment methods and intervention techniques, and strategies for working with families and other professionals. SLPs should also know the process and procedures for identifying, placing, and serving ELs with special needs as well as the role of the SLP in the area of prevention (i.e., RtI). In providing services to ELs, SLPs should follow guidelines, competencies, and definitions outlined in various ASHA position papers, guidelines, and resources on clinical and professional topics found on the ASHA Practice Portal (see https://www.asha.org/practice-portal/). If the provider of speech and language services is a bilingual SLP, then the professional should meet the standards and best practices found in various ASHA policy documents, and guidelines as well as state and federal requirements that guide their practice in their specific work setting.

As stated before, ESOL instruction should be provided only by professionals with appropriate training and experience. The required knowledge, skills, and competencies for providing

ESOL instruction may go beyond those provided in communication sciences and disorders preservice educational training programs. However, SLPs can play a key role by collaborating with providers of ESOL instruction, at any or all stages of service delivery. These ways of collaborating suggested by ASHA (1998a, 2010a) are listed in Table 8–3. These roles are not mandatory but constitute possible avenues that SLPs and ESOL professionals may choose to engage in collaboration.

Interprofessional Collaborative Practice Models

ASHA (2010a, 2017b) recognizes the critical role that SLPs play in school settings and note that collaboration is one of their major responsibilities in working with children across levels and disorders. Yet, interestingly, a mere 27% of SLPs receive preparation in interprofessional collaborative practice in their preprofessional programs (ASHA, 2017c; Hillier, Civetta, & Pridham, 2010; Ludwig & Kerins, 2019; Rosa-Lugo, Mihai, & Nutta, 2017). Giess and Serianni (2018) point out that while SLPs and educators are skilled in working together to meet the needs of children with special needs, each professional continues to focus on their respective practice area with little integration and coordination of goals and objectives, particularly in the development and execution of the Individual Education Plan (IEP). In order to provide appropriate and effective culturally responsive services to ELs with communication disorders, SLPs and classroom teachers will require a different perspective on collaboration and communication that will result in improved student outcomes (Boshoff & Stewart, 2012; Hillier, Civetta, & Pridham, 2010).

Research suggests that an IPP team approach is a very efficient way to promote positive outcomes for children with communication disorders (Moore-Brown & Montgomery, 2018). Collaboration can be defined as the direct interaction between team members engaged in decision making as they work toward achieving a common goal (Friend & Cook, 2016). For example, collaboration between SLPs and ESOL professionals may involve working on a team for a short period of time, for example,

Table 8–3. *SLP-ESOL Collaboration at Assessment, Intervention, and Monitoring Stages for ELs with Communication Disorders*

Stage of Service Delivery	SLP-ESOL Collaboration

Assessment	At this stage, the SLP may:
	
	1. Collaborate with an ESOL professional on issues such as language development and code-switching in ELs who are developing English proficiency
	
	2. Provide information to and gather data from the ESOL professional including, but not limited to:
	   a. ELs' socialization
	   b. Patterns of first and second language development and language use in the classroom and home
	
	3. Play a critical role in RtI efforts to include:
	   a. Assisting general education classroom teachers and ESOL professionals to meet the needs of students in initial RtI tiers with an emphasis on the relevant language underpinnings of learning and literacy
	   b. Collaborating with ESOL professionals to provide their expertise in language, its disorders, and treatment

Intervention	At this stage, the SLP-ESOL collaboration is an essential aspect of the educational and therapeutic process. This collaboration can occur in many ways, ranging from informal conversations to formal, planned activities. By collaborating, the SLP and ESOL professional should: 1. Share ideas and resources as well as plan and work together to coordinate goals and objectives 2. Evaluate progress toward speech and/or language intervention goals and English language development goals

continues

Table 8–3. *continued*

Stage of Service Delivery	SLP-ESOL Collaboration
Intervention *continued*	3. Coordinate the instruction of English language development with the intervention for the communication disorder
	4. Consider cultural and linguistic factors that affect service delivery
	5. Prepare for and participate in IEP reviews
Monitoring	At this stage, the SLP may:
	1. Consult with ESOL professionals on issues such as the EL's performance on testing completed by the ESOL professional and the EL's performance on testing completed by the SLP
	2. Share evaluation results after the assessment regarding the EL's performance
	3. Collaborate with the ESOL professional in developing an appropriate intervention plan, including:
	a. Adapting curricula to meet the EL's specific needs, such as modifying assignments, activities, and tests
	b. Considering the EL's individual needs and learning style
	c. Selecting appropriate materials and instructional strategies
	d. Involving parents and caregivers in the EL's program of instruction

Source: Adapted from *Provision of Instruction in English as a Second Language by Speech-Language Pathologists in School Settings* [Technical Report], by American Speech-Language-Hearing Association, 1998. Retrieved from http://www.asha.org/policy; *Roles and Responsibilities of Speech-Language Pathologists in Schools* [Professional Issues Statement], by American Speech-Language-Hearing Association, 2010. Retrieved from http://www.asha.org/policy

when implementing specific instructional strategies and interventions for ELs who are struggling (RtI—Tier 1), making placement decisions for ELs with communication disorders, or for a more extended period of time, when team members develop and implement interventions for ELs with communication disorders.

Friend and Cook (2016) note that effective teams have a shared purpose, clearly defined roles, and shared leadership. However, effective teams do not occur without effort; they require time, commitment, and nurturing. According to McCartney (1999), successful collaboration can be threatened by several hurdles. First, team members might have individual assumptions concerning the model of collaboration to be used and different perceptions of their roles and responsibilities in participating and implementing a collaborative initiative. Additionally, members of the team may not be aware of the unique roles and responsibilities of each team member (Rosa-Lugo & Fradd, 2000; Solomon-Rice, Soto, & Robinson, 2018). When team members have overlapping responsibilities for only a subset of goals, collaboration may be limited to the shared tasks. Specifically, the ESOL professional may focus more on getting through the curriculum, whereas speech-language services are provided without considering the common core state standards (National Governors Association, 2011).

Given some of the challenges noted with team development, Schrage (1995) offers another description of what organizations need to consider and implement if they want to encourage collaboration. Particularly, he notes that "collaboration isn't necessarily teamwork; and teamwork isn't certainly collaboration" (p. xv). Collaboration is "an act of shared creation and/or shared discovery" that incorporates multiple perspectives to address a task that results in something of value (Schrage, 1995). Thus, collaboration requires individuals from different backgrounds, perspectives, and varied expertise to build a common ground, a shared language, and a shared goal. While each professional has their specialty and responsibilities, it is important that they draw on each other for ideas and knowledge (Rosa-Lugo & Fradd, 2000).

Despite these difficulties, the outcomes of the collaborative team process can be highly beneficial for the team participants and, more important, for ELs with communication disorders and their families. Team formation can be conceptualized as a developmental process that evolves through stages. Tuckman and Jensen (1977) described a five-stage model of team development: forming, storming, norming, performing, and adjourning.

These stages were used to describe the path that most teams follow to attain high performance. Based on the work of Lowe and Herranen (1978, 1982), Peña and Quinn (2003) looked at team development in speech-language pathology in the context of a school environment. The stages of team development they discussed are listed in Table 8–4.

Table 8–4. *Predictable Stages of Team Development*

Stage	Characteristics
Becoming Acquainted	Polite and impersonal, hierarchical interactions, autocratic leadership
Trial and Error	Intrateam alliances/factions, role conflict, attempts to coordinate and facilitate team function, ambiguity about role on team
Collective Indecision	False assumptions of shared responsibility, with little accomplished; avoidance of conflict and maintenance of equilibrium; decisions by default; general indecision and autocratic leadership
Crisis	Internal or external event forces team members to realize they are functioning ineffectively; crisis has function of either unifying or dissolving team; team members may react emotionally, express anger, concern, or uneasiness; productivity remains low
Tentative Purpose	Renegotiation of roles, realization that team members need to assume shared responsibility, consciousness of purpose, productivity remains low
Resolution	Concerted effort to work together as a team; development of effective communication strategies; genuinely shared leadership, decision making, and responsibility
Team Maintenance	Realization of the greater mission—meeting the client's needs, team functioning is effective, dependent on internal group process, conflicts are resolved quickly and with mutual respect

Source: From "Developing Effective Collaboration Teams in Speech-Language Pathology: A Case Study," by E. D. Peña & R. Quinn R, 2003, *Communications Disorders Quarterly, 24*(2), 53–63. Copyright 2003 by Sage. Adapted with permission.

Their observation and data analysis of the interactions between SLPs and ESOL professionals in classrooms generated several recommendations that SLPs and ESOL professionals should consider if they want to have effective teams. First, ESOL professionals need to be included in the preliminary sessions that are conducted at the onset of any SLP initiative; more specifically, they need to be included in the entry, orientation, and problem identification stages. The result of this inclusion is a shared understanding of the model and process of collaboration, on the one hand, and a set of common goals and purpose, on the other hand. Many times, ESOL professionals believe that once the in-class screening, observations, and evaluations are completed, a more traditional pull-out model will be used and the SLPs will work one-on-one with ELs with communication disorders in a different setting. The presence of ESOL professionals at the initial stages of SLPs' program implementation will ensure that their presence in the classroom will be understood and accepted by teachers, thus making collaboration more effective and diffusing potential crises.

Additionally, collaboration needs to be voluntary. School-based professionals should be provided with rewards and incentive for participation and should be given enough time to participate in the collaboration process. Therefore, the administrators' support for the collaborative process is critical and must be demonstrated through meaningful incentives, including the allocation of time to dedicate to the process. Moreover, collaborators must see each other as peers. To ensure this aspect of collaboration and to foster collegiality, initial stages of any SLP project need to include teaching team members to plan collaboratively while being aware of the roles of different professionals in that process. Learning how to give constructive feedback and how to listen to such feedback may be important training in order to evaluate implementation of a given intervention. Finally, developing a shared definition of collaboration as it refers to the team is an important aspect of an effective collaborative effort.

Prelock, Miller, and Reed (1995) describe the key elements for establishing effective collaborative partnerships in the delivery of services to children with communication disorders. In terms of collaboratively planning and implementing lessons, they propose several transdisciplinary components that collaborative lesson plans need to include for effective delivery.

The proposed framework establishes the roles during planned meetings and during lesson implementation, identifies concerns regarding student performance, selects educational goals, teaching techniques, and materials, and explores key vocabulary that needs to be covered during instruction. Special attention is given to data collection that focuses on student performance during class activities and other assessments. All these elements are outlined in Table 8–5.

Based on these lesson plan components, an example of a collaborative lesson plan adapted from Prelock, Miller, and Reed (1995) is presented in Table 8–6. It is an SLP-ESOL collaborative lesson plan designed for an EL with a communication disorder. The lesson plan contains the targeted curriculum, lists the targeted speech-language goals, and describes the facilitating techniques to address those goals. In addition, the lesson plan details the lesson procedures, targeted vocabulary, materials used, and what types of data are to be collected.

Table 8–5. *Components of Collaborative Lesson Plans*

Component	Description
Roles during Planning Meetings	• Typically, a team meets once every 2 or 3 weeks and plans for a 2- to 3-week unit in 30 to 40 minutes. Initially, most teams should meet weekly for 30 minutes to plan single lessons. As teams became more time efficient, the need for weekly planning meetings will probably decrease.
	• The roles team members can take are as time managers/facilitators of the discussion during the meeting or as recorders responsible for writing the collaboratively planned lesson.
	• The time manager keeps the team on task and goal directed.
	• The facilitator ensures that all aspects of the lesson plan are covered and that all members of the team participate in the planning process.
	• The recorder writes the lesson plan.

Table 8–5. *continued*

Component	Description
Roles during Lesson Implementation	• There are three important roles in collaborative intervention: leader, helper, and data collector. • The leader is responsible for introducing the lesson, providing directions, and primarily teaching the lesson. • The helper keeps an eye on the lesson in progress to ensure the clarity of the message, to assist in student comprehension, and to make sure that the stated objectives are addressed. • The data collector verifies that the objectives are measurable and gathers the data during the presentation of the lesson.
Establishment of Collaborative Concerns	• Following role designation, the team identifies concerns regarding student performance for both identified students and total classroom needs. • By establishing collaborative concerns, a team can determine relevant curricular and speech-language goals.
Selection of Goals	• Based on collaborative concerns, the team decides the number and content of lessons that are needed to be planned, emphasizing goals to address the student's performance.
Facilitating Techniques	• To support the communication needs of the identified student while in the classroom, facilitating techniques often are necessary. • Additionally, other students in the classroom have become familiar with these cues and use them in their interactions with the identified child.

continues

Table 8–5. continued

Component	Description
Brainstorming	• Time is allotted for brainstorming the lesson activity (approximately 5–10 minutes). Once the brainstorming period has ended, a team decision for an activity can be made from the list of suggestions. • When making this decision, the team considers goals for the curriculum and for the identified student.
Outline of Procedures	• The procedures for a collaborative lesson are ordered and instructions and/or models to be used are listed.
Key Vocabulary	• In order to ensure student comprehension, it is critical to identify and teach key vocabulary within the collaborative lesson. Many students with communication disorders demonstrate deficits in learning, categorizing, and applying vocabulary within the classroom context. • The ESOL professional's knowledge of the vocabulary specific to the curriculum allows the SLP to predict breakdowns in understanding. Together, they can assist student learning.
Data Collection	• During lesson planning, a collaborative team decides what data are to be collected and in what manner. • Examples include tally data (a + / – system), narrative data useful for qualifying a process (e.g., noting how a student decodes unfamiliar words when reading a passage), videotapes of classroom interaction, journal entries, homework assignments, etc.
Material Preparation	• Preparing materials is divided equally among team members.
Follow-up Planning	• Follow-up can be implemented through homework, class work, or pull-out therapy.

Source: Adapted from "Collaborative Partnerships in a Language in the Classroom Program," by P. A. Prelock, B. E. Miller, & N. L. Reed, 1995, *Language, Speech, and Hearing Services in Schools, 26,* 286–292.

Table 8–6. *Example of Collaborative Lesson Plan*

Collaborative Classroom Lesson Plan

Grade: Kindergarten   Area: ESOL

PLANNING

Roles During Planning for EL with a Communication Disorder

Facilitator/Time Manager: SLP   Recorder: ESOL Professional

CLASSROOM INSTRUCTION/INTERVENTION

Roles During Classroom Instruction/Intervention

Leader: SLP

Partner: ESOL Professional

Data Collector: ESOL Professional

Establishing Current Collaborative Concerns:

need to get identified child involved; need strategies for turn taking and establishing eye contact

all children having difficulty understanding and applying letter-sound knowledge; need to develop metalinguistic skills

Targeted Curriculum Goals	• Students will identify and differentiate between symbols (e.g., letters, numbers).
Targeted Speech-Language Goals	• Students will recognize that symbols have meaning. • Student will increase attention to the speaker and participation in class discussions. • Student will increase use of intelligible speech when answering questions.
Facilitating Techniques	• ESOL professional will sit by student with a communication disorder to prompt attention. • ESOL professional will correct production of back sounds using "hand to throat" cue.

continues

Table 8–6. continued

Brainstorming Activities	
Procedures	1. Discuss the meaning of symbols.
	2. Have students identify the symbol or signs they see (e.g., restroom, street signs, fire drill, etc.).
	3. Walk around school to find various symbols: take photographs or make drawings for inside vs. outside, restrooms, exit, wet floor, arrows for directions, traffic light, crosswalk, and poison.
	4. Define symbols as signs that have meaning and can look like pictures, numbers, or letters.
Targeted Vocabulary	• symbol • letter • sign • sound
Materials	• photos/drawings of signs/symbols
Data Collection	1. Tally the number of times the student raises hand to volunteer and makes eye contact with leader.
	2. Tally the number of times the student produces back sounds and is intelligible
	3. Describe students' understanding of signs/symbols and the application to letters/sounds.
Follow-Up	1. Discuss the words and/or numbers on photos of signs that give the signs meaning.
	2. Prepare a homework assignment that requires student to draw a sign found in their home/neighborhood. Student will provide the meaning of chosen sign.

Source: Adapted from "Collaborative Partnerships in a Language in the Classroom Program," by P. A. Prelock, B. E. Miller, & N. L. Reed, 1995, *Language, Speech, and Hearing Services in Schools, 26,* 286–292.

The Power of Two + : Making Administrators Part of the Collaborative Process

It is true that the major players in an SLP-ESOL collaborative initiative are the SLPs and ESOL professionals, but administrators are important and powerful team members (Ermeling & Graff-Ermeling, 2016). Administrative support is critical to the success of collaboration between SLPs and ESOL professionals. Administrators' engagement in and support of collaboration are constantly cited in research as factors that have a strong influence on the success of professional collaboration (Fullan, 2014; Honigsfield & Dove, 2019). Many elements of effective collaboration, ranging from simple verbal encouragement to release time and money, are contingent on school administrators who are committed to supporting collaborative, inclusive learning environments for ELs. Given the importance of the role of the administrator in developing a school culture that promotes collaborative instructional practices, it is critical to consider how the SLP and ESOL team engages administrators to support interprofessional collaborative practice (IPP).

Rea (2005) has several suggestions that the SLP-ESOL team should consider for the successful integration of administrators in the team's IPP efforts. First, the SLP-ESOL team should involve administrators from the incipient stages of team building and goal setting. The SLP-ESOL team should share with administrators the team's long- and short-term implementation strategies, the research base that supports the instruction, and the anticipated need for resources. SLP and ESOL professionals should not assume that administrators know everything there is to know about collaboration or the practices that the SLP and ESOL professional can engage in to collaboratively ensure the success of ELs and, specifically, ELs with communication disorders. Information about evidence-based practices and successful collaboration models should be shared.

Once the instruction process has started and the goals have been established, the SLP-ESOL team should schedule an observation. A preobservation conference is recommended so that administrators and the team can discuss the purpose of the observation and what the role and responsibility of each professional will be in the specific context. Setting specific times for observations increases the likelihood that the administrator will have an opportunity to see the team combine their competencies, knowledge, and skills to facilitate the success of ELs. The team will also have the opportunity to highlight specific aspects of their initiative. After observations, the teams should ask administrators for feedback on the team's performance and incorporate their suggestions in future collaborative initiatives. If administrators cannot participate in class observations, the team can videotape their class and share particularly interesting segments with their administrator. It's important not only to choose positive instances but also to share problematic examples. This will provide administrators with the opportunity to provide feedback and constructive criticism.

The SLP-ESOL team should also make a special effort to involve parents as collaborators and contributors. To improve participation, collaboration, and service delivery with families from diverse backgrounds, professionals must understand and respect their culturally specific beliefs and values (Garcia, Mendez Pérez, & Ortiz, 2000; Kummerer, Lopez-Reyna, & Hughes, 2007; Lian & Fontanez-Phelan, 2001; Rodriguez & Olswang, 2003; Salas-Provance, Erickson, & Reed, 2002). Barriers to successful parental collaboration have been categorized as logistical or attitudinal (Nathenson-Mejia, 1994; Navarette, 1996; Violand Sanchez, Sutton, & Ware, 1991). When working with diverse parents, it is critical that professionals identify these potential barriers (i.e., language, time, money, safety, child care concerns, and investing in strategies to foster parent decision making).

Professional development is an area where the SLP-ESOL team can involve administrators quite extensively. Numerous professional development opportunities are available at the local, state, or national level. The SLP-ESOL-administrator team can share their initiatives on successful collaborations with other professionals in the field and obtain feedback from their colleagues with similar challenges and initiatives.

Creating interprofessional collaborative practice environments is not an easy task. It requires effort, dedication, and action on everyone's part to include administrators. SLP and

ESOL professionals should encourage administrators to be a leader in collaborative efforts. Without the explicit support of administrators, the success of the SLP-ESOL team is questionable and can be a barrier in creating a supportive learning environment for ELs with a communication disorder.

Summary and Final Thoughts

To illustrate how this text can be used by SLP and ESOL professionals, let's examine the case of a hypothetical student named Alejandro, who is a 7-year-old Spanish-speaking EL in a second-grade English-only classroom. Alejandro has behavior problems and does not always participate in class tasks. His oral language proficiency test results show that he is limited in both English and Spanish. A bilingual general language performance test indicates that his Spanish performance is normal, but his English performance is below average. The various professionals working with Alejandro need to determine if he has a communication disorder, a disability, or if his school performance is related to his limited English proficiency and perhaps other factors. Alejandro's dilemma is offered as an example of circumstances that require professionals to have the valuable information presented in this book. Given the information presented in the book chapters, Alejandro's situation is best addressed through the collaboration of the SLPs and ESOL professionals at his school. Interprofessional collaborative practice partnerships between SLPs and ESOL professionals have very important implications for how school SLPs and ESOL professionals might approach assessment and classroom interventions for ELs and, specifically, ELs with communication disorders in a school setting.

Chapter 1 provides the backdrop for the merging of two particular disciplines, speech-language pathology and English as a second language to address the needs of English learners in general and English learners with communication disorders. Well-prepared professionals in both fields would be familiar with the content of Chapter 2, which describes the general EL population in the United States and offers definitions of the categories of ELs, as well as ELs with communication disorders.

Chapter 3 considers the role and responsibilities of SLPs and ESOL professionals in working with ELs and ELCDs, and Chapter 4 lays the foundational knowledge for analyzing whether Alejandro's English language development shows tendencies of a disorder or if it follows a normal process, offering an in-depth explanation of second language acquisition. In order for SLPs to conduct an accurate assessment of a communication disorder, they must be able to distinguish normal progression in a second language from those aspects of language that are characteristic of a communication disorder. When professionals are familiar with the natural variation in the language acquisition process and the different contexts of acquiring the language, they can begin to identify any traits that fall outside the expected range. Making a decision about a language disorder is a process that should take place over time, with multiple opportunities for observing and analyzing the student's language use. Knowing what to look for and documenting students' strengths and weaknesses is an important step in the identification of potential disorders.

Building on the information learned about general second language acquisition, Chapter 5 offers a definition of literacy and provides an overview of literacy development in ELs. Although there are many commonalities between first and second language reading and writing, several distinctions exist that could affect Alejandro's literacy skills. In this chapter, SLPs and ESOL professionals learn that they should pay attention to Alejandro's literacy in Spanish, oral language proficiency in English, age of arrival to the U.S. mainland, expectations of the school experience, and his parents' educational levels. In addition, the first language issues that affect his literacy development in English include the contrasts between the English and Spanish languages, Alejandro's vocabulary knowledge in both languages, and his awareness of language in both English and Spanish, among other factors (Anderson, 2008). All these variables must be considered to determine if his performance is a result of a communication disorder or related to his stage of second language acquisition.

Understanding the definition of language proficiency and the importance of identification practices and protocols used by SLPs and ESOL professionals to determine language proficiency are the focus of Chapters 6. This chapter introduces our assessment/intervention/monitoring (AIM) model and provides information about procedures and specific standardized tests used to assess ELs and ELs with communication disorders. The chapter concludes with a discussion on the importance of using multiple data sources to determine if Alejandro has a communication disorder or is demonstrating characteristics of a second language learner.

Because one focus of this text is literacy, in Chapter 7, we explore the various approaches and practical strategies in literacy instruction, which is the second component of our AIM model. By combining theory, research, and practice, we have explored several instructional strategies used in the instruction of ELs and adapted for use with ELs with communication disorders. Classroom practices and practical strategies to facilitate and support Alejandro's literacy development are offered as ways that can be used to improve his phonemic awareness, knowledge of phonics, fluency, vocabulary, and text comprehension. Moreover, suggestions were provided to Alejandro's professional team on how they can work together to facilitate his oral language and writing development. Chapter 7 also includes the third element, monitoring of our AIM model. We looked at monitoring from the perspective of large-scale assessments, with special attention on the analysis of test accommodations.

To understand the basis of educational decisions made during the literacy instruction of ELs with communication disorders, we focus on the critical role of the SLP and ESOL professional in working with ELs in Chapter 8. Specifically, we highlight the advantages and importance of interprofessional collaborative practice in the four key components of language and literacy development for ELs with communication disorders (Figure 8–1). For example, one result of SLP-ESOL teamwork is that SLPs know what the literacy curriculum goals and classroom expectations are and ESOL professionals are more aware of how communication disorders affect the classroom performance of ELs. SLPs provide techniques to facilitate language and literacy development in ELs with communication disorders. By building on these techniques, ESOL professionals can continue to address the communication needs of ELs with communication disorders through the provision of modified instruction and feedback.

Finally, the interprofessional collaborative practice between the two professionals, the SLP and the ESOL professional, ensures continuity in practice and across settings, with the goal

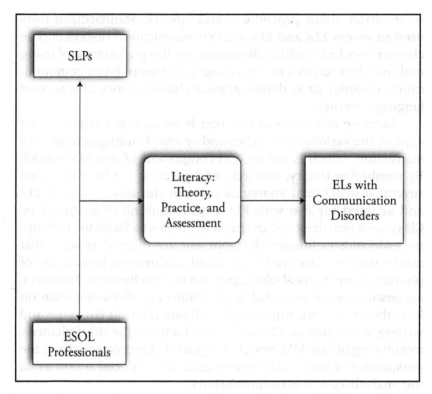

Figure 8–1. Four key components of literacy development for ELs with communication disorders.

of ensuring that ELs with communication disorders succeed in the classroom. By collecting data on effective language and literacy interventions for ELs and collaboration situations, we can base our instructional decisions on evidence-based research. The benefits of this type of research effort are enormous and can only contribute in a positive manner to the success of language development and literacy acquisition for ELs with communication disorders.

References

Abedi, J. (2003). The No Child Left Behind Act and English language learners: Assessment and accountability issues. *Educational Researcher, 33*(1), 4–14.

Abedi, J. (2008). Classification system for English language learners: Issues and recommendations. *Educational Measurement Issues and Practice, 27*(3), 17–31.

Abedi, J. (2009). English language learners with disabilities: Classification, assessment, and accommodation issues. *Journal of Applied Testing Technology, 10*(2), 1–30.

Abedi, J., Courtney, M., & Leon, S. (2003). *Research-supported accommodations for English language learners in the NAEP* (CSE Tech. Rep. No. 586). Los Angeles, CA: University of California's National Center for Research on Evaluation, Standards, and Student Testing.

Abedi, J., Courtney, M., Mirocha, J., Leon, S., & Goldberg, J. (2005). *Language accommodations for English language learners in largescale assessments: Bilingual dictionaries and linguistic modification* (CSE Tech. Rep. No. 666). Los Angeles, CA: University of California's National Center for Research on Evaluation, Standards, and Student Testing.

Abedi, J., Hofstetter, C. H., & Lord, C. (2004). Assessment accommodations for English language learners: Implications for policy-based empirical research. *Review of Education Research, 74*(1), 1–28.

Abella, R., Urritia, J., & Shneyderman, A. (2005). An examination of the validity of English-language achievement test scores in an English language learner population. *Bilingual Research Journal, 29*(1), 127–144.

Accurso, K., Gebhard, M., & Purington, S. B. (2017). Analyzing diverse learners' writing in mathematics: Systemic functional linguistics in secondary pre-service teacher education. *International Journal for Mathematics Teaching & Learning, 18*(1), 84–108.

Acevedo, M. A. (1993). Development of Spanish consonants in preschool children. *Journal of Childhood Communication Disorders, 15*(2), 9–15.

Adler, C. R. (Ed.). (2001). *Put reading first: The research building blocks for teaching children to read.* National Institute for Literacy. Retrieved from http://www.nifl.gov/partnershipforreading/publications/reading_first1text.html

Alatis, J. E. (1987). The growth of professionalism in TESOL: Challenges and prospects for the future. *TESOL Quarterly, 21*(1), 9–19.

Albers, C., Kenyon, D., & Boals, T. (2009). Measures for determining English language proficiency and the resulting implications for instructional provision and intervention. *Assessment for Effective Intervention, 34*(2), 74–85.

Albus, A., Bielinski, J., Thurlow, M., & Liu, K. (2001). *The effect of simplified English language dictionary on a reading test* (LEP Projects Report 1). Minneapolis, MN: University of Minnesota, National Center on Educational Outcomes.

Alderson, J. C. (1984). Reading in a foreign language: A reading problem or a language problem? In J. C. Alderson & A. H. Urquhart (Eds.), *Reading in a foreign language.* London, UK: Longman.

Alexander, K., & Alexander, M. D. (2018). *American public-school law* (9th ed.). St. Paul, MN: West Academic.

Alfano, A. R., & Douglas, M. (2018). Facilitating preliteracy development in children with hearing loss when the home language is not English. *Topics in Language Disorders, 38*(3), 194–201. doi:10.1097/TLD.0000000000000156

Al-Issa, A. (2006). Schema theory and L2 reading comprehension: Implications for teaching. *Journal of College Teaching and Learning, 3*(7), 41–48.

Alvear, S. A. (2018). The additive advantage and bilingual programs in a large urban school district. *American Educational Research Journal.* Advance online publication. doi:10.3102/0002831218800986

American Speech-Language-Hearing Association. (n.d.-a). *2014 Standards and implementation procedures for the certificate of clinical competence in speech-language pathology.* Retrieved from https://www.asha.org/Certification/2014-Speech-Language-Pathology-Certification-Standards/

American Speech-Language-Hearing Association. (n.d.-b). *ASHA practice policy.* Retrieved from http://www.asha.org/policy/type.htm

American Speech-Language-Hearing Association. (n.d.-c). *Bilingual service delivery.* Retrieved from https://www.asha.org/PRPSpecific Topic.aspx?folderid=8589935225&section=Key_Issues

American Speech-Language-Hearing Association. (n.d.-d). *Collaborating with interpreters, transliterators, and translators* [Practice portal]. Retrieved from http://www.asha.org/Practice-Portal/Professional-Issues/Collaborating-With-Interpreters/

American Speech-Language-Hearing Association. (n.d.-e). *Written language disorders* [Practice portal]. Retrieved from https://www.asha.org/PRPSpecificTopic.aspx?folderid=8589942549&section=Roles_and_Responsibilities

American Speech-Language-Hearing Association. (n.d.-f). *Examples of state speech-language eligibility guidelines.* Retrieved from http://www.asha.org/slp/schools/prof-consult/eligibility.htm

American Speech-Language-Hearing Association. (n.d.-g). *Spoken language disorders.* Retrieved from https://www.asha.org/Practice-Portal/Clinical-Topics/Spoken-Language-Disorders/

American Speech-Language-Hearing Association. (1983). Position paper: Social dialects and implications of the position on social dialects. *ASHA, 25*(9), 23–27.

American Speech-Language-Hearing Association. (1985). Clinical management of communicatively handicapped minority language populations. *ASHA, 27*(6), 29–32.

American Speech-Language-Hearing Association. (1987). *Multicultural professional education in communication disorders: Curriculum approaches.* Rockville, MD: Author.

American Speech-Language-Hearing Association. (1989). *Bilingual speech-language pathologists and audiologists: Definition* [Relevant paper]. Retrieved from http://www.asha.org/policy

American Speech-Language-Hearing Association. (1992). *Professional certification standards.* Rockville, MD: Author.

American Speech-Language-Hearing Association. (1993). *Definitions of communication disorders and variations* [Relevant paper]. Retrieved from http://www.asha.org/policy

American Speech-Language-Hearing Association. (1998a). *Provision of instruction in English as a second language by speech-language pathologists in school settings* [Position statement]. Retrieved from http://www.asha.org/policy

American Speech-Language-Hearing Association. (1998b). *Students and professionals who speak English with accents and nonstandard dialects: Issues and recommendations* [Position statement]. Retrieved from http://www.asha.org/policy

American Speech-Language-Hearing Association. (1998c). *Students and professionals who speak English with accents and nonstandard dialects: Issues and recommendation* [Technical report]. Retrieved from http://www.asha.org/policy

American Speech-Language Hearing Association. (2000). *Guidelines for the roles and responsibilities of the school-based speech-language pathologist.* Retrieved from http://www.asha.org/policy

American Speech-Language-Hearing Association. (2001). *Roles and responsibilities of speech-language pathologists with respect to reading and writing in children and adolescents* [Position statement]. Retrieved from http://www.asha.org/policy

American Speech-Language-Hearing Association. (2002a). *Knowledge and skills needed by speech-language pathologists with respect to reading and writing in children and adolescents* [Knowledge and skills]. Retrieved from http://www.asha.org/policy

American Speech-Language-Hearing Association. (2002b). *A workload analysis approach for establishing speech-language caseload standards in the schools* [Guidelines, position statement, and technical report]. Retrieved from http://www.asha.org/policy

American Speech-Language-Hearing Association. (2003a). *American English dialects* [Technical report]. Retrieved from http://www.asha .org/policy

American Speech-Language-Hearing Association. (2003b). *Implementation guide: A workload analysis approach for establishing speech language caseload standards in the schools.* Rockville, MD: Author.

American Speech-Language-Hearing Association. (2004a). *Evidence-based practice in communication disorders: An introduction* [Technical report]. Retrieved from http://www.asha.org/policy

American Speech-Language-Hearing Association. (2004b). *Knowledge and skills needed by speech-language pathologists and audiologists to provide culturally and linguistically appropriate services* [Knowledge and skills]. Retrieved from http://www.asha.org/policy

American Speech-Language-Hearing Association. (2004c). *Admission/discharge criteria in speech-language pathology* [Guidelines]. Retrieved from http://www.asha.org/policy

American Speech-Language-Hearing Association. (2005a). *Cultural competence* [Issues in ethics]. Retrieved from http://www.asha.org/ policy

American Speech-Language-Hearing Association. (2005b). *Evidence based practice in communication disorders* [Position statement]. Retrieved from http://www.asha.org/policy

American Speech-Language-Hearing Association. (2005c). *Standards and implementation procedures for the certificate of clinical competence in speech-language pathology.* Retrieved from http://www .asha.org/certification/2005SLPStdRevisions.htm

American Speech-Language-Hearing Association. (2006). *Professional performance review process for the school-based speech-language pathologist.* Retrieved from http://www.asha.org/policy

American Speech-Language-Hearing Association. (2007). *Scope of practice in speech-language pathology* [Scope of practice]. Retrieved from http://www.asha.org/policy

American Speech-Language-Hearing Association. (2008a). *Bylaws of the American Speech-Language-Hearing Association* [Bylaws]. Retrieved from http://www.asha.org/policy

American Speech-Language-Hearing Association. (2008b). *Communication facts: Special populations: Literacy—2008 edition*. Retrieved from http://www.asha.org/research/reports/literacy.htm

American Speech-Language-Hearing Association. (2010a). *Code of ethics* [Ethics]. Retrieved from http://www.asha.org/policy and http://www.asha.org/docs/html/ET2010-00309.html

American Speech-Language-Hearing Association. (2010b). *Employment settings*. Retrieved from http://www.asha.org/careers/professions/EmploymentSettings.htm

American Speech-Language-Hearing Association. (2010c). *Highlights and trends: ASHA counts for year-end 2010*. Retrieved from http://www.asha.org/uploadedFiles/2010-Member-Counts.pdf

American Speech-Language-Hearing Association. (2010d). *Roles and responsibilities of speech-language pathologists in schools* [Professional issues statement]. Retrieved from http://www.asha.org/policy

American Speech-Language-Hearing Association. (2011a). *CAA-accredited academic program statistics*. Retrieved from http://www.asha.org/academic/accreditation/CAA_Program_Stats.htm

American Speech-Language-Hearing Association. (2011b). *The clinical education of students with accents* [Professional issues statement]. Retrieved from https://www.asha.org/policy/pi2011-00324/

American Speech-Language-Hearing Association. (2011c). *Cultural competence in professional service delivery* [Professional issues statement]. Retrieved from http://www.asha.org/policy

American Speech-Language-Hearing Association. (2013). *Cultural and linguistic competence*. Retrieved from http://www.asha.org/Practice/ethics/Cultural-and-Linguistic-Competence/

American Speech-Language-Hearing Association. (2016a). *Code of ethics* [Ethics]. Retrieved from http://www.asha.org/policy/

American Speech-Language-Hearing Association. (2016b). *Every student succeeds act analysis*. Retrieved from https://www.asha.org/uploadedFiles/Every-Student-Succeeds-Act-Key-Issues.pdf

American Speech-Language-Hearing Association. (2016c). *Roles and responsibilities of speech-language pathologists in schools* [Policy documents]. Retrieved from https://www.asha.org/uploadedFiles/Roles-Responsibilities-SLPs-Schools-Poster.pdf

American Speech-Language-Hearing Association. (2016d). *Scope of practice in speech-language pathology* [Scope of practice]. Retrieved from http://www.asha.org/policy/

American Speech-Language-Hearing Association. (Ed.). (2016e). *Interprofessional education and interprofessional practice in communication sciences and disorders: An introduction and case-based examples of implementation in education and health care settings*.

Rockville, MD: American Speech-Language-Hearing Association. Retrieved from http://www.asha.org/uploadedFiles/IPE-IPP-Reader-eBook.pdf

American Speech-Language-Hearing Association. (2017a). *Bylaws of the American speech-language-hearing association* [Bylaws]. Retrieved from http://www.asha.org/policy

American Speech-Language-Hearing Association. (2017b). *Data snapshot: ASHA bilingual service providers, year-end 2016.* Retrieved from http://www.asha.org/uploadedFiles/Demographic-Profile-Bilingual-Spanish-Service-Members.pdf

American Speech-Language-Hearing Association. (2017c). *Practice and curriculum analysis for the profession of speech-language pathology.* Rockville, MD: Author.

American Speech-Language-Hearing Association. (2017d). *Issues in ethics: Cultural and linguistic competence.* Retrieved from https://www.asha.org/Practice/ethics/Cultural-and-Linguistic-Competence/

American Speech-Language-Hearing Association. (2017e). *Bilingual service delivery* [Practice portal]. Retrieved from http://www.asha.org/Practice-Portal/Professional-Issues/Bilingual-Service-Delivery/

American Speech-Language-Hearing Association. (2018). *2020 Standards for the certificate of clinical competence in speech-language pathology.* Retrieved from https://www.asha.org/certification/2020-SLP-Certification-Standards

American Speech-Language-Hearing Association. (2019a). *Cultural competence.* Retrieved from https://www.asha.org/practice-portal/

American Speech-Language-Hearing Association. (2019b). *ASHA/N-CEP evidence-based systematic reviews.* Retrieved from https://www.asha.org/Research/EBP/EBSRs/

American Speech-Language-Hearing Association. (2019c). *ASHA summary membership and affiliation counts, year-end 2018.* Retrieved from http://www.asha.org

American Speech-Language-Hearing Association. (2019d). *Demographic profile of ASHA members providing bilingual services, year-end 2018.* Retrieved from http://www.asha.org

Anaby, D. R., Campbell, W. N., Missiuna, C., Shaw, S. R., Bennett, S., Khan, S., . . . GOLDS (Group for Optimizing Leadership and Delivering Services). (2019). Recommended practices to organize and deliver school-based services for children with disabilities: A scoping review. *Child Care Health Development, 45,* 15–27.

Anaya, J., Peña, E., & Bedore, L. (2018). Conceptual scoring and classification accuracy of vocabulary testing in bilingual children. *Language, Speech, and Hearing Services in Schools, 49*(1), 85–97.

Anderson, M., Liu, K., Swierzbin, B., Thurlow, M., & Bielinski, J. (2000). *Bilingual accommodations for limited English proficient students on statewide reading rests: Phase 2* (Minnesota Rep. No. 31). Minneapolis, MN: National Center for Educational Outcomes.

Anderson, N. B. (1992). Understanding cultural diversity. *American Journal of Speech-Language Pathology, 1,* 11–12.

Anderson, N. J. (2008a). *Practical English language teaching: Reading.* New York, NY: McGraw-Hill.

Anderson, N. J. (2008b). *Active skills for reading, Book 3* (2nd ed.). Boston, MA: Heinle Cengage.

Anderson, N. J. (2009). ACTIVE reading: The research base for a pedagogical approach in the reading classroom. In Z. Han & N. J. Anderson (Eds.), *Second language reading research and instruction: Crossing the boundaries.* Ann Arbor, MI: University of Michigan Press.

Anderson, N. J., & Nunan, D. (2008). *Practical English language teaching: PELT.* New York, NY: McGraw-Hill.

Anderson, R. (1995). Spanish morphological and syntactic development. In H. Kayser (Ed.), *Bilingual speech-language pathology: An Hispanic focus* (pp. 41–74). San Diego, CA: Singular.

Antunez, B. (2002a). Implementing reading first with English language learners. *Directions in Language and Education, 15.* Retrieved from http://www.ncela.gwu.edu/pubs/directions/15.pdf

Antunez, B. (2002b). *The preparation and professional development of teachers of English language learners.* Washington, DC: ERIC Clearinghouse on Teaching and Teacher Education (ERIC Document Reproduction Service No. ED 477 724).

Archibald, L. (2017). SLP-educator classroom collaboration: A review to inform reason-based practice. *Autism & Developmental Language Impairments, 2,* 1–17.

Arias, G., & Friberg, J. (2017). Bilingual Language Assessment: Contemporary versus recommended practice in American schools. *Language, Speech, and Hearing Services in Schools, 48*(1), 1–15.

Artiles, A. J., & Klingner, J. K. (Eds.). (2006). Forging a knowledge base on English language learners with special needs: Theoretical, population, and technical issues. *Teachers College Record, 108,* 2187–2438.

Asaad Daana, H. (2018). Phonological development and phonological processes in the speech of an English-Arabic bilingual child. *International Journal of Applied Linguistics and English Literature, 7*(5), 197–206. doi:10.7575/aiac.ijalel.v.7n.5p.197

ASHA Leader. (2007). The state of the evidence: ASHA develops levels of evidence for communication sciences and disorders. *ASHA Leader, 12*(3), 8–9, 24–25.

August, D. (2003). *Supporting the development of English literacy in English language learners: Key issues and promising practices* (Rep. No. 61). Baltimore, MD: CRESPAR/Johns Hopkins University. Retrieved from http://www.csos.jhu.edu/crespar/techReports/ Report61.pdf

August, D., Carlo, M., Dressler, C., & Snow, C. (2005). The critical role of vocabulary development for English language learners. *Learning Disabilities Research and Practice, 20*(1), 50–57.

August, D., & Shanahan, T. (Eds.). (2006). *Developing literacy on second language learners: Report of the National Literacy Panel on language minority children and youth.* Mahwah, NJ: Lawrence Erlbaum.

August, D., Shanahan, L., & Shanahan, T. (2006). *Developing literacy in second language learners: Lessons from the Report of the National Literacy Panel on language minority children and youth.* New York, NY: Routledge.

Ausubel, D. P. (1968). *Educational psychology, a cognitive view.* New York, NY: Holt, Rinehart and Winston.

Baker, C. (2001). *Foundations of bilingual education and bilingualism* (3rd ed.). Clevedon, UK: Multilingual Matters.

Ballantyne, K. G., Sanderman, A. R., & Levy, J. (2008). *Educating English language learners: Building teacher capacity.* Washington, DC: National Clearinghouse for English Language Acquisition. Retrieved from http://www.ncela.gwu.edu/practice/mainstream_teachers.htm

Bardack, S. (2010). *Common ELL terms and definitions.* Washington, DC: English Language Learner Center, American Institutes for Research. Retrieved from https://www.air.org/sites/default/files/downloads/report/NEW_-_Common_ELL_TERMS_AND_DEFINITIONS_6_22_10_0.pdf

Barragan, B., Castilla-Earls, A., Martinez-Nieto, L., Restrepo, M. A., & Gray, S. (2018). Performance of low-income dual language learners attending English-only schools on the Clinical Evaluation of Language Fundamentals–Fourth Edition, Spanish. *Language, Speech, and Hearing Services in Schools, 49*(2), 292–305.

Barron, V., & Menken, K. (2002, August). What are the characteristics of the shortage of teachers qualified to teach English language learners? *AskNCELA, 14.* Retrieved from http://www.ncela.gwu.edu/expert/faq/14shortage.htm

Bartlett, F. C. (1932). *Remembering: A study in experimental and social psychology.* Cambridge, UK: Cambridge University Press.

Bartolomé, L. (2002). Creating an equal playing field: Teachers as advocates, border crossers, and cultural brokers. In Z. F. Beykont (Ed.), *The power of culture: Teaching across language difference* (pp. 167–191). Cambridge, MA: Harvard Education Publishing Group.

Batsche, G., Elliott, J., Graden, J., Grimes, J., Kovaleski, J., & Prasse, D. (2005). *Response to intervention: Policy considerations and imple-*

mentation. Alexandria, VA: National Association of State Directors of Special Education.

Battle, D. (2002). *Communication disorders in multicultural populations* (3rd ed.). Woburn, MA: Butterworth-Heinemann.

Bauer, K. L., Iyer, S. N., Boon, R. T., & Fore, C. (2010). 20 ways for classroom teachers to collaborate with speech-language pathologists. *Intervention in School and Clinic, 45*(5), 333–337.

Bear, D. R., Invernizzi, M., Templeton, S., & Johnston, F. (2019). *Words their way: Word study for phonics, vocabulary, and spelling instruction* (7th ed.). Upper Saddle River, NJ: Pearson Prentice-Hall.

Beare, S. (2000) *Differences in content generating and planning processes of adult L1 and L2 proficient writers* (PhD thesis). University of Ottawa, Canada.

Beck, A. R. (1995). Language assessment methods for three age groups of children. *Journal of Communication Development, 17*(2), 51–56.

Beck, I. L., McKeown, M. G., & Kucan, L. (2002). *Bringing words to life: Robust vocabulary instruction.* New York, NY: Guilford Press.

Bedore, L. M., & Peña, E. D. (2008). Assessment of bilingual children for identification of language impairment: Current findings and implications for practice. *International Journal of Bilingual Education and Bilingualism, 11*(1), 1–29.

Bedore, L. M., Peña, E. D., Garcia, M., & Cortez, C. (2005). Conceptual versus monolingual scoring: When does it make a difference? *Language, Speech, and Hearing Services in Schools, 36*, 188–200.

Beers, K. (2003). *When kids can't read—What teachers can do.* Portsmouth, NH: Heinemann.

Berko-Gleason, J. (1958). The child's learning of English morphology. *Word, 14*, 150–177.

Berman, R. (1994). Learner's transfer of writing skills between languages. *TESL Canada Journal, 12*(1), 29–46.

Bernhardt, E. (2005). Progress and procrastination in second language reading. *Annual Review of Applied Linguistics, 25*, 133–150.

Bernhardt, E., & Kamil, M. L. (1995). Interpreting relationships between L1 and L2 reading: Consolidating the linguistic threshold and the linguistic interdependence hypotheses. *Applied Linguistics, 16*, 15–34.

Berninger, V. W. (2015). *Interdisciplinary frameworks for schools: Best professional practices for serving the needs of all students.* Washington, DC: American Psychological Association.

Berube, B. (2000). *Managing ESL programs in rural and small urban schools.* Arlington, VA: TESOL.

Berube, B. (2002). The three R's for ESL instruction in U.S. rural schools: A test of commitment. *TESOL Matters, 12*(4). Retrieved from http://www.tesol.org/s_tesol/sec_document.asp?CID=193& DID=955

Betz, S., Eickhoff, J., & Sullivan, S. (2013). Factors influencing the selection of standardized tests for the diagnosis of specific language impairment. *Language, Speech, and Hearing Services in Schools, 44,* 133–146.

Bialik, K., Scheller, A., & Walker, K. (2018, October 25). *6 facts about English language learners in U.S. public schools.* Pew Research Center. Retrieved from http://www.pewresearch.org/fact-tank/2018/10/25/6-facts-about-english-language-learners-in-u-s-public-schools/

Bialystok, E. (2001). *Bilingualism in development: Language, literacy, and cognition.* New York, NY: Cambridge University Press.

Bialystok, E., Luk, G., & Kwan, E. (2005). Bilingualism, biliteracy, and learning to read: Interactions among languages and writing systems. *Scientific Studies of Reading, 9,* 43–61.

Bilingual Education Act. (1968). Pub. L. No. 90-247, 81 Stat. 816 (1968).

Birnbaum, B. W. (2008). *English language learners with disabilities: A resource guide for educators.* Lewiston, NY: Edwin Mellen Press.

Blake, H., & McLeod, S. (2019). Speech-language pathologists support for multilingual speakers' English intelligibility and participation informed by the ICF. *Journal of Communication Disorders, 77,* 56–70.

Bland, J., & Krashen, S. D. (2014). Compelling comprehensible input, academic language and school libraries. *Children's Literature in English Language Education Journal, 2*(2), 1–12.

Bliss, L. S. (2002). *Discourse impairments: Assessment and intervention applications.* Boston, MA: Allyn & Bacon.

Blood, G., Mamett, C., Gordon, R., & Blood, I. (2010). Written language disorders: Speech-language pathologists' training, knowledge, and confidence. *Language, Speech, and Hearing Services in Schools, 41*(4), 416–428.

Bloome, D., Champion, T., Katz, L., Morton, M., & Muldrow, R. (2001). Spoken and written narrative development: African American preschoolers as storytellers and story makers. In J. Harris, A. Kamhi, & K. Pollock (Eds.), *Literacy in African American communities* (pp. 45–76). Mahwah, NJ: Erlbaum.

Bloomfield, L. (1942). *Outline guide for the practical study of foreign languages.* Baltimore, MD: Linguistic Society of America.

Blosser, J. (2006). *Partnering with teachers for speech-language service delivery.* Available from http://www.speechpathology.com/

Blosser, J. L., & Kratcoski, A. (1997). PACs: A framework for determining appropriate service delivery option. *Language, Speech, and Hearing Services in Schools, 28,* 99–107.

Bolt, S. E., & Thurlow, M. L. (2004). Five of the most frequently allowed testing accommodations in state policy. *Remedial and Special Education, 25*(3), 141–152.

Boshoff, K., & Stewart, H. (2012). Key principles for confronting the challenges of collaboration in educational settings. *Australian Occupational Therapy Journal, 60,* 144–147.

Bossers, B. (1991). On thresholds, ceilings, and short circuits: The relation between L1 reading, L2 reading, and L1 knowledge. *AILA Review, 8,* 45–60.

Boyle, A., Golden, L., LeFloch, K. C., & O'Day, J. (2014). *Building teacher capacity to support English language learners in schools receiving school improvement grants* (NCEE 2015-4004). Washington, DC: U.S. Department of Education, Institute of Education Sciences, National Center for Education Evaluation and Regional Assistance. Retrieved from https://ies.ed.gov/ncee/pubs/20154004/pdf/20154004.pdf

Brandel, J., & Loeb, D. F. (2011). Program intensity and service delivery models in the schools: SLP survey results. *Language, Speech, and Hearing Services in Schools, 42*(4), 461–490.

Brea-Spahn, M. R., & Dunn Davison, M. (2012). Writing intervention for Spanish speaking English language learners: A review of research. *EBP Briefs, 7*(2), 1–11.

Brice, A., Brice, R., & Kester, E. (2010). *Language loss in English language learners (ELLs).* Retrieved from http://www.pediastaff.com/resources-language-loss-in-english-language-learners-ells--february-2010

Briggs, M. (1991). Team development: Decision-making for early intervention. *Infant-Toddler Intervention, 1*(1), 1–9.

Brisbois, J. (1995). Connections between first and second-language reading. *Journal of Reading Behavior, 24*(4), 565–584.

Brisk, M., Barnhardt, R., Herrera, S., & Rochon, R. (2002). *Educators' preparation for cultural and linguistic diversity: A call to action 2002.* Washington, DC: American Association of Colleges for Teacher Education. Retrieved from https://files.eric.ed.gov/fulltext/ED477737.pdf

Brisk, M. E. (Ed.). (2008). *Language, culture, and community in teacher education.* Mahwah, NJ: Lawrence Erlbaum.

Brisk, M. E., & Harrington, M. (2007). *Literacy and bilingualism: A handbook for all teachers.* Mahwah, NJ: Lawrence Erlbaum.

Britton, J. (1975). *The development of writing abilities.* London, UK: Macmillan.

Brown, H. D. (2014). *Principles of language learning and teaching* (6th ed.). White Plains, NY: Pearson Education.

Brown, J. E., & Doolittle, J. (2008). A cultural, linguistic, and ecological framework for response to intervention with English language learners. *Teaching Exceptional Children, 40*(5), 66–72.

Brown, J. E., & Campbell Ault, P. (2015). Disentangling language differences from disability: A case study of district-preservice collaboration. *Journal of Multilingual Education Research*, *6*, Article 7. Retrieved from https://fordham.bepress.com/jmer/vol6/iss1/7

Brown, J. E., & Sanford, A. (2011, March). *RTI for English language learners: Appropriately using screening and progress monitoring tools to improve instructional outcomes.* Washington, DC: U.S. Department of Education, Office of Special Education Programs, National Center on Response to Intervention. Retrieved from http://www.rti4success.org/sites/ default/files/rtiforells.pdf

Brown, R. (1973). *A first language: The early stages.* Cambridge, MA: Harvard University Press.

Brown, S., & Attardo, S. (2014). *Understanding language structure, interaction, and variation: An introduction to linguistics and sociolinguistics for nonspecialists* (3rd ed.). Ann Arbor: Michigan University Press.

Brownell, R. (2010a). *Expressive One-Word Picture Vocabulary Test—Fourth Edition manual.* San Antonio, TX: Pearson.

Brownell, R. (2010b). *Receptive One-Word Picture Vocabulary Test—Fourth Edition manual.* San Antonio, TX: Pearson.

Bruce, K. L., Lara-Alecio, R., Parker, R., Hasbrouck, J. E., Weaver, L., & Irby, B. (1997). Accurately describing the language. *Bilingual Research Journal*, *21*(2–3), 123–145.

Bruck, M. (1985). Predictors of transfer out of early French immersion programs. *Applied Psycholinguistics*, *6*, 39–61.

Bunch, G. C., Kibler, A., & Pimentel, S. (2013). *Realizing opportunities for English learners in the common core English language arts and disciplinary literacy standards.* Retrieved from http://ell.stanford.edu/sites/default/files/pdf/academicpapers/01_Bunch_Kibler_Pimentel_RealizingOpp%20in%20ELA_FINAL_0.pdf

Burns, M. K., Appleton, J. J., & Stehouwer, J. D. (2005). Meta-analysis of response-to-intervention research: Examining field-based and research-implemented models. *Journal of Psychoeducational Assessment*, *23*, 381–394.

Burns, M. K., Griffiths, A. J., Parson, L. B., Tilly, W. D., & W. D., & VanDerHeyden, A. (2007). *Response to intervention: Research to practice.* Alexandria, VA: National Association of State Directors of Special Education.

Burrus, A. E., & Haynes, W. O. (2009). *Professional communication in speech-language pathology: How to write, talk, and act like a clinician.* San Diego, CA: Plural Publishing.

Butler, F. A., & Stevens, R. (1997). *Accommodation strategies for English language learners on large-scale assessments: Student characteristics and other considerations* (CSE Tech. Rep. No. 448). Los Angeles, CA: University of California's National Center for Research on Evaluation, Standards, and Student Testing.

Butler, K. (1997). Dynamic assessment at the millennium: A transient tutorial for today! *Journal of Children's Communication Development, 19,* 43–54.

Caesar, L. G., & Kohler, P. D. (2007). The state of school-based bilingual assessment: Actual practice versus recommended guidelines. *Language, Speech, and Hearing Services in Schools, 38,* 190–200.

Calderón, M. (2007). *Teaching reading to English language learners, Grades 6–12: A framework for improving achievement in the content areas.* Thousand Oaks, CA: Corwin Press.

Calderón, M. (2018). *Teaching reading to English language learners, Grades 6–12: A framework for improving achievement in the content areas* (2nd ed.). Thousand Oaks, CA: Corwin Press.

Calderon, M., Slavin, R., & Sanchez, M. (2011). Effective instruction for English learners. *Immigrant Children, 21*(1). Retrieved from http://www.futureofchildren.org/futureofchildren/publications/journals/article/index.xml?journalid=74&articleid=542

California Department of Education. (n.d.). *California English language development.* Retrieved from http://www.cde.ca.gov/ta/tg/el/ cefceldt.asp

Callahan, R. (2013, February). *The English learner dropout dilemma: Multiple risks and multiple resources* (California Dropout Research Project Report #19). Santa Barbara, CA: Gevirtz Graduate School of Education, University of California. Retrieved from http://cdrpsb.org/pubs_reports.htm

Campbell, L. R., Brennan, D. G., & Steckol, K. F. (1992). Preservice training to meet the needs of people from diverse cultural backgrounds. *ASHA, 34,* 27–32.

Campbell, W. N., & Douglas, N. F. (2017) Supporting evidence-based practice in speech-language pathology: A review of implementation strategies for promoting health professional behavior change. *Evidence-Based Communication Assessment and Intervention, 11,* 3–4, 72–81. doi:10.1080/17489539.2017.1370215

Capps, R. (2015, May 28). *Trends in immigration and migration of English and dual language learners.* Paper presented at the National Research Council Committee on Fostering School Success for English Learners, Washington, DC. Retrieved from http://www.nationalacademies.org/hmd/~/media/Files/Activity%20Files/Children/DualLanguageLearners/2015-MAY-28/1Capps%20Randy.pdf

Capps, R., Fix, M., Murray, J., Ost, J., Passel, J., & Herwantoro, S. (2005). *The new demography of America's schools: Immigration and the No Child Left Behind Act.* Washington, DC: The Urban Institute. Retrieved from http://www.urban.org/publications/311230.html

Cardenas-Hagan, E., Carlson, C. D., & Pollard-Durodola, S. D. (2007). The cross-linguistic transfer of early literacy skills: The role of initial

L1 and L2 skills and language of instruction. *Language, Speech, and Hearing Services in Schools, 38,* 249–259.

Carlo, M. S., August, D., McLaughlin, B., Snow, C. E., Dressler, C., Lippman, D. N., . . . White, C. E. (2004). Closing the gap: Addressing the vocabulary needs of English language learners in bilingual mainstream classrooms. *Reading Research Quarterly, 39,* 188–215.

Carrell, P. L. (1981). Culture-specific schemata in L2 comprehension. In R. Orem & J. Haskell (Eds.), *Selected papers from the Ninth Illinois TESOL/BE Annual Convention, First Midwest TESOL Conference* (pp. 123–132). Chicago, IL: TESOL/BE.

Carrell, P. L. (1983). Some issues in studying the role of schemata or background knowledge in second language comprehension. *Reading in a Foreign Language, 1,* 81–92.

Carrell, P. L. (1991). Second language reading: Reading ability or language proficiency? *Applied Linguistics, 12,* 159–179.

Casteel, C. J., & Ballantyne, K. G. (Eds.). (2010). *Professional development in action: Improving teaching for English learners.* Washington, DC: National Clearinghouse for English Language Acquisition. Retrieved from http://www.ncela.gwu.edu/files/uploads/3/PD_in_Action.pdf

Catts, H. W. (1993). The relationship between speech-language impairments and reading disabilities. *Journal of Speech and Hearing Research, 36,* 948–958.

Catts, H. W., & Kamhi, A. G. (2004). *Language and reading disabilities* (2nd ed.). Needham Heights, MA: Allyn & Bacon.

Catts, H. W., & Kamhi, A. G. (2017). Prologue: Reading comprehension is not a single ability. *Language, Speech, and Hearing Services in Schools, 48,* 73–76.

CELF Technical Report. (2008). Retrieved from http://www.pearson assessments.com/NR/rdonlyres/F7DBBC32-B63E-4B8E-B1C4-59D 8358E5CA5/0/CELF_4_Tech_Report.pdf

Centeno, J. G., Anderson, R. T., & Obler, L. K. (2007). *Communication disorders in Spanish speakers: Theoretical, research and clinical aspects. Communication disorders across languages.* Clevedon, UK: Multilingual Matters.

Center for Applied Linguistics. (2007). *What's different about teaching reading to students learning English? Trainer's manual.* Washington, DC: Center for Applied Linguistics. Retrieved from http://www .cal.org/solutions/resources/index.html#1

Chabon, S., Esparza-Brown, J. E., & Gildersleeve-Neumann, C. (2010, August 3). Ethics, equity, and English-language learners: A decision making framework. *ASHA Leader.*

Chabon, S., & Lee-Wilkerson, D. (2007). Dialogues on diversity in speech-language pathology: Not for the faint of heart. In J. Branche,

J. Mullennix, & E. Cohen (Eds.), *Diversity across the curriculum: A guide for faculty in higher education*. Bolton, MA: Anker.

Chall, J. S. (1983). *Stages of reading development*. New York, NY: McGraw-Hill.

Chall, J. S., & Jacobs, V. A. (2003). Poor children's fourth-grade slump. *American Educator, 27*(1), 14–15.

Chamberlain, S. P. (2005). Recognizing and responding to cultural differences in the education of culturally and linguistically diverse learners. *Intervention in School and Clinic, 40*, 195–211.

Champion, T., & Mainess, K. (2003). Typical and disordered narration in African American children. In A. McCabe & L. S. Bliss (Eds.), *Patterns of narrative discourse: A multicultural lifespan approach* (pp. 55–70). Boston, MA: Allyn & Bacon.

Champion, T., & Seymour, H. (1995). Narrative discourse among African American children. *Journal of Narrative and Life History, 5*, 333–352.

Chomsky, N. (1965). *Aspects of a theory of syntax*. Cambridge, MA: MIT Press.

Chomsky, N. (2005). *Rules and representations* (2nd ed.). New York, NY: Columbia University Press.

Chow, B. W., McBride-Chang, C., & Burgess, S. (2005). Phonological processing skills and early reading abilities in Hong Kong Chinese kindergarteners learning to read English as a second language. *Journal of Educational Psychology, 97*(1), 81–87.

Chu, S.-Y., & Flores, S. (2011). Assessment of English language learners with learning disabilities. *Clearing House: A Journal of Educational Strategies, Issues and Ideas, 84*(6), 244–248.

Cirrin, F., Schooling, T., Nelson, N., Diehl, S., Flynn, P., Staskowski, M., . . . Adamczyk, D. (2010). Evidence-based systematic review: Effects of different service delivery models on communication outcomes for elementary school-age children. *Language, Speech, and Hearing Services in Schools, 41(3)*, 233–264.

Civil Rights Act of 1964 § 7, 42 U.S.C. § 2000e et seq (1964).

Clair, N., & Adger, C. T. (1999). *Professional development for teachers in culturally diverse schools*. Washington, DC: ERIC Clearinghouse on Teaching and Teacher Education (ERIC Document Reproduction Service No. ED 435 185).

Clark, E. V. (2016). *First language acquisition* (3rd ed.). New York, NY: Cambridge University Press.

Clarke, M. A. (1980). The short circuit hypothesis of ESL reading or when language competence interferes with reading performance. *Modern Language Journal, 64*, 203–209.

Cloud, N., Genesee, F., & Hamayan, E. (2000). *Dual language instruction: A handbook for enriched education*. Boston, MA: Heinle and Heinle.

Cloud, N., Genesee, F., & Hamayan, E. (2009). *Literacy instruction for English language learners.* Portsmouth, NH: Heinemann.

Cohen, D. K. (1995). What is the system in systemic reform? *Educational Researcher, 24*(9), 11–31.

Coleman, R., & Goldenberg, C. (2012, February). The common core challenge for English language learners. *Principal Leadership,* pp. 46–51.

Coleman, T. (2000). *Clinical management of communication disorders in culturally diverse children.* Boston, MA: Allyn & Bacon.

Coleman, T., & McCabe-Smith, L. (2000). Key terms and concepts. In T. Coleman (Ed.), *Clinical management of communication disorders in culturally diverse children* (pp. 3–12). Boston, MA: Allyn & Bacon.

Collier, C. (2000). *Separating difference and disability: Strategies for identification and instruction.* Ferndale, WA: Cross-Cultural Developmental Education Services.

Collier, C. (2008). *Handbook for second language acquisition.* Ferndale, WA: Cross-Cultural Developmental Education Services.

Collier, C. (2010). *RtI for diverse learners.* Thousand Oaks, CA: Corwin.

Collier, C. (2011). *Seven steps to separating difference from disability.* Thousand Oaks, CA: Corwin Press.

Collier, V. (1998). *Promoting academic success for ESL students: Understanding second language acquisition.* New York, NY: Bastos.

Collier, V., & Thomas, W. P. (1995). *Language minority student achievement and program effectiveness: Research summary on ongoing study.* Fairfax, VA: George Mason University.

Collier, V., & Thomas, W. P. (2004). The astounding effectiveness of dual language education for all. *NABE Journal of Research and Practice, 2,* 1–20.

Collier, V., & Thomas, W. P. (2014). *Creating dual language schools for a transformed world: Administrators speak.* Albuquerque, NM: Dual Language Education of New Mexico-Fuente Press.

Collier, V., & Thomas, W. P. (2017). *Why dual language schooling.* Albuquerque, NM: Dual Language Education of New Mexico—Fuente Press.

Cook, V. (2001). Using the first language in the classroom. *Canadian Modern: Language Review, 57*(3), 402–423.

Cook, V. (2008). *Second language learning and language teaching* (4th ed.). London, UK: Hodder Education.

Congress.Gov. (2015). S.1177—Every student succeeds act. Retrieved from https://www.congress.gov/bill/114th-congress/senate-bill/1177

Core, C., Hoff, E., Rumiche, R., & Senor, M. (2013). Total and conceptual vocabulary in Spanish-English bilinguals from 22 to 30 months: Implications for assessment. *Journal of Speech, Language, and Hearing Research, 56*(5), 1637–1649.

Coret, M., & McCrimmon, A. (2015). Test review: Wiig, E.H., Semel, E., & Secord, W. A. (2013). Clinical Evaluation of Language Fundamentals—Fifth Edition (CELF-5). *Journal of Psychoeducational Assessment, 33*(5), 495–500.

Cornejo, R. J., Weinstein, A., & Najar, C. (1983). *Eliciting spontaneous speech in bilingual students: Methods and techniques.* Las Cruces, NM: Educational Resources Information Center (ERIC), Clearinghouse on Rural Education and Small Schools (CRESS), New Mexico State University.

Cosentino de Cohen, C., Deterding, N., & Clewell, B. C. (2005). *Who's left behind? Immigrant children in high and low LEP schools.* Washington, DC: The Urban Institute.

Council for Clinical Certification in Audiology and Speech-Language Pathology of the American Speech-Language-Hearing Association. (2013). *2014 Standards for the Certificate of Clinical Competence in Speech-Language Pathology.* Retrieved from http://www.asha .org/Certification/2014-Speech-Language-Pathology-Certification-Standards/

Council for Clinical Certification in Audiology and Speech-Language Pathology of the Council of Chief State School Officers. (2010). *Common core state standards.* Retrieved from http://www.corestandards .org/ELA-Literacy/

Council on Academic Accreditation in Audiology and Speech-Language Pathology. (2017). *Standards for accreditation of graduate education programs in audiology and speech-language pathology.* Retrieved from https://caa.asha.org/wp-content/uploads/Accreditation-Stan dards-for-Graduate-Programs.pdf

Crawford, J. (2003). Hard sell: Why is bilingual education so unpopular with the American public? In O. Garcia & C. Baker (Eds.), *Bilingual education: An introductory reader* (pp. 145–164). Clevedon, UK: Multilingual Matters.

Cross, C. T. (2015). *The shaping of federal education policy over time.* Retrieved from http://www.ecs.org/clearinghouse/01/19/16/11916.pdf

Cross, T., Bazrn, B., Dennis, K., & Isaacs, M. (1989). *Toward a culturally competent system of care* (Vol. 1). Washington, DC: CAASP Technical Assistance Center, Georgetown University Child Development Center.

Crowley, C. J. (2003, October). Diagnosing communication disorders in culturally and linguistically diverse students. *ERIC Digest,* p. E650.

Crowley, C. J., Guest, K., & Sudler, K. (2015). Cultural competence needed to distinguish disorder from difference: Beyond Kumbaya. *Perspectives on Communication Disorders and Sciences in Culturally and Linguistically Diverse (CLD) Populations (SIG 14), 22*(2), 64–76.

Cummins, J. (1976). The influence of bilingualism on cognitive growth: A synthesis of research findings and explanatory hypotheses. *Working Papers on Bilingualism, 9,* 1–43.

Cummins, J. (1979). Linguistic interdependence and the educational development of bilingual children. *Review of Educational Research, 49*, 222–251.

Cummins, J. (1980). The construct of language proficiency in bilingual education. In J. E. Alatis (Ed.), *Georgetown University round table on languages and linguistics*. Washington, DC: Georgetown University Press.

Cummins, J. (1984). *Bilingualism and special education*. Clevedon, UK: Multilingual Matters.

Cummins, J. (1991). Interdependence of first- and second-language proficiency in bilingual children. In E. Bialystok (Ed.), *Language processing in bilingual children* (pp. 70–89). Cambridge, UK: Cambridge University Press.

Cummins, J. (1992). The role of primary language development in promoting educational success of language minority students. In California State Department of Education (Ed.), *Schooling and language minority students: A theoretical framework*. Los Angeles, CA: California State University, Evaluation, Dissemination, and Assessment Center.

Cummins, J. (1998, February). *Beyond adversarial discourse: Searching for common ground in the education of bilingual students*. Paper presented at the California State Board of Education, Sacramento.

Cummins, J. (2000). *Language, power, and pedagogy: Bilingual children in the crossfire*. Philadelphia, PA: Multilingual Matters.

Cummins, J. (2008). Teaching for transfer: Challenging the two solitudes assumption in bilingual education. In J. Cummins & N. H. Hornberger (Eds.), *Encyclopedia of language and education: Vol. 5. Bilingual education* (2nd ed., pp. 65–75). New York, NY: Springer Science Business Media.

Cummins, J. (2017). Teaching minoritized students: Are additive approaches legitimate? *Harvard Educational Review, 87*(3), 404–425. doi:10.17763/1943-5045-87.3.404

Cummins, J., Chow, P., & Schecter, S. R. (2006). Community as curriculum. *Language Arts, 83*, 297–307.

Cummins, J., & Corson, D. (1997). *Bilingual education*. Boston, MA: Kluwer Academic.

Curtin, E. M. (2009). *Practical strategies for teaching English language learners*. Upper Saddle River, NJ: Pearson.

Custodio, B., & O'Loughlin, J. (2017). *Students with interrupted formal education: Bridging where they are and what they need*. Thousand Oaks, CA: Corwin.

D'Amour, D., & Oandasan, I. (2005). Interprofessionality as the field of interprofessional practice and interprofessional education: An emerging concept. *Journal of Interprofessional Care, 19* (Suppl. 1), 8–20.

Dawson, J. I., Stout, C. E., & Elyer, J. A. (2003). *The Structured Photographic Expressive Language Test (SPELT-3)* (3rd ed.). DeKalb, IL: Janelle.

Davidson, S., & Denton, D. (2010). Ethics compliance: Enforcing ASHA's Code of Ethics. *Perspectives on Fluency and Fluency Disorders, 20*(3), 71–75.

Davis, J. N., & Bistodeau, L. (1993). How do L1 and L2 reading differ? Evidence from think aloud protocols. *Modern Language Journal, 77*, 459–470. Retrieved from http://educationnorthwest.org/re sources/what-research-says-instruction-english-learners-across-subject-areas

Davis, P. M. (1991). *Cognition and learning: A review of the literature with reference to ethnolinguistic minorities.* Dallas, TX: Summer Institute of Linguistics.

De Houwer, A. (1990). *The acquisition of two languages from birth: A case study.* Cambridge, UK: Cambridge University Press.

de Jong, E., & Harper, C. (2005). Preparing mainstream teachers for English language learners: Is being a good teacher good enough? *Teacher Education Quarterly, 32*(2), 101–124. Retrieved from https://files.eric.ed.gov/fulltext/EJ795308.pdf

de Jong, E., & Harper, C. (2011). "Accommodating diversity": Preservice teachers' views on effective practices for English language learners. In T. Lucas (Ed.), *Teacher preparation for linguistically diverse classrooms. A resource for teacher educators* (pp. 73–90). New York, NY: Routledge.

de Schonewise, E. A., & Klingner, J. K. (2012). Linguistic and cultural issues in developing disciplinary literacy for adolescent English language learners. *Topics in Language Disorders, 32*(1), 51–68.

Deaux, K., & Wrightman, L. S. (1988). *Social psychology* (5th ed.). Pacific Grove, CA: Brooks/Cole.

DeGuerrero, M. C., & Villamil, O. S. (2000). Exploring ESL teachers' roles through metaphoranalysis. *TESOL Quarterly, 34*, 341–351.

Denman, D., Speyer, R., Munro, N., Pearce, W. M., Chen, Y. W., & Cordier, R. (2017). Psychometric properties of language assessments for children aged 4–12 years: A systematic review. *Frontiers in Psychology, 8*, 1515.

Diaz-Rico, L. T. (2004). *Teaching English learners: Strategies and methods.* Boston, MA: Pearson.

Diaz-Rico, L. T., & Weed, K. Z. (2006). *The cross-cultural, language, and academic development handbook: A complete K–12 reference guide* (3rd ed.). Boston, MA: Pearson.

Dixon, C. N., & Nessel, D. (2008). *Using the language experience approach with English language learners: Strategies for engaging students and developing literacy.* Thousand Oaks, CA: Sage.

Dollaghan, C. A., & Horner, E. A. (2011). Bilingual language assessment: A meta-analysis of diagnostic accuracy. *Journal of Speech, Language, and Hearing Research, 54,* 1077–1088.

Douglas, N. F., & Burshnic, V.L. (2019). Implementation science: Tackling the research to practice gap in communication sciences and disorders. *Perspectives of the ASHA Special Interest Groups, 4*(1), 23–27. doi:10.1044/2018_PERS-ST-2018-0000

Dornyei, Z. (2005). *The psychology of the language learner: Individual differences in second language acquisition.* Mahwah, NJ: Lawrence Erlbaum.

Duchan, J. (2002, December 24). What do you know about your profession's history: And why is it important? *The ASHA Leader.* Retrieved from http://www.asha.org/publications/leader/2002/021224/021224a.htm

Duffy, K. R., Stephens-Pisecco, T. L., & Schultz, E. K. (2018). *WMLS III: Comprehensive assessment, intervention and application* (WMLA Assessment Service Bulletin No. 1). Itasca, IL: Houghton Mifflin Harcourt.

Dufva, M., & Voeten, M. J. M. (1999). Native language literacy and phonological memory as prerequisites for learning English as a foreign language. *Applied Psycholinguistics, 20,* 329–348.

Dulay, H., & Burt, M. K. (1974). Natural sequences in child second language acquisition. *Language Learning, 24,* 37–53.

Dulay, H., & Burt, M. K. (1980). On acquisition orders. In S. Felix (Ed.), *Second language development: Trends and issues.* Tubingen, Germany: Narr.

Dulay, H., Burt, M. K., & Krashen, S. (1982). *Language two.* New York, NY: Oxford University Press.

Durgunoglu, A. Y. (1998). Acquiring literacy in English and Spanish in the United States. In A. Y. Durgunoglu & L. Verhoeven (Eds.), *Literacy development in a multilingual context: Cross-cultural perspective* (pp. 135–146). Mahwah, NJ: Lawrence Erlbaum.

Durgunoglu, A. Y., Nagy, W. E., & Hancin-Bhatt, B. J. (1993). Cross-language transfer of phonological awareness. *Journal of Educational Psychology, 85,* 453–465.

Echevarría, J., Richards-Tutor, C., & Vogt, M. (2015). *Response to intervention (RTI) and English learners: Using the SIOP Model* (2nd ed.). Saddle River, NJ: Pearson.

Echevarría, J., Short, D., & Powers, K. (2006) School reform and standards-based education: A model for English-language learners. *Journal of Educational Research, 99*(4), 195–211. doi:10.3200/JOER.99.4.195-211

Echevarría, J., & Vogt, M. E. (2011). *Response to Intervention (RTI) and English learners.* Boston, MA: Pearson.

Echevarría, J., Vogt, M., & Short, D. (2008). *Making content comprehensible for English Learners: The SIOP model* (3rd ed.). Boston, MA: Allyn & Bacon.

Echevarría J., Vogt M., & Short D. J. (2010). *Making content comprehensible for secondary English language learners.* Boston, ME: Allyn & Bacon.

Echevarría, J., Vogt, M. E., & Short, D. (2017). *Making content comprehensible for English Learners: The SIOP model* (5th ed.). New York, NY: Pearson.

Edelsky, C. (1981). From "JIMOSALCO" to "7 naranjas se calleron e el arbol-est-trite en lagrymas": Writing development in a bilingual program. In B. Cronnel (Ed.), *The writing needs of linguistically different students* (pp. 63–98). Los Alamitos, CA: Southwest Regional Laboratory.

Edelsky, C. (1986). *Writing in a bilingual program: Habia una vez.* Norwood, NJ: Ablex.

Edgar, D., & Rosa-Lugo, L. I. (2007). The critical shortage of speech language pathologists in the public-school setting: Features of the work environment that affects recruitment and retention. *Language, Speech, and Hearing Services in Schools, 38,* 1–16.

Education Commission of the States (ECS). (2014). *50-State comparison. What ELL training, if any is required of general classroom teachers?* Retrieved from http://ecs.force.com/mbdata/mbquest NB2?rep=ELL1415

Edwards, J., Gross, M., Chen, J., MacDonald, M., Kaplan, D., Brown, M., & Seidenberg, M. (2014). Dialect awareness and lexical comprehension of mainstream American English in African American English-speaking children. *Journal of Speech, Language and Hearing Research, 57,* 1883–1895.

Eggington, W. (1987). Written academic discourse in Korea. In U. Connor & R. B. Kaplan (Eds.), *Implications for effective communication in writing across languages: Analysis of L2 text* (pp. 153–167). Reading, MA: Addison-Wesley.

Ehren, B. (Ed.). (2005). Responsiveness to intervention and the speech-language pathologist [Special issue]. *Topics in Language Disorders, 25*(2), 120–131.

Ehren, B. (2006). Partnerships to support reading comprehension for students with language impairment. *Topics in Language Disorders, 26*(1), 41–53.

Ehren, B., & Ehren, T. C. (2001). New or expanded literacy roles for speech-language pathologists: Making it happen in the schools. *Seminars in Speech and Language, 22,* 233–243.

Ehren, B., Montgomery, J., Rudebusch, J., & Whitmire, K. (2009). *Responsiveness to intervention: New roles for speech-language pathol-*

ogists. Retrieved from http://www.asha.org/SLP/schools/prof-consult/ NewRolesSLP/

Ehren, B., Montgomery, J., & Whitmire, K. (2006). Responsiveness to intervention: New roles for speech-language pathologists. In ASHA (Ed.), *New roles in response to intervention: Creating successful schools and children* (pp. 3–8). Rockville, MD: ASHA. Retrieved from http://www.asha.org/uploadedFiles/slp/schools/prof-consult/ rtiroledefinitions.pdf

Ehren, B., & Murza, K. (2010). The urgent need to address workforce readiness in adolescent literacy intervention. *Perspectives on Language Learning and Education, 17,* 93–99.

Ehren, B., Murza, K. A., & Malani, M. D. (2012). Disciplinary literacy from a speech–language pathologist's perspective. *Topics in Language Disorders, 32*(1), 85–98.

Ehren, B., Nelson, N., Staskowski, M., & Davis, K. (2012, November). *SLPs helping students with language disabilities to acquire disciplinary literacy.* Paper presented at the American Speech-Language-Hearing Association Conference, Atlanta, GA.

Ehren, T., Lefkowitz, N., & Roth, C. (1997, October). Developing, evaluating, and managing competencies across work settings. *ASHA Special Interest Division 11 Newsletter, 7*(3), 3–4.

Elementary and Secondary Education Act [ESEA] (No Child Left Behind Act of 2001). (2010, December 6). Retrieved March 28, 2018, from http://www2.ed.gov

Ellis, R. (1997). *Second language acquisition.* Oxford, UK: Pergamon.

Ellis, R. (2003). *Task-based language learning and teaching.* Oxford, UK: Oxford University Press.

Ellis, R. (2008a). *The study of second language acquisition* (2nd ed.). Oxford, UK: Oxford University Press.

Ellis, R. (2008b). Principles of instructed second language acquisition. *Center for Applied Linguistics Digest.* Retrieved from http://www.cal .org/resources/digest/digest_pdfs/ Instructed2ndLangFinalWeb.pdf

Ermeling, B. A., & Graff-Ermeling, G. (2016). *Teaching better: Igniting and sustaining instructional improvement.* Thousand Oaks, CA: Corwin.

Esparza-Brown, J., & Doolittle, J. (2008). *A cultural, linguistic, and ecological framework for response to intervention with English language learners.* National Center for Culturally Responsive Educational Systems (NCCRESt) Practitioner Briefs. Retrieved from http:// www.nccrest.org/publications/briefs.html

Esparza-Brown, J., & Sanford, A. (2011, March). *RTI for English language learners: Appropriately using screening and progress monitoring tools to improve instructional outcomes.* Washington, DC: U.S.

Department of Education, Office of Special Education Programs, National Center on Response to Intervention.

Esquinca, A., Yaden, D., & Rueda, R. (2005). Current language proficiency tests and their implications for preschool English language learners. In *Proceedings of the 4th international symposium on bilingualism* (pp. 674–680). Somerville, MA: Cascadilla Press.

Estrada, P., & Wang, H. (2018). Making English learner reclassification to fluent English proficient attainable or elusive: When meeting criteria is and is not enough. *American Educational Research Journal*, *155*(2), 207–242.

Evans, K., Munson, B., & Edwards, J. (2018). Does speaker race affect the assessment of children's speech accuracy? A comparison of speech-language pathologists and clinically untrained listeners. *Language, Speech, and Hearing Services in Schools*, *49*(4), 906–921.

Every Student Succeeds Act (ESSA), Public Law No: 114-95, S.1177. (2015).

Fang, Z., & Schleppegrell, M. J. (2010). Disciplinary literacies across content areas: Supporting secondary reading through functional language analysis. *Journal of Adolescent and Adult Literacy*, *53*(7), 587–597. doi:10.1598/JAAL.53.7.6

Fang, Z., Schleppegrell, M., & Cox, B. (2006). Understanding the language demands of schooling: Nouns in academic registers. *Journal of Literacy Research*, *38*(3), 247–273.

Fantini, A. (1985). *Language acquisition of a bilingual child: A sociolinguistic perspective (to age 10)*. San Diego, CA: College-Hill Press.

Farrell, G. (2009). *Teaching reading to English language learners*. Thousand Oaks, CA: Corwin Press.

Farrugia-Bernard, A. M. (2018). Speech-language pathologists as determiners of the human right to diversity in communication for school children in the U.S. *International Journal of Speech-Language Pathology*, *20*(1), 170–173.

Fenner, D., & Kuhlman, N. (2012). *Preparing effective teachers of English language learners: Practical applications for the TESOL P-12 professional teaching standards*. Alexandria, VA: TESOL Press.

Fernandez, A. T. (1992). Legal support for bilingual education and language-appropriate related services for limited English proficient students with disabilities. *Bilingual Research Journal*, *16*(3–4), 117–140.

Field, R. (2008). Keeping pace in suburbia and rural America. *School Administrator*, *65*(10), 2–26.

Fitton, L., Bustamante, K., Wofford, M., Brown, D., Gabas, C., Hoge, R., & Wood, C. (2016). Intensifying English vocabulary instruction for English language learners. *Perspectives of the ASHA Special Interest Groups*, *1*(16), 4–14.

Flores, S., Park, T., Viano, S., & Coca, V. (2017). State policy and the educational outcomes of English Learner and immigrant students: Three administrative data stories. *American Behavioral Scientist*, *61*(14), 1824–1844.

Florida Department of Education (FLDOE). (n.d.). *League of United Latin American Citizens (LULAC) et al. v. State Board of Education Consent Decree.* United States District Court for the Southern District of Florida, August 14, 1990. Retrieved from http://www.fldoe.org/academics/eng-language-learners/consent-decree.stml

Florida Department of Education (FLDOE). (2001). *Preparing Florida teachers to work with limited English proficient students.* Retrieved from http://www.fldoe.org/profdev/pdf/final_esol.pdf

Florida Department of Education (FLDOE). (2010). *Approved Florida teacher standards for teacher endorsement.* Retrieved from http://www.fldoe.org/aala

Florida Department of Education (FLDOE). (2011). *Consent decree.* Retrieved from http://www.fldoe.org/aala/cdpage2.asp

Florida Department of Education (FLDOE). (2015). *Technical assistance paper: Evaluation, determination of eligibility reevaluation and the provision of exceptional student education services.* Retrieved from https://info.fldoe.org/docushare/dsweb/Get/Document-7505/dps-2015-152.pdf

Florida Department of Education (FLDOE). (2019). *League of United Latin American Citizens (LULAC) et al. v. State Board of Education Consent Decree.* United States District Court for the Southern District of Florida, August 14, 1990. Retrieved from http://www.fldoe.org/academics/eng-language-learners/consent-decree.stml

Flynn, K., & Hill, J. (2005). *English language learners: A growing population.* Denver, CO: Mid-continent Research for Education and Learning.

Flynn, P. (2010, August 31). New service delivery models: Connecting SLPs with teachers and curriculum. *ASHA Leader.*

Francis, D., Rivera, M., Lesaux, N., Kieffer, M., & Rivera, H. (2006). *Practical guidelines for the education of English language learners: Research-based recommendations for instruction and academic interventions.* Portsmouth, NH: RMC Research Corporation, Center on Instruction. Retrieved from https://www.centeroninstruction.org/files/ELL1-Interventions.pdf

Freeman, D. E., & Freeman, Y. S. (2014). *Essential linguistics: What you need to know to teach ESL, reading, spelling, and grammar* (2nd ed.). Portsmouth, NH: Heinemann.

Freeman, Y. S., Freeman, D. E. & Mercuri, S. (2002). *Closing the achievement gap: How to reach limited formal schooling and long term English language learners.* Portsmouth, NH: Heinemann.

Freeman, Y. S., Freeman, D. E., & Ramirez, R. (2008). *Diverse learners in the mainstream classroom: Strategies for supporting all students across content areas, English language learners, students with disabilities, gifted/talented students.* Portsmouth, NH: Heinemann.

Frey, W. H. (2015). *Diversity explosion: How new racial demographics are remaking America.* Washington, DC: Brookings Institution Press.

Friend, M., & Cook, L. (2010). *Interactions: Collaboration skills for school professionals* (6th ed.). Boston, MA: Pearson.

Friend, M., & Cook, L. (2017). *Interactions: Collaboration skills for school professionals, Enhanced Pearson eText with Loose-Leaf Version—Access Code Package* (8th ed.). Upper Saddle River, NJ: Pearson.

Frisby, C. L. (1992). Issues and problems in the influence of culture on the psychoeducational needs of African-American children. *School Psychology Review, 21*(4), 532–551.

Fuchs, D., & Deshler, D. D. (2007). What we need to know about responsiveness to intervention (and shouldn't be afraid to ask). *Learning Disabilities Research and Practice, 22,* 129–136.

Fuchs, D., Mock, D., Morgan, P. L., & Young, C. L. (2003). Responsiveness-to-intervention: Definitions, evidence, and implications for the learning disabilities construct. *Learning Disabilities Research and Practice, 18,* 157–171.

Fulcher-Rood, K., Castilla-Earls, A. P., & Higginbotham, J. (2019). Diagnostic decisions in child language assessment: Findings from a case review assessment task. *Language, Speech, and Hearing Services in Schools, 50*(3), 385–398.

Fullan, M. (2014). *The principal: Three keys to maximizing impact.* San Francisco, CA: Jossey-Bass.

Garcia, E. E. (1991). *The education of linguistically and culturally diverse students: Effective instructional practices* (NCRCDSLL Educational Practice Reports, Paper EPR01). Santa Cruz, CA: Center for Research on Education, Diversity & Excellence. Retrieved from http://repositories.cdlib.org/crede/ncrcdslleducational/EPR01

Garcia, G. E., & Godina, H. (2004). Addressing the literacy needs of adolescent English language learners. In T. Jetton & J. Dole (Eds.), *Adolescent literacy: Research and practice* (pp. 304–320). New York, NY: Guilford Press.

Garcia, O., & Kleifgen, J. (2018). *Educating emergent bilinguals: Policies, programs, and practices for English language learners* (2nd ed.). New York, NY: Teachers College Press.

Garcia, R. (1982). *Teaching in a pluralistic society: Concept, models, strategies.* New York, NY: Harper and Row.

Garcia, S. B. (2002). Parent-professional collaboration in culturally sensitive assessment. In A. J. Artiles & A. A. Ortiz (Eds.), *English lan-*

guage learners with special education needs (pp. 87–103). McHenry, IL: Center for Applied Linguistics and Delta Systems.

Garcia, S. B., & Guerra, P. L. (2004). Deconstructing deficit thinking: Working with educators to create more equitable learning environments. *Education and Urban Society, 36*(2), 150–168.

Garcia, S. B., Mendez-Perez, A. M., & Ortiz, A. A. (2000). Mexican American mothers' beliefs about disabilities: Implications for early childhood intervention. *Remedial and Special Education, 21*, 90–100.

Gardner, R. (1980). On the validity of affective variables in second language acquisition: Conceptual, contextual, and statistical considerations. *Language Learning, 30*(2), 255–270.

Gardner, R. C. (2001). Integrative motivation and second language acquisition. In Z. Dornyei & R. Schmidt (Eds.), *Motivation and second language acquisition* (pp. 69–90). Honolulu: University of Hawaii, Second Language Teaching and Curriculum Center.

Genesee, F., Lindholm-Leary, K., Saunders, W., & Christian, D. (2005). English language learners in U.S. schools: An overview of research findings. *Journal of Education for Student Placed at Risk, 10*(4), 363–385.

Genesee, F., Lindholm-Leary, K., Saunders, W., & Christian, D. (2006). *Educating English language learners.* New York: Cambridge University Press.

Geva, E. (2006). Second-language oral proficiency and second-language literacy. In D. August & T. Shanahan (Eds.), *Developing literacy on second-language learners: Report of the National Literacy Panel on language-minority children and youth.* Mahwah, NJ: Lawrence Erlbaum.

Gibbons, P. (2002). *Scaffolding language, scaffolding learning: Teaching second language learners in the mainstream classroom.* Portsmouth, NH: Heinemann.

Giess, S. A. (2010). *Implementing a workload approach to caseload: Methods and strategies.* Rockville, MD: American Speech-Language Hearing Association.

Giess, S. A., & Serianni, R. (2018). Interprofessional practice in schools. *Perspectives of the ASHA Special Interest Groups, 3*(16), 88–94.

Gildersleeve-Neumann, C., & Goldstein, B. A. (2012). Intervention for multilingual children with speech sound disorders. In S. McLeod & B. A. Goldstein (Eds.), *Multilingual aspects of speech sound disorders in children* (pp. 214–227). Bristol, UK: Multilingual Matters.

Gill, S., Posamentier, J., & Hill, P. (2016). *Suburban schools: The unrecognized frontier in public education.* University of Washington: Center on Reinventing Public Education. Retrieved from https://www.crpe.org/sites/default/files/crpe.suburban_schools_5.2016.pdf

Gillam, R. B., & Johnston, J. R. (1992). Spoken and written language relationships in language/learning impaired and normally achieving school-age children. *Journal of Speech and Hearing Research, 25,* 1303–1315.

Gillam, R. B., & Marquardt, T. (2015). *Communication sciences and disorders* (3rd ed.). Burlington, MA: Jones and Bartlett.

Gillam, S. L., & Gillam, R. B. (2006). Making evidence-based decisions about child language intervention in schools. *Language, Speech, and Hearing Services in Schools, 37,* 304–315.

Girolametto, L., Weitzman, E., & Greenberg, J. (2012). Facilitating emergent literacy: Efficacy of a model that partner's speech-language pathologists and educators. *American Journal of Speech-Language Pathology, 21*(1), 47–63.

Goldenberg, C. (2008). Teaching English language learners: What the research says and does not say. *American Educator, 32*(2), 8–44. Retrieved from http://homepages.ucalgary.ca/~hroessin/documents/Goldenberg,_2008,_America_Ed_Summary_of_research.pdf

Goldenberg, C., & Coleman, R. (2010). *Promoting academic achievement among English learners: A guide to the research.* Thousand Oaks, CA: Corwin.

Goldman, S., & McDermott, R. (1987). The culture of competition in American schools. In G. Spindler (Ed.), *Education and cultural process* (2nd ed., pp. 282–299). Prospect Heights, IL: Waveland Press.

Goldman, S., Snow, C., & Vaughn, S. (2016). Common themes in teaching reading for understanding: Lessons from three projects. *Journal of Adolescent & Adult Literacy, 60*(3), 1–10.

Goldstein, B. (2000). *Cultural and linguistic diversity resource guide for speech-language pathologists.* San Diego, CA: Singular/Thompson Learning.

Goldstein, B. (Ed.). (2004a). *Bilingual language development and disorders in Spanish-English speakers.* Baltimore, MD: Brookes.

Goldstein, B. (2004b). Bilingual language development and disorders: Introduction and overview. In B. A. Goldstein (Ed.), *Bilingual language development and disorders in Spanish-English speakers* (pp. 3–20). Baltimore, MD: Brookes.

Goldstein, B., & Iglesias, A. (1996). Phonological patterns in normally developing Spanish-speaking 3- and 4-year-olds of Puerto Rican descent. *Language, Speech, and Hearing Services in Schools, 27*(1), 82–90.

Goldstein, B., & Washington, P. (2001). An initial investigation of phonological patterns in 4-year-old typically developing Spanish English bilingual children. *Language, Speech, and Hearing Services in Schools, 32,* 153–164.

Goldfarb, R., & Serpanos, Y. (2009). *Professional writing in speech language pathology and audiology workbook*. San Diego, CA: Plural Publishing.

Gonzales, D. (2007). *Evaluating bilingual students for eligibility as speech/language impaired: A handbook for evidence-based decision making*. Houston, TX: Region 4 Education Service Center.

Gonzalez-Barrera, A., & Lopez, M. (2013). *Spanish is the most spoken non-English language in U.S. homes, even among non-Hispanics*. Washington, DC: Pew Research Center. Retrieved from http://www.pewresearch.org/fact-tank/2013/08/13/spanish-is-the-most-spoken-non-english-language-in-u-s-homes-even-among-non-hispanics/

Goodman, K. S. (1979). Psycholinguistics universals in the reading process. *Journal of Typographic Research, 4*, 103–110.

Goodman, K. S., & Goodman, Y. (1994). To err is human: Learning about language processes by analyzing miscues. In R. B. Ruddell, M. R. Ruddell, & H. Singer (Eds.), *Theoretical models and processes of reading* (pp. 104–123). Newark, DE: International Reading Association.

Gorman, B. (2015). Dynamic assessment with bilingual: A focus on increasing clinician's confidence. *Perspectives on Communication Disorders and Sciences in Culturally and Linguistically Diverse (CLD) Populations, 22*(3), 112–121.

Gorman, B. K., & Gillam, R. B. (2003). Phonological awareness in Spanish: A tutorial for speech-language pathologists. *Communication Disorders Quarterly, 25*, 13–22.

Gorman, C. (2007). Are doctors just playing hunches? *Time, 169*(9), 52–54.

Gottardo, A. (2002). Language and reading skills in bilingual Spanish English speakers. *Topics in Language Disorders, 23*, 42–66.

Grabe, W. (2001). Notes toward a theory of second language writing. In T. J. Silva & P. K. Masuda (Eds.), *On second language writing*. Mahwah, NJ: Lawrence Erlbaum.

Grabe, W. (2009). *Reading in a second language: Moving from theory to practice*. New York, NY: Cambridge University Press.

Graham, C. (1978). *Jazz chants*. New York, NY: Oxford University Press.

Graham, C. (2000). *Jazz chants: Old and new*. New York, NY: Oxford University Press.

Graham, S. V. (1998). *Quality treatment indicators: A model for clinical expertise in speech-language pathology* (Doctoral dissertation). University of South Florida, Tampa.

Graham, S. V., & Guilford, A. M. (2000, November). *Beyond competence: Development of a model of clinical expertise*. Paper presented at the American Speech-Language-Hearing Association annual conference, Washington, DC.

Green, J. (1982). *Cultural awareness in the human services*. Englewood Cliffs, NJ: Prentice-Hall.

Greenfield, P. M. (1997). You can't take it with you: Why ability assessments don't cross cultures. *American Psychologist, 52*(10), 1115–1124.

Guiberson, M., & Atkins, J. (2012). Speech-language pathologists' preparation, practices, and perspectives on serving culturally and linguistically diverse children. *Communication Disorders Quarterly, 33*(3), 169–180.

Guiberson, M., & Feris, K.P. (2019). Early language interventions for young dual language learners: A scoping review. *American Journal of Speech-Language Pathology, 28*(3), 945–963.

Guiberson, M., Rodriguez, B., & Dale, P. (2011). Classification accuracy of brief parent report measures of language development in Spanish-speaking toddlers. *Language, Speech, and Hearing Services in Schools, 42*, 536–549. doi:10.1044/0161-1461(2011/10-0076)

Guilford, A. (2003). Communication sciences and disorders. In M. A. Richard & W. G. Emener (Eds.), *I'm a people person: A guide to human services professions.* Springfield, IL: Charles C Thomas.

Guilford, A. M., Graham, S. J., & Scheuerle, J. (Eds.). (2007). *The speech language pathologist: From novice to expert.* Upper Saddle River, NJ: Pearson.

Gutierrez-Clellan, V. (1994). Syntactic complexity in Spanish narratives: A developmental study. *Journal of Speech and Hearing Research, 37*, 645–654.

Gutierrez-Clellan, V. (1999). Language choice in intervention with bilingual children. *American Journal of Speech-Language Pathology, 8*, 291–302.

Gutierrez-Clellen, V. F. (2000). Dynamic assessment: An approach to assessing children's language learning potential. *Seminars in Speech and Language, 21*(3), 215–222.

Gutiérrez-Clellen, V. F., Calderón, J., & Ellis Weismer, S. (2004). Verbal working memory in bilingual children. *Journal of Speech, Language, and Hearing Research, 47*, 863–877.

Gutierrez-Clellen, V. F., & DeCurtis, L. (1999). Word definition skills in Spanish-speaking children with language impairment. *Communication Disorders Quarterly, 21*(1), 23–31.

Gutiérrez-Clellen, V. F., & Peña, E. (2001). Dynamic assessment of diverse children: A tutorial. *Language, Speech, and Hearing Services in Schools, 32*, 212–224.

Gutiérrez-Clellen, V. F., & Quinn, R. (1993). Assessing narratives of children from diverse cultural/linguistic groups. *Language, Speech, and Hearing Services in Schools, 24*(1), 2–9.

Gutierrez-Clellen, V. F., Restrepo, M. A., Bedore, L., Peña, L., & Anderson, R. (2000). Language sample analysis: Methodological considerations. *Language, Speech, and Hearing Services in Schools, 31*, 88–98.

Gutierrez-Clellen, V. F., Simon-Cereijido, G., & Leone, A. E. (2009). Code-switching in bilingual children with specific language impairments. *International Journal of Bilingualism, 13*, 91–109.

Haas, E., & Esparza Brown, J. (2019). *Supporting English learners in the classroom: Best practices for distinguishing language acquisition from learning disabilities.* New York, NY: Teachers College Press.

Hacquebord, H. (1989). *Reading comprehension of Turkish and Dutch students attending secondary schools.* Groningen, Germany: RUG.

Hafner, A. L. (2000). *Evaluating the impact of test accommodations on test scores of LEP students and non-LEP students.* Dover, DE: Delaware Department of Education.

Hakuta, K. (1986). *Mirror of language: The debate on bilingualism.* New York, NY: Basic Books.

Halls-Mills, S. (2018). Language progress monitoring for elementary students. *Perspectives of the ASHA Special Interest Groups, SIG 1, 3*(1), 170–179.

Hamayan, E., & Damico, J. (1991). *Limiting bias in the assessment of bilingual students.* Austin, TX: Pro-Ed.

Hammer, C. S., Detwiler, J. S., Detwiler, J., Blood, G. W., & Dean Qualls, C. (2004). Speech-language pathologists' training and confidence in serving Spanish–English bilingual children. *Journal of Communication Disorders, 37*(2), 91–108.

Hammer, C. S., Jia, G., & Uchikoshi, Y. (2011). Language and literacy development of dual language learners growing up in the United States: A call for research. *Child Development Perspectives, 5*(1), 4–9.

Hammett Price, L., Hendricks, S., & Cook, C. (2010). Language sample analysis into clinical practice. *Language, Speech, and Hearing Services in the Schools, 41*, 206–222.

Hanson, M. J. (1992). Ethnic, cultural, and language diversity in intervention settings. In M. J. Hanson & E. W. Lynch (Eds.), *Developing cross-cultural competence: A guide for working with young children and their families* (pp. 3–18). Baltimore, MD: Brookes.

Hanushek, E., Peterson, P., & Woessmann, L. (2012). *Achievement growth: International and state trends in student achievement* (Harvard's Program on Education Policy and Governance & Education Next Report No. 12–03). Retrieved from https://files.eric.ed.gov/full text/ED534652.pdf

Harley, B., & Hart, D. (1997). Language aptitude and second language proficiency in classroom learners of different starting ages. *Studies in Second Language Acquisition, 19*, 379–400.

Harry, B., & Klingner, J. (2006). *Why are so many minority students in special education?* New York, NY: Teachers College Press.

Haskins, R., & Rouse, C. (2005). *Closing achievement gaps. The future of children policy brief.* Washington, DC: The Future of Children.

Hasson, N., Camilleri, B., Jones, D., Smith, J., & Dodd, B. (2013). Discriminating disorder from difference using dynamic assessment with bilingual children. *Child Language Teaching and Therapy, 29*(1), 57–75.

Hegde, M. N., & Davis, D. (1995). *Clinical methods and practicum in speech-language pathology.* San Diego, CA: Singular.

Hegde, M. N., & Maul, C. A. (2006). *Language disorders in children: An evidenced-based approach to assessment and treatment.* Boston, MA: Allyn & Bacon.

Heilmann, J., Miller, J. F., Iglesias, A., Fabiano-Smith, L., Nockerts, A., & Digney-Andriacchi, K. (2008). Narrative transcription accuracy and reliability in two languages. *Topics in Language Disorders, 28,* 178–187.

Heilmann, J., Nockerts, A., & Miller, J. F. (2010). Language sampling: Does the length of the transcript matter? *Language, Speech, and Hearing Services in Schools, 41*(4), 393–404.

Hengst, J., & Johnson, C. J. (2008). Writing and communication disorders across the life span. In C. Bazerman (Ed.), *Handbook of research on writing: History, society, school, individual, text* (pp. 471–484). New York, NY: Lawrence Erlbaum.

Herrell, A., & Jordan, M. (2020). *50 Strategies for teaching English language learners* (6th ed.). Saddle River, NJ: Pearson.

Herrera, G. H., Murry, K. G., & Cabral, R. M. (2007). *Assessment accommodations for classroom teachers of culturally and linguistically diverse students.* Boston, MA: Pearson.

Hester, E. J. (2010). Narrative correlates of reading comprehension in African America children. *Contemporary Issues in Communication Science and Disorders, 37,* 73–85.

Hillier, S. L., Civetta, L., & Pridham, L. (2010). A systematic review of collaborative models for health and education professionals working in school settings and implications for training. *Education for Health, 23*(3), 393.

Hinds, J. (1990). Inductive, deductive, quasi-inductive: Expository writing in Japanese, Korean, Chinese & Tai. In U. Connors & A. Johns (Eds.), *Coherence in writing: Research and pedagogical perspectives* (pp. 87–109). Alexandria, VA: TESOL.

Hoffman, L., & Ireland, M. C. (2018). A panoramic introduction to language intervention progress monitoring. *Perspectives of the ASHA Special Interest Groups, 3*(1), 161–169.

Honigsfeld, A., & Dove, M. (2019). *Collaborating for English learners: A foundational guide to integrated practices* (2nd ed.). Thousand Oaks, CA: Corwin.

Hoover, J., Klingner, J., Baca, L., & Patton, J. M. (2008). *Methods for teaching culturally and linguistically diverse exceptional learners.* Upper Saddle River, NJ: Pearson.

Hoover, J., Mendez Barletta, L., & Klingner, J. K. (2016). Multi-tiered system of supports (MTSS) and English learners. In J. Hoover, L. Baca, & J. Klingner (Eds.), *Why do English language learners struggle with reading?* (2nd ed., pp. 25–56). Thousand Oaks, CA: Corwin.

Hopstock, P. J., & Stephenson, T. G. (2003). *Descriptive study of services to LEP students and LEP students with disabilities. Special Topic Report #2. Analysis of Office of Civil Rights Data related to LEP students.* Washington, DC: U.S. Department of Education, OELA. Retrieved from http://www.ncela.gwu.edu

Horton-Ikard, R., Munoz, M., Thomas-Tate, S., & Keller-Bell, Y. (2009). Establishing a pedagogical framework for the multicultural course in communication sciences and disorders. *American Journal of Speech-Language Pathology, 18,* 192–206.

Horwitz, E. (1987). Linguistic and communicative competence: Reassessing foreign language aptitude. In B. Van Patten, T. Dvorak, & J. Lee (Eds.), *Foreign language learning: A research perspective.* New York, NY: Newbury House.

Howard, E. R., Lindholm-Leary, K. J., Rogers, D., Olague, N., Medina, J., Kennedy, B., . . . Christian, D. (2007). *Guiding principles for dual language education* (3rd ed.). Washington, DC: Center for Applied Linguistics.

Howatt, A. P. R., & Widdowson, H. G. (2004). *A history of English language teaching* (2nd ed.). Oxford, UK: Oxford University Press.

Hudelson, S. (1984). "Kan yu ret an rayt en ingles": Children become literate in English as a second language. *TESOL Quarterly, 18,* 221–238.

Hudelson, S. (1986). Children's writing in ESL: What we've learned, what we're learning. In P. Rigg & D. S. Enright (Eds.), *Children and ESL: Integrating perspectives.* Washington, DC: TESOL.

Hudelson, S. (1987). The role of native language literacy in the education of language minority children. *Language Arts, 64,* 827–841.

Hudelson, S. (1988). *Children's writing in ESL.* Washington, DC: ERIC Clearinghouse on Languages and Linguistics.

Hunt, K. W. (1965). *Grammatical structures written at three grade levels* (Research Rep. No. 3). Champaign, IL: National Council of Teachers of English.

Hutchinson, T. (1996). What to look for in the technical manual: Twenty questions for users. *Language, Speech, and Hearing Services in Schools, 27,* 109–121.

Hux, K. (1993). Language sampling practices: A survey of nine states. *Language, Speech, and Hearing Services in Schools, 2,* 84–91.

Hux, K., Morris-Friehe, M., & Sanger, D. D. (1993). Language sampling practices: A survey of nine states. *Language, Speech, and Hearing Services in Schools, 24,* 84–91.

IDEA Language Proficiency Tests (IPT). (2005). Brea, CA: Ballard & Tighe. Retrieved from http://www.ballard-tighe.com/products/la/iptFamilyTests.asp

IDEA Proficiency Test (IPT). (2016). Brea, CA: Ballard & Tighe. Retrieved from http://www.ballard-tighe.com/ipt/about/

Indiana Department of Education. (2006). *Language Assessment Scales Links (LAS Links)*. Monterey, CA: CB/McGraw-Hill. Retrieved from http://www.doe.in.gov/lmmp/las-links.html

Individuals with Disabilities Education Act (IDEA). (1997). *Federal Register, 62*(204). Part V, Department of Education, 34 CFR PARTSW 300, 303.

Individuals with Disabilities Education Act (IDEA). (2004). Pub. L. No. 108-446, 118 Stat. 2647.

Individuals with Disabilities Education Improvement Act (IDEA). (2004). PL 108-446, 20 U.S.C. §§ 1400 et seq.

Institute of Education Science. (2006). Vocabulary improvement program for English language learners and their classmates. *IES What Works Clearinghouse Intervention Report*. Washington, DC: Author. Retrieved from http://www.asha.org/members/compendiumSearch Results.aspx?type=1&searchtext=Literacy

Institute of Education Science. (2007a). *Effective literacy and English language instruction for English learners in the elementary grades*. Washington, DC: Author. Retrieved from http://ies.ed.gov/ncee/wwc/pdf/practiceguides/20074011.pdf

Institute of Education Science. (2007b). English language learners. *IES What Works Clearinghouse Intervention Report*. Washington, DC: Author. Retrieved from http://www.asha.org/members/compendium SearchResults.aspx?type=1&searchtext=Literacy

Institute of Education Science. (2010). Improving reading comprehension in kindergarten through 3rd grade. *IES Practice Guide*. Washington, DC: Author.

Institute of Education Science. (2016). Foundational skills to support reading for understanding in kindergarten through 3rd grade. *IES Practice Guide*. Washington, DC: Author.

Institute of Education Science. (2018). Teaching elementary school students to be effective writers. *IES Practice Guide*. Washington, DC: Author.

Interprofessional Education Collaborative Expert Panel. (2011). *Core competencies for interprofessional collaborative practice: Report of an expert panel*. Washington, DC: Interprofessional Education Collaborative.

Ireland, M., & Conrad, B. (2016). Evaluation and eligibility for speech-language services in schools. *Perspectives of the ASHA Special Interest Group, SIG 16, 1*(4), 78–90.

Jacobson, P. F., & Schwartz, R. G. (2002). Morphology in incipient bilingual Spanish-speaking preschool children with specific language impairment. *Applied Psycholinguistics, 23,* 23–41.

Jimenez, B. (1987). Acquisition of Spanish consonants in children aged 3–5 years, 7 months. *Language, Speech, and Hearing Services in Schools, 18,* 357–363.

Jimerson, S. R., Burns, M. K., & VanDerHeyden, A. M. (Eds.). (2016). *Handbook of response to intervention: The science and practice of multi-tiered systems of support* (2nd ed.). New York, NY: Springer.

Johannessen, G., Thorsos, N., & Dickinson, G. (2016). Current conditions of bilingual teacher preparation programs in public universities in USA. *Education and Society, 34*(2), 27–48.

Johnson, A. F., Prelock, P., & Apel, K. (2016). *IPE 101: Introduction to interprofessional education and practice for speech-language pathology.* Rockville, MD: American Speech-Language-Hearing Association.

Johnson, K., & Johnson, H. (1999). *Encyclopedic dictionary of applied linguistics: A handbook for language teaching.* Oxford, UK: Blackwell.

Johnson, P. (1981). Effects on reading comprehension of language complexity and cultural background of a text. *TESOL Quarterly, 15*(2), 169–181.

Juárez, M. (1983). Assessment and treatment of minority language handicapped children: The role of the monolingual speech-language pathologist. *Topics in Language Disorders, 3,* 57–65.

Jusczyk, P. W. (1985). The high-amplitude sucking technique as a methodological tool in speech perception research. In G. Gottlieb & N. Krasnegor (Eds.), *Measurement of audition and vision in the first year of postnatal life.* Norwood, NJ: Ablex.

Justice, L. (2006). Evidence-based practice, response to intervention, and the prevention of reading difficulties. *Language, Speech, and Hearing Services in Schools, 37*(4), 284–297.

Justice, L. M., & Fey, M. E. (2004, September 21). Evidence-based practice in schools: Integrating craft and theory with science and data. *ASHA Leader,* pp. 4–5, 30–32.

Kagan, S. (1994). *Cooperative learning.* San Clemente, CA: Resources for Teachers.

Karabenick, S. A., & Clemens Noda, P. A. (2004). Professional development implications of teachers' beliefs and attitudes toward English language learners. *Bilingual Research Journal, 28*(1), 55–75.

Kamhi, A., Allen, J., & Catts, H. (2001). The role of the speech-language pathologist in improving decoding skills. *Seminars in Speech and Language, 22,* 175–185.

Kamhi, A. G., & Catts, H. W. (2012). *Language and reading disabilities* (3rd ed.). Boston, MA: Pearson Education.

Kammey, K. C. W., Ritzer, G., & Yetman, N. R. (1990). *Sociology: Experiences changing society.* Boston, MA: Allyn & Bacon.

Kan, P. F., & Kohnert, K. (2005). Preschoolers learning Hmong and English: Lexical-semantic skills in L1 and L2. *Journal of Speech, Language and Hearing Research, 48,* 372–383.

Kangas, S. (2014). When special education trumps ESL: An investigation of service delivery for ELLs with disabilities. *Critical Inquiry in Language Studies, 11*(4), 273–306.

Kangas, S. (2018). Why working apart doesn't work at all: Special Education and English learner teacher collaborations. *Intervention in School and Clinic, 54*(1), 31–39.

Kangas, S. (2019). English learners with disabilities: Linguistic development and educational equity in jeopardy. In: X. Gao (Ed.), *Second Handbook of English Language Teaching* (pp. 919-937). New York, NY: Springer.

Kapantzoglou, M., Fergadiotis, G., & Restrepo, M. A. (2017). Language sample analysis and elicitation technique effects in bilingual children with and without language impairment. *Journal of Speech, Language, and Hearing Research, 60*(10), 2852–2864.

Kaplan, R. B. (1966). Cultural patterns in intercultural education. *Language Learning, 16,* 1–20.

Kaplan, R. B. (2000). Contrastive rhetoric and discourse analysis: Who writes what to whom? When? In what circumstances? In S. Sarangi & M. Coulthard (Eds.), *Discourse and social life.* Edinburgh, UK: Pearson Education.

Karabenick, S. A., & Clemens Noda, P. A. (2004). Professional development implications of teachers' beliefs and attitudes toward English language learners. *Bilingual Research Journal, 28*(1), 55–75.

Karniol, R. (1992). Stuttering out of bilingualism. *First Language, 12,* 255–283.

Katz, L. A., Maag, A., Fallon, K. A., Blenkarn, K., & Smith, M. K. (2010). What makes a caseload (un)manageable? School-based speech language pathologists speak. *Language, Speech, and Hearing Services in Schools, 41,* 139–151.

Kayser, H. (1995a). Assessment of speech and language impairments in bilingual children. In H. Kayser (Ed.), *Bilingual speech*-language *pathology: An Hispanic focus* (pp. 243–264). San Diego, CA: Singular.

Kayser, H. (Ed.). (1995b). *Bilingual speech-language pathology: An Hispanic focus.* San Diego, CA: Singular.

Kayser, H. (1996). Cultural/linguistic variation in the United States and its implications for assessment and intervention in speech-language pathology: An epilogue. *Language, Speech, and Hearing Services in the Schools, 27*(4), 385–387.

Kayser, H. (1998). *Assessment and intervention resource for Hispanic children*. San Diego, CA: Singular.

Kayser, H. (2002). Bilingual language development and language disorders. In D. E. Battle (Ed.), *Communication disorders in multicultural populations* (3rd ed., pp. 205–232). Woburn, MA: Butterworth-Heinemann.

Kayser, H. (2008). *Educating Latino preschool children*. San Diego, CA: Plural Publishing.

Kayser, H., & Restrepo, M. (1995). Language samples: Elicitation and analysis. In H. Kayser (Ed.), *Bilingual speech-language pathology: An Hispanic focus* (pp. 265–286). San Diego, CA: Singular.

Keller-Allen, C. (2006). *English language learners with disabilities: Identification and other state policies and issues*. Alexandria, VA: Project Forum, National Association of State Directors of Special Education.

Kemp, K., & Klee, T. (1997). Clinical language sampling practices: Results of a survey of speech-language pathologists in the United States. *Child Language Teaching and Therapy, 13*(2), 161–176.

Kena, G., Hussar W., McFarland J., de Brey C., Musu-Gillette, L., Wang, X., . . . Dunlop Velez, E. (2016). *The condition of education 2016* (NCES 2016-144). Washington, DC: U.S. Department of Education, National Center for Education Statistics.

Kena, G., Musu-Gillette, L., Robinson, J., Wang, X., Rathbun, A., Zhang, J., . . . Dunlop Velez, E. (2015). *The condition of education 2015* (NCES 2015-144). Washington, DC: U.S. Department of Education, National Center for Education Statistics.

Kendall, D. (1997). *Race, class, and gender in a diverse society: A text reader*. Upper Saddle River, NJ: Pearson.

Kennedy, B., & Medina, J. (2017). *Dual language education: Answers to questions from the field* (CAL Practitioner Brief). Washington, DC: Center for Applied Linguistics. Retrieved from http://www.cal.org/resource-center/briefs

Kieffer, M. J. (2008). Catching up or falling behind? Initial English proficiency, concentrated poverty, and the reading growth of language minority learners in the United States. *Journal of Educational Psychology, 100*, 851–868.

Kieffer, M. J. (2010). Socioeconomic status, English proficiency, and late-emerging reading difficulties. *Educational Researcher, 39*, 484–486.

Kimble, C. (2013). Speech-language pathologists' comfort levels in English language learner service delivery. *Communication Disorders Quarterly, 35*(1), 21–27.

Kindler, A. L. (2002). *Survey of the states' limited English proficient students and available educational program and services: 2000–2001 summary report*. Washington, DC: National Clearinghouse for

English Language Acquisition and Language Instruction Educational Programs.

Kinneavy, J. E. (1969). The basic aims of discourse. *College Composition and Communication, 20*(5), 297–304.

Kiplinger, V. L., Haug, C. A., & Abedi, J. (2000, June). *A math assessment should test math, not reading: One state's approach to the problem.* Paper presented at the 30th annual National Conference on Large-Scale Assessment, Snowbird, UT.

Kirkpatrick, A. (1997). Traditional Chinese text structures and their influence on the writing in Chinese and English of contemporary mainland Chinese students. *Journal of Second Language Writing, 6*(3), 223–244.

Klecan-Aker, J., & Hedrick, D. (1985). A study of the syntactic language skills of normal school-age children. *Language, Speech, and Hearing Services in Schools, 16*, 187–198.

Klingner, J. K., Artiles, A. J., & Barletta, L. M. (2006). English language learners who struggle with reading: Language acquisition or LD? *Journal of Learning Disabilities, 39*, 108–128.

Klingner, J. K., Artiles, A. J., Kozleski, E., Harry, B., Zion, S., Tate, W., . . . Riley, D. (2005). Addressing the disproportionate representation of culturally and linguistically diverse students in special education through culturally responsive educational systems. *Education Policy Analysis Archives, 13*(38). Retrieved from http://epaa.asu.edu/epaa/v13n38/

Klingner, J. K., & Edwards, P. A. (2006). Cultural considerations with response to intervention models. *Reading Research Quarterly, 41*, 108–117.

Klingner, J. K., & Eppolito, A. E. (2014). *English language learners: Differentiating between language acquisition and learning disabilities.* Arlington, VA: Council for Exceptional Children.

Klingner, J. K., & Harry, B. (2006). The special education referral and decision-making process for English language learners: Child study team meetings and placement conferences. *Teachers College Record, 108*(11), 2247–2281.

Klingner, J. K., Hoover, J., & Baca, L. (Eds.). (2008). *Why do English language learners struggle with reading?* Thousand Oaks, CA: Corwin Press.

Koda, K. (2007). Reading and language learning: Cross-linguistic constraints on second language reading development. *Language Learning Supplement, 57*, 1–44.

Koda, K., & Miller, R. (2018). Cross-linguistic interaction in L2 word meaning inference in English as a foreign language. In H. Pae (Ed.), *Writing systems, reading processes, and cross-linguistic influences: Reflections from the Chinese, Japanese and Korean languages* (pp. 293–312). Philadelphia, PA: John Benjamins.

Kohnert, K. (2008). *Language disorders in bilingual children and adults*. San Diego, CA: Plural Publishing.

Kohnert, K. (2010). Bilingual children with primary language impairment: Issues, evidence and implications for clinical actions. *Journal of Communication Disorders, 43*, 456–473.

Kohnert, K., & Derr, A. (2004). Language intervention with bilingual children. In B. Goldstein (Ed.), *Bilingual language development and disorders in Spanish–English speakers* (pp. 311–338). Baltimore, MD: Brookes.

Kohnert, K., Kennedy, M. R. T., Glaze, L., Kan, P. F., & Carney, E. (2003). Breadth and depth of diversity in Minnesota: Challenges to clinical competency. *American Journal of Speech-Language Pathology, 12*, 259–272.

Kohnert, K., & Medina, A. (2009). Bilingual children and communication disorders: A 30-year research retrospective. *Seminars in Speech and Language, 30*, 219–233. doi:10.1055/s-0029-1241721

Koutsoftas, A., Maffucci, D., & Dayalu, V. (2018). Evaluation of a program to increase classroom based speech and language intervention in an elementary school. *Perspectives of the ASHA Special Interest Groups, 3*(16), 95–109.

Krashen, S. D. (1981). Bilingual education and second language acquisition theory. In California State Department of Education (Ed.), *Schooling and language minority students: A theoretical framework* (pp. 51–79). Los Angeles, CA: California State University, Evaluation, Dissemination, and Assessment Center.

Krashen, S. D. (1987). *Principles and practices in second language acquisition*. New York, NY: Prentice-Hall.

Krashen, S. D. (1993). *The power of reading: Insights from the research*. Englewood, CO: Libraries Unlimited.

Krashen, S. D. (1994). The input hypothesis and its rivals. In N. Ellis (Ed.), *Implicit and explicit learning of languages* (pp. 45–77). London, UK: Academic Press.

Krashen, S. D. (2003). *Explorations in language acquisition and use*. Portsmouth, NH: Heinemann.

Krashen, S. D. (2008). The comprehension hypothesis extended. In T. Piske & M. Young-Scholten (Eds.), *Input matters in SLA* (pp. 81–94). Bristol, UK: Multilingual Matters.

Krashen, S. D. (2011). The compelling (not just interesting) input hypothesis. *The English Connection: A Publication of KOTESOL, 15*(3). Retrieved from https://koreatesol.org/sites/default/files/pdf_publications/TECv15n3-11Autumn

Krashen, S. D. (2017). The case for comprehensible input. *Language Magazine*. Retrieved from https://www.languagemagazine.com/2017/07/17/case-for-comprehension/.pdf

Krashen, S. D., Scarcella, R., & Long, M. (Eds.). (1982). *Child-adult differences in second language acquisition.* Rowley, MA: Newbury House.

Krashen, S. D., & Terrell, T. (1983). *The natural approach: Language acquisition in the classroom.* Oxford, UK: Pergamon Press.

Kritikos, E. (2003). SLPs' beliefs about language assessment of bilingual/bicultural individuals. *American Journal of Speech-Language Pathology, 12,* 73–91.

Kroll, J. F., & Tokowicz, N. (2001). The development of conceptual representation for words in a second language. In J. Nicol (Ed.), *One mind, two languages* (pp. 49–71). Oxford, UK: Blackwell.

Kummerer, S. E., Lopez-Reyna, N. A., & Hughes, M. T. (2007). Mexican immigrant mothers' perceptions of their children's communication disabilities, emergent literacy development, and speech-language therapy program. *American Journal of Speech-Language Pathology, 16*(3), 271–282.

Laing, S. P., & Kamhi, A. (2003). Alternative assessment of language and literacy in culturally and linguistically diverse populations. *Language, Speech, and Hearing Services in Schools, 34,* 44–55.

Langdon, H. W. (1989). Language disorder or difference? Assessing the skills of Hispanic students. *Exceptional Children, 56,* 160–167.

Langdon, H. W. (1992). Language communication and sociocultural patterns in Latino families. In H. W. Langdon & L. L. Cheng (Eds.), *Hispanic children and adults with communication disorders: Assessment and intervention* (pp. 99–131). Gaithersburg, MD: Aspen.

Langdon, H. W. (1999). Foreign accent: Implications for delivery of speech and language services. *Topics in Language Disorders, 19*(4), 49–65.

Langdon, H. W. (2012). *Spanish Structured Photographic Expressive Language Test 3* (SPANISH SPELT®- 3). DeKalb, IL: Janelle.

Langdon, H. W., & Cheng, L. L. (2002). *Collaborating with interpreters and translators: A guide for communication disorders professionals.* Austin, TX: Pro-Ed.

Langdon, H. W., & Irvine Saenz, T. (1996). *Language assessment and intervention with multicultural students.* Oceanside, CA: Academic Communication Associates.

Langdon, H. W., & Saenz, T. I. (2016). Working with interpreters to support students who are English language learners. *Perspectives of the ASHA Special Interest Groups SIG 16*(1), 15–27.

Larkin, E., Restrepo, M. A., & Morgan, G. (2007, November). *How the bilingual syntax measure measures up: A comparison of Spanish/English proficiency scores to the Stanford English Language Proficiency Test and parent report.* Paper presented at the annual convention of the American Speech-Language-Hearing Association, Boston, MA.

Law, J., Boyle, J., Harris, F., Harkness, A., & Nye, C. (2000). Prevalence and natural history of primary speech and language delay: Findings from a systematic review of the literature. *International Journal of Language and Communication Disorders, 35*(2), 165–188.

Lazewnik, R., Creaghead, N., Smith, A., Prendeville, J., Raisor-Becker, L., & Silbert, N. (2019). Identifiers of language impairment for Spanish-English dual language learners. *Language, Speech, and Hearing Services in Schools, 50*(1), 126–137.

Leaders. (2013). *Test review: Preschool language scales* (5th ed.). Retrieved from https://cpb-us-w2.wpmucdn.com/edblogs.columbia.edu/dist/d/730/files/2015/05/PLS5-English-finaldraft-2dgptop.pdf

Leafstedt, J. M., & Gerber, M. M. (2005). Crossover of phonological processing skills: A study of Spanish-speaking students in two instructional settings. *Remedial and Special Education, 26*, 226–235.

League of United Latin American Citizens (LULAC) et al. v. State Board of Education et al. Consent Decree. (1990).

Lee, J. S., & Oxelson, E. (2006). "It's not my job": K–12 teacher attitudes toward students' heritage language maintenance. *Bilingual Research Journal, 30*(2), 453–477.

Lee, J. S., & Schallert, D. L. (1997). The relative contribution of L2 language proficiency and L1 reading ability to L2 reading performance: A test of the threshold hypothesis in an EFL context. *TESOL Quarterly, 31*, 713–739.

Lesaux, N. K., & Siegel, L. S. (2003). The development of reading in children who speak English as a second language. *Developmental Psychology, 36*, 1005–1019.

Letts, C. (1999). Becoming bilingual. In B. Spolsky & R. E. Asher (Eds.), *Concise encyclopedia of educational linguistics*. Oxford, UK: Pergamon.

Letts, C., & Sinka, I. (2013). Research and practice in working with children who are bilingual or have English as an additional language and who have language and communication needs. *Child Language Teaching and Therapy, 29*(1), 7–9.

Leung, B. (1993, November). *Assessment considerations with culturally and linguistically diverse students.* Paper presented at the National Association for Multicultural Education, Los Angeles, CA.

Lewis, L., Parsad, B., Carey, N., Bartfai, N., Smerdon, B., & Green, B. (1999). *Teacher quality: A report on the preparation and qualifications of public-school teachers* (NCES 199-080). Washington, DC: National Center for Education Statistics.

Lhamon, C., & Gupta, V. (2015). *Dear colleague letter: English learner students and limited English proficient parents.* U.S. Department of Education. Retrieved from https://www2.ed.gov/about/offices/list/ocr/ellresources.html

Li, G., & Edwards, P. (Eds.). (2010). *Best practices in ELL instruction.* New York, NY: Guilford Press.

Lian, M., & Fantanez-Phelan, S. (2001). Perceptions of Latino parents regarding cultural and linguistic issues and advocacy for children with disabilities. *Journal of the Association for Persons with Severe Handicaps, 26,* 189–194.

Lidz, C. S. (1991). *Practitioner's guide to dynamic assessment.* New York, NY: Guilford Press.

Lidz, C. S., & Peña, E. (1996). Dynamic assessment: The model, its relevance as a nonbiased approach, and its application to Latino American preschool children. *Language, Speech, and Hearing Services in the Schools, 27,* 367–372.

Lidz, C. S. & Peña, E. D. (2009). Response to intervention and dynamic assessment: Do we just appear to be speaking the same language? *Seminars in Speech and Language, 30,* 121–133.

Lightbown, P., & Spada, N. M. (2013). *How languages are learned* (4th ed.). Oxford, UK: Oxford University Press.

Lin, C. Y., Cheng, C., & Wang, M. (2018). The contribution of phonological and morphological awareness in Chinese-English bilingual reading acquisition. *Reading and Writing: An Interdisciplinary Journal, 31*(1), 99–132. doi:10.1007/s11145-017-9775-8

Linan-Thompson, S. (2010). Response to instruction, English language learners and disproportionate representation: The role of assessment. *Psichothema, 22*(4), 970–974.

Linan-Thompson, S., & Ortiz, A. (2009). Response to intervention and English language learners: Instructional and assessment considerations. *Seminars in Speech and Language, 30,* 105–120.

Linares, N. (1981). Rules for calculating mean length of utterance in morphemes for Spanish. In J. Erickson & D. Omark (Eds.), *Communication assessment of the bilingual bicultural child* (pp. 291–295). Baltimore, MD: University Park Press.

Lindholm-Leary, K. J., & Borsato, G. (2006). Academic achievement. In F. Genesee, K. Lindholm-Leary, W. Saunders, & D. Christian (Eds.), *Educating English language learners* (pp. 157–179). New York, NY: Cambridge University Press.

Lindholm-Leary, K. J., & Genesee, F. (2010). Alternative educational programs for English language learners. In California Department of Education (Ed.), *Improving education for English learners: Research-based approaches* (pp. 323–382). Sacramento, CA: CDE Press. Retrieved from https://www.cde.ca.gov/sp/el/er/documents/chapter6.pdf

Linquanti, R., & Cook, G. (2013). *Toward a "common definition of English learner": Guidance for states and state assessment consortia in defining and addressing policy and technical issues and options.* Washington, DC: Council of Chief State School Officers.

Liu, K., Ward, J., Thurlow, M., & Christensen, L. (2017). Large scale assessment and English language learners with disabilities. *Educational Policy*, *3*(5), 551–583.

Liu, K., Watkins, E., Pompa, D., McLeod, P., Elliott, J., & Gaylord, V. (Eds.). (2013, Winter/Spring). *Impact: Feature issue on educating K–12 English language learners with disabilities.* Minneapolis, MN: University of Minnesota, Institute on Community Integration.

Long, M. H. (1983). Native speaker/non-native speaker conversation and negotiation of comprehensible input. *Applied Linguistics*, *4*(2), 126–141.

Long, M. H. (1990). Maturational constraints on language development. *Studies on Second Language Acquisition*, *12*(3), 251–285.

Long, S. H., & Channell, R. W. (2001). Accuracy of four language analysis procedures performed automatically. *American Journal of Speech-Language Pathology*, *10*, 180–188.

Long, S. H., Fey, M. E., & Channell, R. W. (2000). *Computerized Profiling (CP)* (Version 9.2.7, MS-DOS) [Computer software]. Cleveland, OH: Department of Communication Sciences, Case Western Reserve University.

Lonigan, J., Christopher, J., & Shanahan, T. (2009). *Developing early literacy: Report of the National Early Literacy Panel. Executive Summary. A Scientific Synthesis of Early Literacy Development and Implications for Intervention.* Washington, DC: National Institute for Literacy.

Loop, C. (2002). *Which tests are commonly used to determine English and/or Spanish language proficiency?* Washington, DC: National Clearinghouse for English Language Acquisition.

Lowe, J., & Herranen, M. (1978). Conflict in teamwork: Understanding roles and relationship. *Social Work in Health Care*, *3*, 323–331.

Lowe, J., & Herranen, M. (1982). Understanding teamwork: Another look at the concepts. *Social Work in Health Care*, *7*, 1–11.

Lubinski, R., & Fratelli, C. (Eds.). (2001). *Professional issues in speech language pathology and audiology.* San Diego, CA: Singular.

Ludwig, D., & Kerins, M. (2019). Interprofessional education: application of interprofessional education collaborative core competencies to school settings. *Perspectives of the ASHA Special Interest Groups*, *4*(2), 269–274.

Lynch, E. W., & Hanson, M. J. (Eds.). (1998). *Developing cross-cultural competence: A guide for working with young children and their families.* Baltimore, MD: Brookes.

MacGregor-Mendoza, P. (2000). Aquí no se habla Español: Stories of linguistic repression in Southwest schools. *Bilingual Research Journal*, *24*(4), 333–345.

MacSwan, J., & Pray, L. (2005). Learning English bilingually: Age of onset of exposure and rate of acquisition among English language learners in a bilingual education program. *Bilingual Research Journal, 29*, 653–678.

MacSwan, J., & Rolstad, K. (2006). How language proficiency tests mislead us about ability: Implications for English language learner placement in special education. *Teachers College Record, 108*(11), 2304–2328.

MacWhinney, B. (1996). The CHILDES system. *American Journal of Speech-Language Pathology, 5*, 5–14.

MacWhinney, B. (2000a). *The CHILDES project: Tools for analyzing talk* (3rd ed.). Mahwah, NJ: Erlbaum.

MacWhinney, B. (2000b). CLAN [Computer software]. Pittsburgh, PA: Carnegie Mellon University.

Mancilla-Martinez, J., Kieffer, M. J., Biancarosa, G., Christodoulou, J. A., & Snow, C. E. (2011). Investigating English reading comprehension growth in adolescent language minority learners: Some insights from the simple view. *Reading and Writing, 24*, 339–354.

Mann, N. (2018). *Collaboration among professionals working with English learners with disabilities in a newcomer school: A case study.* Retrieved from https://etd.ohiolink.edu/

Martin, N. (2013a). *Expressive one-word picture vocabulary test: Spanish-bilingual edition* (4th ed.). Novato, CA: Academic Therapy Publications.

Martin, N. (2013b). *Receptive one-word picture vocabulary test: Spanish-bilingual edition* (4th ed.). Novato, CA: Academic Therapy Publications.

Martínez-Álvarez, P. (2019). Dis/ability labels and emergent bilingual children: Current research and new possibilities to grow as bilingual and biliterate learners. *Race Ethnicity and Education, 22*(2), 174–193. doi:10.1080/13613324.2018.1538120

Masgoret, A., & Gardner, R. (2003). Attitudes, motivation, and second language learning: A meta-analysis of studies conducted by Gardner and associates. *Language Learning, 53*, 123–163.

Master, B., Loeb, S., Whitney, C., & Wyckoff, J. (2016). Different skills? Identifying differentially effective teachers of English language learners. *Elementary School Journal, 117*(2), 261–284.

Mathes, P. G., Pollard-Durodola, S., Cardenas-Hagen, E., Linan-Thompson, S., & Vaugh, S. (2007). Teaching struggling readers who are native Spanish speakers: What do we know? *Language, Speech, and Hearing Services in Schools, 38*, 260–271.

Matsuda, M., & O'Connor, L. (1993, April). *Creating an effective partnership: Training bilingual communication aides.* Paper presented at the annual conference of the California Speech-Language-Hearing Association, Palm Springs, CA.

Matsuda, P. K. (1997). Contrastive rhetoric in context: A dynamic model of L2 writing. *Journal of Second Language Writing, 6*(1), 45–60.

Matsumoto, K. (1995). Research paper writing strategies of professional Japanese EFL writers. *TESL Canada Journal, 13*(1), 17–27.

Mattes, L. J., & Saldana-Illingworth, C. (2008). *Bilingual communication assessment resource: Tools for assessing speech, language, and learning.* Oceanside, CA: Academic Communication Associates.

Matthews, H., & Ewen, D. (2006). *Reaching all children? Understanding early care and education participation among immigrant families.* Washington, DC: Center for Law and Social Policy. Retrieved from https://files.eric.ed.gov/fulltext/ED489574.pdf

McAnally, P. L., Rose, S., & Quigley, S. P. (1994). *Language learning practices with deaf children.* Austin, TX: Pro-Ed.

McCarthy, M. P. (2003, October). Promoting problem-solving and self-evaluation in clinical education through a collaborative approach to supervision. *Perspectives on Administration and Supervision,* pp. 20–26.

McCartney, E. (1999). Barriers to collaboration: An analysis of systemic barriers to collaboration between teachers and speech and language therapists. *International Journal of Language and Communication Disorders, 34,* 431–440.

McCauley, R. J. (1996). Familiar strangers: Criterion-referenced measures in communication disorders. *Language, Speech, and Hearing Services in Schools, 27,* 122–131.

McCauley, R. J., & Swisher, L. (1984). Psychometric review of language and articulation tests for preschool children. *Journal of Speech and Hearing Disorders, 49,* 34–42.

McCombs, M., & McCombs, Z. (1969). Descriptive style of deaf children. *Volta Review, 71,* 23–26.

McConnell-Stephen, P. L., Weiler, E. M., Sandman, D. E., & Dell'aira, A. (1994). Survey of speech-language psychologists regarding training in dialects. *Hearsay, 9,* 15–19.

McDonnell, L. M., McLaughlin, M. J., & Morison, P. (Eds.). (1997). *Educating one and all: Students with disabilities and standards-based reform.* Washington, DC: National Academy Press.

McFarland, J., Hussar, B., de Brey, C., Snyder, T., Wang, X., Wilkinson-Flicker, S., . . . Hinz, S. (2018). *The condition of education 2018* (NCES 20181444). Retrieved from https://nces.ed.gov/pubsearch/pubsinfo.asp?pubid=2018144

McFarland, J., Hussar, B., Wang, X., Zhang, J., Wang, K., Rathbun, A., . . . Bullock Mann, F. (2018). *The condition of education 2018* (NCES 2018-144). Washington, DC: National Center for Education Statistics.

Retrieved from https://nces.ed.gov/pubsearch/pubsinfo.asp?pubid =2018144

McLeod, V., & International Expert Panel on Multilingual Children's Speech. (2017). Tutorial: Speech assessment for multilingual children who do not speak the same language(s) as the speech-language pathologist. *American Journal of Speech-Language Pathology, 26*(3), 691–708.

Mehler, J., Bertoncini, J., Barriere, M., & Jassik-Gerschenfeld, D. (1978). Infant recognition of mother's voice. *Perception, 7,* 491–497.

Mellard, D. F., & Johnson, E. (2007). *RTI: A practitioner's guide to implementing Response to Intervention.* Thousand Oaks, CA: Corwin Press.

Menken, K., & Atunez, B. (2001). *An overview of the preparation and certification of teachers working with limited English proficient students.* Washington, DC: National Clearinghouse of Bilingual Education. Retrieved from http://www.ericsp.org/pages/digests/ncbe.pdf

Menyuk, P., & Brisk, M. E. (2005). *Language development and education: Children with varying language experience.* Hampshire, UK: Palgrave MacMillan.

Merino, B. (1992). Acquisition of syntactic and phonological features in Spanish. In H. W. Langdon & L. Cheng (Eds.), *Hispanic children and adults with communication disorders: Assessment and intervention.* Gaithersburg, MD: Aspen.

Meyer, A., Rose, D. H., & Gordon, D. (2014). *Universal design for learning: Theory and Practice.* Wakefield, MA: CAST Professional Publishing.

Mihai, F. (2010). *Assessing English language learners in the content areas.* Ann Arbor, MI: University of Michigan Press.

Mihai, F. M. (2017). *Assessing English learners in the content areas: A research-into-practice guide for educators* (2nd ed.). Ann Arbor, MI: University of Michigan Press.

Miller, J., & Iglesias, A. (2006). *Systematic Analysis of Language Transcripts (SALT),* English & Spanish (Version 9) [Computer software]. Madison: Language Analysis Lab, University of Wisconsin–Madison.

Miller, J., & Iglesias, A. (2016). *Systematic analysis of language transcripts (SALT):* Research Version 16 [Computer software]. Middleton, WI: SALT Software, LLC.

Miller, J. F., Andriacchi, K., & Nockerts, A. (2016). Using language sample analysis to assess spoken language production in adolescents. *Language, Speech, and Hearing Services in Schools, 47,* 99–112.

Miller, J. F., Freiberg, C., Rolland, M.-B., & Reeves, M. A. (1992). Implementing computerized language sample analysis in the public school. *Topics in Language Disorders, 12*(2), 69–82.

Minnesota Department of Education. (2017). *English learner education program guidelines: Identification and program basics.*

Retrieved from http://search.education.state.mn.us/search?q=identi fication+and+placement+procedures+for+ELs+&searchbutton=Go &output=xml_no_dtd&oe=UTF-8&ie=UTF-8&client=New_frontend& proxystylesheet=New_frontend&site=default_collection

Mitchell, R., & Myles, F. (2013). *Second language learning theories* (3rd ed.). New York, NY: Routledge.

Moats, L. C. (2010). *Speech to print: Language essentials for teachers* (2nd ed.). Baltimore, MD: Brookes.

Moeller, D. (1976). *Speech pathology and audiology: Iowa organization of a discipline.* Iowa City, IA: University of Iowa Press.

Monroy, R., & Scheu, D. (1997). Reflejo cultural en los estilos de his-panohablantes estudiantes de inglés como LE. Consideraciones pedagógicas (Cultural reflection in the styles of Spanish-speaking English learners. Pedagogical considerations). In F. Gutiérrez, (Ed.), *Estudios de Lingüística Aplicada y Literatura. Homenaje Póstumo al profesor Juan Conesa Sánchez* (pp. 189–201). Murcia, Spain: Uni-versidad de Murcia.

Montone, C. L. (1995, June). *Piecing linguistically and culturally diverse learners: Effective programs and practices.* Paper presented at National Center for Research on Cultural Diversity and Second Language Learn-ing, Santa Cruz, CA. Retrieved from ERIC database (ED381036)

Moore, B., & Montgomery, J. K. (2018). *Making a difference for America's children: Speech-language pathologists in public schools* (3rd ed.). Austin, TX: Pro-Ed.

Morgan, P. L., Farkas, G., Hillemeier, M. M., Mattison, R., Maczuga, S., Li, H., & Cook, M. (2015). Minorities are disproportionately under-represented in special education: Longitudinal evidence across five disability conditions. *Educational Researcher, 44*(5), 278–292. doi:10 .3102/0013189X15591157

Moughamian, A. C., Rivera, M. O., & Francis, D. J. (2009). *Instruc-tional models and strategies for teaching English language learners.* Portsmouth, NH: RMC Research Corporation, Center on Instruction. Retrieved from https://files.eric.ed.gov/fulltext/ED517794.pdf

Muljani, D., Koda, K., & Moates, D. (1998). The development of word recognition in a second language. *Applied Psycholinguistics, 19,* 99–113.

Mullen, R. (2007, March 6). The state of the evidence: ASHA develops levels of evidence for communication sciences and disorders. *ASHA Leader.*

Muñoz, M., White, M., & Horton-Ikard, R. (2014). The identification conundrum. *ASHA Leader, 19*(11), 48–53.

Murdick, N., Gartin, B., & Crabtree, T. (2014). *Special education law* (3rd ed.). Upper Saddle River, NJ: Pearson Education.

Murza, K. A., Malani, M. D., & Hahs-Vaughn, D. L. (2014). Using the Common Core State Standards to guide therapy in the schools: Confidently accepting the challenge. *Perspectives on School-Based Issues, 15*(4), 125–133. doi:10.1044/sbi15.4.125

Nathenson-Mejia, S. (1994). Bridges between home and school: Literacy building activities for non-native English speaking homes. *Journal of Educational Issues of Language Minority Students, 14*, 149–164.

National Academies of Sciences, Engineering, and Medicine. (2017). *Promoting the educational success of children and youth learning English: Promising futures*. Washington, DC: National Academies Press.

National Assessment of Educational Progress. (2008). *Reading framework for the 2009 national assessment of educational progress*. Washington, DC: National Assessment Governing Board. Retrieved from https://www.nagb.gov/assets/documents/publications/frame works/reading/2009-reading-framework.pdf

National Association for Bilingual Education (NABE) & ILIEAD Project. (2002). *Determining appropriate referrals of English language learners to special education: A self-assessment guide for principals*. Arlington, VA: Council for Exceptional Children.

National Center for Education Statistics. (2009). *The nation's report card: Reading 2009* (NCES 2010–458). Washington, DC: Institute of Education Sciences, U.S. Department of Education.

National Center on Educational Outcomes. (2011). *Understanding subgroups in common state assessments: Special education students and ELLs* (NCEO Brief No. 4). Minneapolis, MN: National Center on Educational Outcomes, University of Minnesota.

National Clearinghouse for English Language Acquisition. (2011, February). *The growing number of English learner students*. Retrieved from http://www.ncela.gwu.edu/files/uploads/9/growingLEP_0809 .pdf

National Council of Teachers of English. (2008). *English Language Learners: An NCTE Policy Research Brief*. Washington, DC: Author. Retrieved from https://secure.ncte.org/library/NCTEFiles/Resources/ Positions/Chron0308PolicyBrief.pdf?_ga=2.155591416.232623478 .1575582054-432028660.1575582054

National Early Literacy Panel. (2008). *Developing early literacy: Report of the National Early Literacy Panel*. Washington, DC: National Institute for Literacy. Retrieved from http://www.nifl.gov/earlychild hood/NELP/NELPreport.html

National Governors Association. (2011). *Realizing the potential: How governors can lead effective implementation of the Common Core State Standards*. Retrieved from https://files.eric.ed.gov/fulltext/ED 532524.pdf

National Institute for Literacy. (n.d.). *Frequently asked questions.* Retrieved from http://www.nifl.gov/nifl/faqs.html

National Reading Panel. (2000a). *Report of the National Reading Panel: Teaching children to read: An evidenced-based assessment of the scientific research literature on reading and its implications for reading instruction* (NIH Publication No. 00-4769). Washington, DC: U.S. Government Printing Office.

National Reading Panel. (2000b, April). *Teaching children to read: An evidence-based assessment of the scientific research literature on reading and its implications for reading instruction—reports of the subgroups.* Retrieved from http://www.nationalreadingpanel.org/Publications/subgroups.htm

Navarette, Y. G. (1996). Family involvement in a bilingual school. *Journal of Educational Issues of Language Minority Students, 6,* 77–84.

Nelson, N. W. (2010). *Language and literacy disorders: Infancy through adolescence.* Boston, MA: Allyn & Bacon.

New York State Education Department. (2018). *New York State Identification Test for English Language Learners: Guide to the NYSITELL, Levels I–VIII.* Retrieved from http://www.p12.nysed.gov/assessment/nysitell/2018/nysitellguide18rev.pdf

Nippold, M. (2012). Different service delivery models for different communication disorders. *Language, Speech, and Hearing Services in Schools, 43,* 117–120.

Nixon, S., McCardle, P., & Leos, K. (2007). Epilogue: Implications of research on English language learners for classroom and clinical practice. *Language, Speech, and Hearing Services in Schools, 38,* 272–277.

No Child Left Behind (NCLB). (2001a). Pub. L. No. 107-110, § 115, Stat. 1425.

No Child Left Behind (NCLB). (2001b). 20 U.S.C. (2001 & Supp 2002). Washington, DC: U.S. Department of Education.

No Child Left Behind Act of 2001. (2002). Pub. L. No. 107-110, 115 Stat. 1446.

Nutta, J., Bautista, N., & Butler, M. (2010). *Teaching sciences to English language learners.* New York, NY: Routledge.

Nutta, J., Mokhtari, K, & Strebel, C. (Eds.). (2012). *Preparing every teacher to reach English learners: A practical guide for teacher educators.* Cambridge, MA: Harvard Education Press.

Nutta, J., Strebel, C., Mihai, F., Crevecoeur-Bryant, E., & Mokhtari, K. (2018). *Show, tell, build: Twenty key instructional tools and techniques for educating English learners.* Cambridge, MA: Harvard Educational Press.

Office of English Language Acquisition (OELA). (2016). *English learner toolkit.* Washington, DC: U.S. Department of Education.

Ortiz, A., & Robertson, P. (2018). Preparing teachers to serve English learners with language-and/or learning difficulties and disabilities. *Teacher Education and Special Education (TESE)*, *41*(3), 176–187.

Ortiz, A. A. (1997). Learning disabilities occurring concomitantly with linguistic differences. *Journal of Learning Disabilities*, *30*, 321–332.

Ortiz, A. A., & Artiles, A. J. (2010). Meeting the needs of English language learners with disabilities: A linguistically and culturally responsive model. In G. Li & P. Edwards (Eds.), *Best practices in ELL instruction* (pp. 247–272). New York, NY: Guilford.

Ortiz, A. A., & Yates, J. R. (2001). A framework for serving English language learners with disabilities. *Journal of Special Education Leadership*, *14*(2), 72–80.

Ortiz, A. A., & Yates, J. R. (2002). Considerations in the assessment of English language learners referred to special education. In A. Artiles & A. Ortiz (Eds.), *English language learners with special education needs: Identification, assessment and instruction* (pp. 65–86). McHenry, IL: Center for Applied Linguistics and Delta Systems.

Oschwald, J., Schättin, A., von Bastian, C. C., & Souza, A. S. (2018). Bidialectalism and bilingualism: Exploring the role of Language similarity as a link between linguistic ability and executive control. *Frontiers in Psychology*, *9*, 1997.

Ovando, C. J. (2003). Bilingual education in the United States: Historical development and current issues. *Bilingual Research Journal*, *27*, 1–24.

Ovando, C. J., & Combs, M. C. (2018). *Bilingual and ESL classrooms: Teaching in multicultural contexts*. Lanham, MD: Rowman & Littlefield.

Owens, R. E. (2004). *Language development: A functional approach to assessment and intervention* (4th ed.). Boston, MA: Allyn & Bacon.

Pae, T. I. (2019). A simultaneous analysis of relations between L1 and L2 skills in reading and writing. *Reading Research Quarterly*, *54*(1), 109–124.

Paez, M. M., Tabors, P. O., & Lopez, L. M. (2007). Dual language and literacy development of Spanish-speaking preschool children. *Journal of Applied Developmental Psychology*, *28*(2), 85–102.

Paradis, J. (2005). Grammatical morphology in children learning English as a second language: Implications of similarities with specific language impairment. *Language, Speech, and Hearing Services in Schools*, *36*, 172–187.

Paradis, J. (2007). Bilingual children with specific language impairment: Theoretical and applied issues. *Applied Psycholinguistics*, *28*, 551–564.

Paradis, J. (2016). The development of English as a second language with and without specific language impairment: Clinical implications. *Journal of Speech, Language and Hearing Research*, *59*(1), 171–182.

Paradis, J. (2018). Language-level input factors are not enough to explain child bilingual acquisition. *Linguistic Approaches to Bilingualism, 8*(6), 753–757.

Paradis, J., Crago, M., Genesee, F., & Rice, M. (2003). French-English bilingual children with SLI: How do they compare with their monolingual peers? *Journal of Speech, Language, and Hearing Research, 46,* 113–127.

Paradis, J., & Genesee, F. (1996). Syntactic acquisition in bilingual children. *Studies in Second Language Acquisition, 18,* 1–25.

Paradis, J., Genesee, F., & Crago, M. (2011). *Dual language development and disorders: A handbook on bilingualism and second language learning* (2nd ed.). Baltimore, MD: Brookes.

Paradis, J., Schneider, P., & Duncan, T. (2013). Discriminating children with language impairment among English language learners from diverse first-language backgrounds. *Journal of Speech, Language, and Hearing Research, 56*(3), 971–981.

Parker, F., & Riley, K. (2010). *Linguistics for non-linguists: A primer with exercises* (5th ed.). Upper Saddle River, NJ: Pearson.

Patterson, J. L., & Pearson, B. Z. (2004). Influences, contexts and processes. In B. A. Goldstein (Ed.), *Bilingual language development and disorders in Spanish-English speakers* (pp. 77–104). Baltimore, MD: Brookes.

Paul, D., Blosser, J., & Jakubowitz, M. (2006). Principles and challenges for forming successful literacy partnerships. *Topics in Language Disorders, 26*(1), 5–23.

Pavelko, S. L., Owens, R. E., Ireland, M., & Hahs-Vaughn, D. L. (2016). Use of language sample analysis by school-based SLPs: Results of a nationwide survey. *Language, Speech, and Hearing Services in Schools, 47,* 246–258.

Pawan, F., & Ortloff, J. H. (2011). Sustaining collaboration: English-as-a-second-language, and content-area teachers. *Teaching and Teacher Education: An International Journal of Research and Studies, 27*(2), 463–471.

Payne, K. (1986). Cultural and linguistic groups in the United States. In O. Taylor (Ed.), *Nature of communication disorders in culturally and linguistically diverse populations.* San Diego, CA: College-Hill Press.

Pearson, B. Z., Fernández, S., & Oller, D. K. (1993). Lexical development in bilingual infants and toddlers: Comparison to monolingual norms. *Language and Learning, 43*(1), 93–120.

Peercy, M. M., & Martin-Beltran, M. (2011). Envisioning collaboration: Including ESOL students and teachers in the mainstream classroom. *International Journal of Inclusive Education, 16*(7), 657–673. doi:10.1080/13603116.2010.495791

Peña, E., Gillam, R., & Bedore, L. (2014). Dynamic assessment of narrative ability in English accurately identifies language impairment in English language learners. *Journal of Speech, Language and Hearing Research, 57* (6), 2208–2220.

Peña, E., Gutierrez-Clellen, V., Iglesias, A., Goldstein, B., & Bedore, L. (2018). *Bilingual English-Spanish Assessment™ (BESA™) manual.* Baltimore, MD: Brookes.

Peña, E., Iglesias, A., & Lidz, C. S. (2001). Reducing test bias through assessment of children's word learning ability. *American Journal of Speech-Language Pathology, 10,* 138–151.

Peña, E. D., & Kester, E. S. (2004). Semantic development in Spanish-English bilinguals: Theory, assessment, and intervention. In Goldstein B. A. (Ed.), *Bilingual language development and disorders in Spanish–English speakers* (pp.105–130). Baltimore, MD: Brookes.

Peña, E. D., & Quinn, R. (2003). Developing effective collaboration teams in speech-language pathology: A case study. *Communication Disorders Quarterly, 24,* 53–63.

Peña, E. D., Quinn, R., & Iglesias, A. (1992). The application of dynamic methods to language assessment: A nonbiased procedure. *Journal of Special Education, 26*(3), 269–280.

Peregoy, S., & Boyle, O. (1991). Second language oral proficiency characteristics of low, intermediate and high second language readers. *Hispanic Journal of Behavioral Sciences, 13*(1), 35–47.

Peregoy, S., & Boyle, O. F. (2005). *Reading, writing, and learning in ESL: A resource book for K–12 teachers.* New York, NY: Pearson Education.

Peregoy, S., & Boyle, O. (2008). *Reading, writing, and learning in ESL: A resource book for teaching K–12 English learners.* Boston, MA: Pearson.

Peregoy, S., & Boyle, O. F. (2017). *Reading, writing and learning in ESL: A resource book for teaching K–12 English learners* (7th ed.). Upper Saddle River, NJ: Pearson.

Perfetti, C. A. (2003). The universal grammar of reading, *Scientific Studies of Reading, 7*(1), 3–24. doi:10.1207/S1532799XSSR0701_02

Perkins, K., Brutten, S., & Pohlman, J. (1989). First and second language reading comprehension. *RELC Journal, 20,* 1–9.

Perona, K., Plante, E., & Vance, R. (2005). Diagnostic accuracy of the Structured Photographic Expressive Language Test: Third edition (SPELT-3). *Language, Speech, and Hearing Services in Schools, 36,* 103–115.

Perozzi, J. (1992). The effect of instruction in L1 on receptive acquisition of L2 for bilingual children with language delay. *Language Speech and Hearing Services in Schools, 23*(4), 348–352. doi:10.1044/0161-1461.2304.348

Pershey, M. G., & Rapking, C. I. (2003). A survey of collaborative speech-language service delivery under large caseload conditions in an urban school district in the United States. *Journal of Speech-Language Pathology and Audiology, 27,* 211–220.

Peters-Johnson, C. (1998). Action: School services, survey of speech language pathology services in school-based settings national study report. *Language, Speech, and Hearing Services in Schools, 29,* 120–126.

Petersen, D., Chantthongthip, H., Ukrainetz, T., Spenser, T., & Steeve, R. (2017). Dynamic assessment of narratives: Efficient, accurate identification of language impairment in bilingual students. *Journal of Speech Language and Hearing Research, 60*(4), 983–998.

Petersen, D., & Spencer, T. (2014). Narrative assessment and intervention: A clinical tutorial on extending explicit language instruction and progress monitoring to all students. *Perspectives on Communication Disorders and Sciences in Culturally and Linguistically Diverse Populations, 21*(1), 5–21.

Pham, G., Kohnert, K., & Mann, D. (2011). Addressing clinician-client mismatch: A preliminary intervention study with a bilingual Vietnamese-English preschooler. *Language Speech and Hearing Services in Schools, 42*(4), 408–422.

Phuntsog, N. (2001). Culturally responsive teaching: What do select United States elementary school teachers think? *Intercultural Education, 12*(1), 51–64.

Pica, T. (1994). Questions from the language classroom: Research perspectives. *TESOL Quarterly, 28,* 49–79.

Pieretti, R., & Roseberry-McKibbin, C. (2015). Assessment and intervention for English language learners with primary language impairment: Research-based best practices. *Communication Disorders Quarterly, 37*(2), 117–128.

Pinker, S. (1994). *The language instinct: How the mind creates language.* New York, NY: William Morrow.

Pinker, S. (1999). *Words and rules: The ingredients of language.* London, UK: Weidenfeld & Nicholson.

Pinker, S. (2007). *The stuff of thought: Language as window into human nature.* New York, NY: Viking.

Plante, E., & Vance, B. (1994). Selection of preschool language tests: A data-based approach. *Language Speech and Hearing Services in Schools, 25,* 15–24.

Pompa, D., & Villegas, L. (2017). *Analyzing state ESSA plans for English learner accountability: A framework for community stakeholder.* Washington, DC: Migration Policy Institute. Retrieved from https://www.migrationpolicy.org/

Potochnick, S. (2018). The academic adaptation of immigrant students with interrupted schooling. *American Educational Research Journal, 55*(4), 859–892.

Powell, R. (2018). Unique contributions to the curriculum: From research to practice for speech-language pathologists in schools. *Language, Speech, and Hearing in the Schools, 49*(2), 140–147.

Power deFur, L. (2016). *Common core state standards and the speech-language pathologist: Standards-based intervention for special populations.* San Diego, CA: Plural Publishing.

Pray, L. (2003, April). *A comparison of the rate of English acquisition of general education and special education second language learners.* Paper presented at the national conference of the American Educational Research Association, Chicago, IL.

Pray, L. (2005). How well do commonly used language instruments measure English oral-language proficiency? *Bilingual Research Journal, 29*(2), 387–409.

Pray, L. (2009). Comparison of oral language usage among English language learners diagnosed with a learning disability and those in general education. *International Multilingual Research Journal, 3,* 110–119.

Preis, J. (2013). The effects of teaching about white privilege in speech-language pathology. *Perspectives on Communication Disorders and Sciences in Culturally and Linguistically Diverse (CLD) Populations, 20*(2), 72–83.

Prelock, P. A., Hutchins, T., & Glascoe, F. P. (2008). Speech-language impairment: How to identify the most common and least diagnosed disability of childhood. *Medscape Journal of Medicine, 10*(6), 136–149.

Prelock, P. A., Miller, B. E., & Reed, N. L. (1995). Collaborative partnerships in a language in the classroom program. *Language, Speech, and Hearing Services in Schools, 26,* 286–292.

President's Advisory Commission on Educational Excellence for Hispanic Americans. (2003). *From risk to opportunity: Fulfilling the educational needs of Hispanic Americans in the 21st century.* Washington, DC: Author.

Pretto, A. (2012). Integrating an interpreter. *ASHA Leader, 17*(9), 40–41.

Proctor, C. P., August, D., Carlo, M. S., & Snow, C. (2006). The intriguing role of Spanish language vocabulary knowledge in predicting English reading comprehension. *Journal of Educational Psychology, 98,* 159–169.

Proietti Ergün, A. L. (2018). Age and input effect in simultaneous bilingual: Turkish and Italian. *Dil Eğitimi ve Araştırmaları Dergisi, 3*(3), 152–163.

Pye, C. (1987). The Pye analysis of language. *Working Papers in Language Development, 3,* 1–37.

Quiocho, A. L., & Ulanoff, S. H. (2009). *Differentiated literacy instruction for English language learners.* Boston, MA: Allyn & Bacon.

Quiroga, T., Lemos-Britten, Z., Mostafapour, E., Abbott, R. D., & Berninger, V. W. (2002). Phonological awareness and beginning Spanish speaking ESL first graders. Research into practice. *Journal of School Psychology, 40*(1), 85–111.

Ralabate, P. K., & Nelson, L. L. (2017). *Culturally responsive design for English learners: The UDL approach.* Wakefield, MA: CAST Professional Publishing.

Rea, P. J. (2005). Engage your administrator in your collaboration initiative. *Intervention in School and Clinic, 40*(5), 312–316.

Reeves, J. (2006). Secondary teacher attitudes toward including English-language learners in mainstream classrooms. *Journal of Educational Research, 99*(3), 131–143.

Reid, J. (1996). U.S. academic readers, ESL writers, and second sentences. *Journal of Second Language Writing, 5*(2), 129–161.

Rennie, J. (1993). ESL and bilingual program models. *ERIC Digest.* ERIC Clearinghouse on Languages and Linguistics. Digest based on an article in *Streamlined Seminar, 12*(1). National Association of Elementary School Principals. Retrieved from http://www.cal.org/resources/digest/rennie01.html

Restrepo, M. A. (1997). Guidelines for identifying primarily Spanish speaking preschool children with language impairment. *Communication Disorders and Sciences in Culturally and Linguistically Diverse Populations, 3*(1), 11–13.

Restrepo, M. A. (1998). Identifiers of predominantly Spanish-speaking children with language impairment. *Journal of Speech, Language, and Hearing Research, 41,* 1398–1411.

Restrepo, M. A., Castilla, A., Schwanenflugel, P., Neuharth-Pritchitt, S., Hamilton, C., & Arboleda, A. (2010). Effects of a supplemental Spanish oral language program on sentence length, complexity, and grammaticality in Spanish speaking children attending English only preschools. *Language Speech and Hearing Services in Schools, 41,* 3–13.

Restrepo, M. A., & Gutierrez-Clellen, V. (2004). Grammatical impairment in Spanish-English bilingual children. In B. Goldstein (Ed.), *Bilingual language development and disorders in Spanish-English speakers* (pp. 213–234). Baltimore, MD: Brookes.

Restrepo, M. A., & Kruth, K. (2000). Grammatical characteristics of a bilingual student with specific language impairment. *Journal of Children's Communication Development, 21,* 66–76.

Restrepo, M. A., & Silverman, S. W. (2001). Validity of the Spanish Preschool Language Scale-3 for use with bilingual children. *American Journal of Speech-Language Pathology, 10,* 382–393.

Restrepo, M. A., & Towle-Harmon, M. (2008, September 23). Addressing emergent literacy skills in English-Language Learners. *ASHA Leader.*

Retherford, K. (2000). *Guide to analysis of language transcripts* (3rd ed.). Eau Claire, WI: Thinking.

Rhodes, R. L., Ochoa, S. H., & Ortiz, S. O. (2005). *Assessing culturally and linguistically diverse students: A practical guide.* New York, NY: Guilford Press.

Richards, J. C., & Rodgers, T. S. (1986). *Approaches and methods in language teaching.* New York, NY: Cambridge Press.

Richards-Tutor, C., Baker, D. L., Gersten, R., Baker, S. K., & Smith, J. M. (2016). The effectiveness of reading interventions for English learners: A research synthesis. *Exceptional Children, 82*(2), 144–169.

Rinaldi, C., & Samson, J. (2008). English language learners and response to intervention. *Teaching Exceptional Children, 40*(5), 6–14.

Riquelme, L. (2013). Cultural competence for everyone: A shift in perspectives. *Perspectives on Dysphagia, 18,* 42–49. doi:10.1044/gero18.2.42

Ritter, M. (2009). The speech-language pathologist and reading: Opportunities to extend services for the children we serve. *Perspectives on School-Based Issues, 10*(2), 38–44.

Rivers, K., Rosa-Lugo, L. I., & Hedrick, D. (2004). Performance of African-American adolescents on a measure of language proficiency. *Negro Educational Review, 55*(2–3), 117–127.

Roache, M., Shore, J., Gouleta, E., & Butkevich, E. (2003). An investigation of collaboration among school professionals in serving culturally and linguistically diverse students with exceptionalities. *Bilingual Research Journal, 27*(1), 117–136.

Robb, L. (2002). Multiple text: Multiple opportunities for teaching and learning. *Voices from the Middle, 9*(4), 28–32.

Robson, G. (1992). *Individual learner differences and classroom participation: A pilot study* (Unpublished paper). Temple University, Japan.

Rodina, Y. (2018). Narrative abilities of preschool bilingual Norwegian-Russian children. *International Journal of Bilingualism, 21*(5), 617–635. doi:10.1177/1367006916643528

Rodriguez, B. L., & Olswang, L. B. (2003). Mexican-American and Anglo-American mothers' beliefs and values about child rearing, education, and language impairment. *American Journal of Speech-Language Pathology, 12*(4), 452–462.

Rodriguez, E., Bustamante, K., Wood, C., & Sunderman, G. (2017). A comparison of the grammatical production of child heritage speakers of Spanish across language and grade: Kindergarten and Grade 1. *Languages, 2*(4), 27.

Rodriquez, A., & Rodriguez, D. (2017). English learners with learning disabilities: What is the current state? *Insights Into Learning Disabilities, 14*(1), 97–112.

Rojas, R., & Iglesias, A. (2013). The language growth of Spanish-speaking English language learners. *Child Development, 84,* 630–646.

Rollins, P. R., McCabe, A., & Bliss, L. (2000). Culturally sensitive assessment of narrative in children. *Seminars in Speech and Language, 21,* 223–234.

Romaine, S. (1995). *Bilingualism.* Boston, MA: Blackwell.

Roninson, O. Z. (2003). "But they don't speak English!" Bilingual students and speech-language services in public schools. *Newsletter of the ASHA Special Interest Division 16: Perspectives on School-Based Issues, 4*(1), 42–46.

Roos, P. (1978). Bilingual education: The Hispanic response to unequal educational opportunity. *Law and Contemporary Problems, 42*(4), 111–140.

Rosa-Lugo, L. I., & Abreu, R. (2017). *Live webinar: Working with interpreters: Best practices for Audiologists and SLPs.* Rockville, MD; ASHA. Retrieved from https://www.asha.org/eWeb/OLSDynamic Page.aspx?Webcode=olsdetails&title=Working+with+Interpreters% 3a+Best+Practices+for+Audiologists+and+SLPs

Rosa-Lugo, L. I., & Champion, T. (2007). The influence of knowledge and experience on responding to diversity in speech-language pathology. In A. Guilford, S. Graham, & J. Scheuerle (Eds.), *The speech-language pathologist. From novice to expert* (pp. 89–104). Upper Saddle River, NJ: Pearson.

Rosa-Lugo, L. I., & Esparza-Brown, J. (2011). *Response to intervention with English learners.* Video lecture. Retrieved from http://tapestry .usf.edu/video-lectures.html

Rosa-Lugo, L. I., & Fradd, S. (2000). Preparing professionals to serve English language learners with communication disorders. *Communication Disorders Quarterly, 22*(1), 29–42.

Rosa-Lugo, L. I., Mihai, F. M., & Nutta, J. W. (2012). *Language and literacy development: An interdisciplinary focus on English learners with communication disorders.* San Diego, CA: Plural Publishing.

Rosa-Lugo, L. I., Mihai, F., & Nutta, J. (2017). Preparation of speech-language pathologists to work with English learners (ELs): Incorporating interprofessional education (IPE) and interprofessional collaborative practice (IPP) competencies. *Perspectives of the ASHA*

Special Interest Groups, SIG 14, 2(14), 103–121. doi:10.1044/persp2.SIG14.103

Rosa-Lugo, L. I., Rivera, E. A., & McKeown, S. W. (1998). Meeting the critical shortage of speech-language pathologists to serve the public schools: Collaborative rewards. *Language, Speech, and Hearing Services in Schools, 29*, 232–242.

Rosa-Lugo, L. I., Rivera, E., & Rierson, T. K. (2010, October). The role of dynamic assessment within the response to intervention model in school-age English language learners. *Perspectives on School-Based Issues, ASHA Division 16, 11*(3), 91–106.

Roseberry-McKibbin, C. (1993). *Bilingual classroom communication profile*. Oceanside, CA: Academic Communication Associates.

Roseberry-McKibbin, C. (2000). Distinguishing language differences from language disorders in linguistically and culturally diverse students. In K. Fieiberg (Ed.), *Educating exceptional children* (pp. 78–81). Guilford, CT: Dushkin/McGraw-Hill.

Roseberry-McKibbin, C. (2003). *Assessment of bilingual learners: Language difference or disorder? Video and workbook*. Rockville, MD: American Speech-Language-Hearing Association.

Roseberry-McKibbin, C. (2007). *Language disorders in children: A multicultural and case perspective*. Boston, MA: Allyn & Bacon.

Roseberry-McKibbin, C. (2008a). *Increasing the language and academic skills of children in poverty: Practical strategies for professionals*. San Diego, CA: Plural Publishing.

Roseberry-McKibbin, C. (2008b). *Increasing language skills of students with low income backgrounds*. San Diego, CA: Plural Publishing.

Roseberry-McKibbin, C. (2008c). *Multicultural students with special language needs* (3rd ed.). Oceanside, CA: Academic Communication Associates.

Roseberry-McKibbin, C. (2013). *Increasing the language skills of students in poverty: Practical strategies for professionals* (2nd ed.). San Diego, CA: Plural Publishing.

Roseberry-McKibbin, C. (2014). *Multicultural students with special language needs* (4th ed.). Oceanside, CA: Academic Communication Associates.

Roseberry-McKibbin, C. (2015). English language learners and the common core standards: Meeting the needs of students with low socioeconomic status and language impairment. *Perspectives on Communication Disorders and Sciences in Culturally and Linguistically Diverse (CLD) Populations, 22*(1), 4–14.

Roseberry-McKibbin, C. (2018). *Multicultural students with special language needs: Practical strategies for assessment and intervention* (5th ed.). Oceanside, CA: Academic Communication Associates.

Roseberry-McKibbin, C., Brice, A., & O'Hanlon, L. (2005). Serving English language learners in public schools: A national survey. *Language, Speech, and Hearing Services in Schools, 36,* 48–61.

Roseberry-McKibbin, C., & Eicholtz, G. E. (1994). Serving LEP children in schools: A national survey. *Language, Speech, and Hearing Services in Schools, 25*(3), 156–164.

Roseberry-McKibbin, C., & O'Hanlon, I. (2005). Nonbiased assessment of English language learners: A tutorial. *Communication Disorders Quarterly, 26,* 178–185.

Roseberry-McKibbin, C., O'Hanlon, L., & Brice, A. (2004). Service delivery to English language learners in the public schools: A national survey. *ASHA Leader, 9*(17), 8–35.

Roth, F. (2015). The 21st century educational landscape: Implications for the academic and clinical preparation of SLPs. *Perspectives on Issues in Higher Education, 18,* 55–61.

Rowe, B. M., & Levine, D. P. (2006). *A concise introduction to linguistics.* Boston, MA: Pearson Education.

Rumbaut, R. G., & Massey, D. S. (2013). Immigration and language diversity in the United States. *Daedalus, 142*(3), 141–154.

Rumelhart, D. (1980). Schemata: The building blocks of cognition. In R. J. Spiro & W. F. Brewer (Eds.), *Theoretical issues in reading comprehension.* Hillsdale, NJ: Erlbaum.

Saad, C., & Polovoy, C. (2009, May 5). Differences or disorders? In the 1980s, research focused on culturally and linguistically diverse populations. *ASHA Leader.*

Saenz, T. I., & Huer, M. B. (2003). Testing strategies involving least biased assessment of bilingual children. *Communication Disorders Quarterly, 24*(4), 184–193.

Salas-Provance, M., Erickson, J., & Reed, J. (2002). Disabilities as viewed by four generations of one Hispanic family. *American Journal of Speech-Language Pathology, 11,* 151–162.

Samson, J. F., & Collins, B. A. (2012). *Preparing all teachers to meet the needs of English language learners: Applying research to policy and practice for teacher effectiveness.* Washington, DC: Center for American Progress. Retrieved from https://www.americanprogress.org/issues/education-k-12/reports/2012/04/30/11372/preparing-all-teachers-to-meet-the-needs-of-english-language-learners/

Samson, J. F., & Lesaux, N. K. (2009). Language-minority learners in special education: Rates and predictors of identification for services. *Journal of Learning Disabilities, 42,* 248–162.

Samway, K. (1987). *The writing processes of non-native English speaking children in the elementary grades* (Unpublished doctoral dissertation). University of Rochester, New York.

Sanford, A., Brown, J., & Turner, M. (2012). Enhancing instruction for English learners in response to intervention systems: The PLUSS Model. *Multiple Voices for Ethnically Diverse Exceptional Learners, 13*(1), 56–70.

Scarborough, H. (2001). Connecting early language and literacy to later reading (dis)abilities: Evidence, theory, and practice. In S. B. Neuman & D. K. Dickinson (Eds.), *Handbook for research in early literacy* (pp. 97–110). New York, NY: Guilford Press.

Schatz, M. (Ed.). (2010). *Education of English language learners (challenges in language and literacy)*. New York, NY: Guilford.

Schiff-Myers, N. (1992). Considering arrested language development and language loss in the assessment of second language learner. *Language, Speech, and Hearing Services in Schools, 23*, 28–33.

Schnell de Acedo, B. (1994). Early morphological development: The acquisition of articles in Spanish. In J. Sokolov & C. Snow (Eds.), *Handbook of research in language development using CHILDES*. Hillsdale, NJ: Lawrence Erlbaum.

Schooling, T., Venediktov, R., & Leech, H. (2010). *Evidence-based systematic review: Effects of service delivery on the speech and language skills of children from birth to 5 years of age*. Rockville, MD: American Speech-Language-Hearing Association, National Center for Evidence-Based Practice in Communication Disorders.

Schraeder, P. (2008). *A guide to school services in speech-language pathology*. San Diego, CA: Plural Publishing.

Schraeder, T. (2001, October). Three current hot issues related to professional ethics. *School-Based Issues, 2*(1), 28.

Schraeder, T. (2012). Literacy, common core state standards and the school-based speech/language pathologist: Making sense of it all. *Perspectives on School-Based Issues, 1*(1), 3–10.

Schrage, M. (1995). *No more teams! Mastering the dynamics of creative collaboration*. New York, NY: Currency Doubleday.

Schrank, F. A., Alvarado, C. G., & Wendling, B. J. (2010). *Interpretive supplement: Instructional interventions for English language learners related to the Woodcock-Muñoz Language Survey–Revised Normative Update*. Rolling Meadows, IL: Riverside.

Schuele, C. M. (2017). The speech-language pathologist's role in reading and writing: In theory meets in reality. *Perspectives of the ASHA Special Interest Groups, 2*(1), 115–116.

Schuele, C. M., & Larrivee, L. (2004). What's my job? Differential diagnosis of the speech-language pathologist's role in literacy learning. *Perspectives on Language Learning and Education, 11*(3), 4–7.

Schumann, J. H. (1978). The acculturation model for second language acquisition. In R. C. Gingras (Ed.), *Second language acquisition and foreign language learning*. Washington, DC: Center for Applied Linguistics.

Scott, A., Boynton Hauerwas, & Brown, R. (2014). State policy and guidance for identifying learning disabilities in culturally and linguistically diverse students. *Learning Disability Quarterly, 37*(3), 172–185.

Scott, V. M. (1991, October). *Write from the start: A task-oriented developmental writing program for foreign language students*. Paper presented at the Southern Conference on Language Teaching, Valdosta, GA.

Sehlaoui, A. S. (2018). Role of heritage languages in mastering English pronunciation. In J. I. Liontas, TESOL International Association, & M. DelliCarpini (Eds.), *The TESOL encyclopedia of English language teaching*. New York, NY: Wiley. doi:10.1002/9781118784235.eelt0866

Self, T., Coufal, K. L., & Francois, J. (2011). Interprofessional collaborative practice: Preparing future professionals to use the ICF-CY. *Perspectives on Language Learning and Education, 18*, 68–74.

Selin, C. M., Rice, M. L., Girolamo, T., & Wang, C. J. (2019). Speech-language pathologists' clinical decision making for children with specific language impairment. *Language, Speech, and Hearing Services in Schools, 50*(2), 283–307.

Selinker, L. (1972). Interlanguage. *International Review of Applied Linguistics in Language Teaching, 10*, 209–232.

Semel, E., Wiig, E. H., & Secord. W. A. (2003). *Clinical Evaluation of Language Fundamentals–4*. San Antonio, TX: Psych Corp/Harcourt.

Semel, E., Wiig, E. H., & Secord, W. A. (2006). *The Clinical Evaluation of Language Fundamentals—Fourth edition, Spanish edition (CELF-4 Spanish)*. San Antonio, TX: Pearson.

Semel E., Wiig, E. H., & Secord, W. A. (2013). *Clinical Evaluation of Language Fundamentals—Fifth edition (CELF-5 English)*. Bloomington, MN: NCS Pearson.

Senaga, N., & Inglebret, E. (2003, November). *Assessment practices used by bilingual SLPs*. Paper presented at the meeting of the American Speech-Language-Hearing Association, Chicago, IL.

Seymour, H. N., Bland-Stewart, L., & Green, L. J. (1998). Difference versus deficit in child African American English. *Language, Speech, and Hearing Services in Schools, 29*, 96–108.

Shanahan, T., & Shanahan, C. (2012). What is disciplinary literacy and why does it matter? *Topics in Language Disorders, 32*(1), 7–18.

Shipley, K., & McAfee, J., (2016). *Assessment in speech-language pathology. A resource manual*. (5th ed.). Boston, MA: Cengage Learning.

Short, D. J., & Echevarria, J. (1999). *The Sheltered Instruction Observation Protocol: A tool for teacher-research collaboration and professional development* (Educational Practice Report No. 3). Santa Cruz, CA: Center for Research on Education, Diversity and Excellence.

Short, D. J., & Fitzsimmons, S. (2006, January). *Literacy development of bilingual adolescents: Issues and recommendations.* Paper presented at the meeting of National Association of Bilingual Education, Phoenix, AZ.

Short, D., & Fitzsimmons, S. (2007). *Double the work: Challenges and solutions to acquiring language and academic literacy for adolescent English language learners—a report to Carnegie Corporation of New York.* Washington, DC: Alliance for Excellent Education.

Sibold, C. (2011). Building English language learners' academic vocabulary: Strategies & tips. *Multicultural Education, 18*(2), 24–28.

Silva, T. (1993). Toward an understanding of the distinct nature of L2 writing: The ESL research and its implications. *TESOL Quarterly, 27*(4), 657–677.

Silva-Corvalán, C. (2018). Simultaneous bilingualism: Early developments, incomplete later outcomes? *International Journal of Bilingualism, 22*(5), 497–512.

Simon-Cereijido, G., & Gutierrez-Clellen, V. (2007). Spontaneous language markers of Spanish language impairment. *Applied Psycholinguistics, 28*, 317–339.

Simmons, A. (1962). A comparison of type-token ration of spoken and written language in deaf and hard of hearing children. *Volta Review, 84*, 81–95.

Sireci, S. G., Li, S., & Scarpati, S. (2003). *The effects of test accommodation on test performance: A review of the literature* (Center for Educational Assessment Research Report No. 485). Amherst, MA: School of Education, University of Massachusetts.

Skehan, P. (1986a). Cluster analysis and the identification of learner types. In V. Cook (Ed.), *Experimental approaches to second language acquisition.* Oxford, UK: Pergamon.

Skehan, P. (1986b). Where does language aptitude come from? In P. Meara (Ed.), *Spoken language.* London, UK: Centre for Information on Language Teaching.

Skehan, P. (1989). *Individual differences in second language learning.* London, UK: Edward Arnold.

Skehan, P. (1990). The relationship between native and foreign language learning ability: Educational and linguistic factors. In H. Dechert (Ed.), *Current trends in European second language acquisition research.* Clevedon, UK: Multilingual Matters.

Skehan, P. (1998). *A cognitive approach to language learning.* Oxford, UK: Oxford University Press.

Skinner, B. F. (1957). *Verbal behavior.* Acton, MA: Copley.

Smith, K. (2014, October 28). *PLS-5 validity study—a comparison of test scores.* Retrieved from https://community.asha.org/blogs/kristin-smith/2014/10/28/pls-5

Snyder, T. D., de Brey, C., & Dillow, S. A. (2016). *Digest of education statistics 2014* (NCES 2016-006). Washington, DC: National Center for Education Statistics, Institute of Education Sciences, U.S. Department of Education.

Snyder, T. D., & Dillow, S. A. (2015). *Digest of education statistics 2013* (NCES 2015-011). Washington, DC: National Center for Education Statistics, Institute of Education Sciences, U.S. Department of Education.

Solomon-Rice, P., Soto, G., & Robinson, N. (2018). Project building bridges: Training speech-language pathologists to provide culturally and linguistically responsive augmentative and alternative communication services to school-age children with diverse backgrounds. *Perspectives of the ASHA Special Interest Groups, 3*(12), 186–204.

Solorzano, R. W. (2008). High stakes testing: Issues, implication, and remedies for English language learners. *Review of Educational Research, 78*(2), 260–329.

Spaulding, T. J., Plante, E., & Farinella, K. A. (2006). Eligibility criteria for language impairment: Is the low end of normal always appropriate? *Language, Speech, and Hearing Services in Schools, 37*, 61–72.

Spencer, S. (2005). Lynne Cook and June Downing: The practicalities of collaboration in special education service delivery. *Intervention in School and Clinic, 40*(5), 296–300.

Spracher, M. (2000). Learning about literacy SLPs play key role in reading, writing. *ASHA Leader, 5*(8), 1–19.

Stallings, J. A., & Mohlman, G. G. (1988). Classroom observation techniques. In J. P. Keeves (Ed.), *Educational research, methodology, and measurement: An international handbook* (pp. 469–474). Oxford, UK: Pergamon.

Stauffer, R. (1975). *Directing the reading-thinking process.* New York, NY: Harper & Row.

Steinberg, J., Cline, F., Ling, G., Cook, L., & Tognatta, N. (2009). Examining the validity and fairness of a state standards-based assessment of English-language arts for deaf or hard of hearing students. *Journal of Applied Testing Technology, 10*(2), 1–33.

Stein-Rubin, C., & Fabus, R. (2011). *A guide to clinical assessment and professional report writing in speech-language pathology.* Clifton Park, NY: Delmar.

Steppling, M., Quattlebaum, P., & Brady, D. E. (2007). Toward a discussion of issues associated with speech-language pathologists' dismissal practices in public school settings. *Communication Disorders Quarterly, 28*(3), 179–187.

Stewner-Manzanares, G. (1988). *The Bilingual Education Act: Twenty years later* (New Focus, Occasional Papers in Bilingual Education,

Number 6). Washington, DC: Office of Bilingual Education and Minority Affairs.

Stockman, I. J., Boult, J., & Robinson, G. (2004, July 20). Multicultural issues in academic and clinical education: A cultural mosaic. *ASHA Leader*, pp. 6–7, 20.

Strong, M. (1983). Social styles and second language acquisition of Spanish-speaking kindergartners. *TESOL Quarterly*, *17*, 241–258.

Sugarman, J. (2018). *A matter of design. English learner program models in K–12 education*. Washington, DC: Migration Policy Institute. Retrieved from http://www.migrationpolicy.org/research/english-learner-program-models-k-12-education

Suleman, S., McFarlane, L., Pollock, K., Schneider, P., Leroy, C., & Skoczylas, M. (2014). Collaboration: More than 'working together': An exploratory study to determine effect of interprofessional education on awareness and application of models of specialized service delivery by student speech-language pathologists and teachers. *Canadian Journal of Speech Language Pathology and Audiology*, *37*, 298–307.

Sullivan, A. L. (2011). Disproportionality in special education identification and placement of English language learners. *Exceptional Children*, *77*, 317–334.

Sullivan, A. L., & Bal, A. (2013). Disproportionality in special education: Effects of individual and school variables on disability risk. *Exceptional Children*, *79*(4), 475–494.

Summers, C., Smith, V., Mueller, V., Alexander, V., & Muzza, A. (2017). Language of intervention in bilingual children with autism spectrum disorders. *Perspectives of the ASHA Special Interest Groups (SIG 1)*, *2*(Pt 4), 203–211.

Swain, M. (1985). Communicative competence: Some roles of comprehensible input in its development. In S. Gass & C. Madden (Eds.), *Input and second language acquisition* (pp. 235–252). Rowley, MA: Newbury.

Swain, M. (1995). Three functions of output in second language learning. In G. Cook & B. Seidlhofer (Eds.), *Principles and practice in the study of language: Studies in honor of H. G. Widdowson*. Oxford, UK: Oxford University Press.

Swales, J. M. (1990). *Genre analysis: English in academic and research settings*. New York, NY: Cambridge University Press.

Swisher, L. (1994). Learning and generalization components of morphological acquisition by children with specific language impairment: Is there a functional relation? *Journal of Speech and Hearing Research*, *37*(6), 1406–1413.

Taylor, O. (1986). *Treatment of communication disorders in culturally and linguistically diverse populations.* Austin, TX: Pro-Ed.

Teachers of English to Speakers of Other Languages (TESOL). (n.d.-a). *Bylaws and standing rules. SR II. Mission.* Retrieved from http://www.tesol.org/s_tesol/seccss.asp?CID=413&DID=2038

Teachers of English to Speakers of Other Languages (TESOL). (n.d.-b). *The early history of TESOL.* Retrieved from http://www.tesol.org/s_tesol/bin.asp?CID=32&DID=8283&DOC=FILE.PDF

Teachers of English to Speakers of Other Languages (TESOL). (n.d.-c). *Membership statistics.* Retrieved from http://www.tesol.org/s_tesol/seccss.asp?CID=130&DID=1600

Teachers of English to Speakers of Other Languages (TESOL). (n.d.-d). *TESOL's mission and values.* Retrieved from https://www.tesol.org/about-tesol/association-governance/mission-and-values

Teachers of English to Speakers of Other Languages (TESOL). (2001a). *ESL standards into classroom practice: Grades preK–2.* Alexandria, VA: Author.

Teachers of English to Speakers of Other Languages (TESOL). (2001b). *Position statement on language and literacy development for young English language learners.* Retrieved from http://tesol.org/s_tesol/bin.asp?CID=32&DID=371&DOC=FILE.PDF

Teachers of English to Speakers of Other Languages (TESOL). (2003a). *TESOL position statement on preparation of pre-K–12 educators for cultural and linguistic diversity in the United States.* Retrieved from https://www.tesol.org/docs/pdf/1301.pdf?sfvrsn=2&sfvrsn=2

Teachers of English to Speakers of Other Languages (TESOL). (2003b). *TESOL position statement on teacher quality in the field of teaching English to speakers of other languages.* Retrieved from https://www.tesol.org/docs/pdf/374.pdf?sfvrsn=2&sfvrsn=2

Teachers of English to Speakers of Other Languages (TESOL). (2005a). *TESOL position statement on highly qualified teachers under No Child Left Behind.* Retrieved from https://www.tesol.org/docs/pdf/374.pdf?sfvrsn=2&sfvrsn=2

Teachers of English to Speakers of Other Languages (TESOL). (2005b). *TESOL position statement on research and policy.* Retrieved from https://www.tesol.org/docs/pdf/3401.pdf?sfvrsn=2&sfvrsn=2

Teachers of English to Speakers of Other Languages (TESOL). (2006). *PreK–12 English language proficiency standards.* Alexandria, VA: Author.

Teachers of English to Speakers of Other Languages (TESOL). (2007a). *Position statement on teacher credentialing for teachers of English to speakers of other languages in primary and secondary schools.* Retrieved from http://tesol.org/s_tesol/bin.asp?CID=32&DID=8863&DOC=FILE.PDF

Teachers of English to Speakers of Other Languages (TESOL). (2007b). *The identification of English language learners with special educational needs.* Retrieved from http://www.tesol.org/s_tesol/bin.asp ?CID=32&DID=8283&DOC=FILE.PDF

Teachers of English to Speakers of Other Languages. (2008). *Position statement on teacher preparation for content-based instruction (CBI).* Retrieved from https://www.tesol.org/docs/pdf/10882.pdf ?sfvrsn=2&sfvrsn=2

Teachers of English to Speakers of Other Languages (TESOL). (2009a). *Position statement on the rights of deaf learners to acquire full proficiency in a native signed language.* Retrieved from http://www .tesol.org/s_tesol/seccss.asp?CID=32&DID=37

Teachers of English to Speakers of Other Languages (TESOL). (2009b). *Integrating the paper to practice: Using the TESOL ELP standards in preK–12 classrooms.* Alexandria, VA: Author.

Teachers of English to Speakers of Other Languages (TESOL). (2010a). *Position paper on language and literacy development for young English language learners (ages 3–8).* Retrieved from http://tesol.org/ s_tesol/bin.asp?CID=32&DID=13010&DOC=FILE.PDF

Teachers of English to Speakers of Other Languages (TESOL). (2010b). *Position statement on language and literacy development for young English language learners.* Retrieved from https://www.tesol.org/ docs/pdf/371.pdf?sfvrsn=2&sfvrsn=2

Teachers of English to Speakers of Other Languages (TESOL). (2010c). *Standards for the recognition of initial TESOL programs in P–12 ESL teacher education.* Retrieved from https://www.tesol.org/docs/ default-source/advocacy/the-revised-tesol-ncate-standards-for-the-recognition-of-initial-tesol-programs-in-p-12-esl-teacher-education-(2010-pdf).pdf?sfvrsn=4

Teachers of English to Speakers of Other Languages (TESOL). (2010d). *TESOL/NCATE standards for the recognition of initial TESOL programs in P–12 ESL teacher education.* Retrieved from http://www .tesol.org/s_tesol/seccss.asp?CID=219&DID=1689

TESOL International Association. (2013a, March). *Overview of the Common Core State Standards Initiatives for ELLs.* Alexandria, VA: Author.

TESOL International Association. (2013b, April). *Implementing the Common Core State Standards for ELs: The changing role of the ESL teacher.* Alexandria, VA: Author.

TESOL International Association. (2016, February). *The preparation of the ESL educator in the era of college- and career-readiness standards.* Alexandria, VA: Author.

TESOL International Association (TESOL). (2019). *Standards for Initial TESOL Pre-K-12 teacher preparation programs.* Alexandria, VA: Author.

Texas Education Agency. (2019). *TELPAS and TELPAS alternate educator guide*. Retrieved from https://tea.texas.gov/student.assessment/ell/telpas/

Texas English Language Proficiency Assessment System (TELPAS). (2011). Retrieved from https://1.cdn.edl.io/Qtw4T8U7IS4pt1mq35tg vefjlr8hFaZQWXJEARICrOv8DjDf.pdf

Tharp, R. G., & Gallimore, R. (1988). *Rousing minds to life*. New York, NY: Cambridge University Press.

Thistlethwaite, J., Moran, M., & World Health Organization Study Group on Interprofessional Education and Collaborative Practice. (2010). Learning objectives for interprofessional education (IPE): Literature review and synthesis. *Journal of Interprofessional Education, 24*(5), 503–513.

Thomas, W. P., & Collier, V. (1997). *School effectiveness for language minority students*. Washington, DC: National Clearinghouse for Bilingual Education.

Thomas, W. P., & Collier, V. (2002). *A national study of school effectiveness for language minority students' long-term academic achievement*. Santa Cruz, CA: Center for Research on Education, Diversity & Excellence. Retrieved from http://repositories.cdlib.org/crede/finalrpts/1_1_final/and http://crede.berkeley.edu/research/llaa/1.1_final.html

Thomas, W. P., & Collier, V. P. (2012). *Dual language education for a transformed world*. Albuquerque, NM: Dual Language Education of New Mexico—Fuente Press.

Thomason, K. M., Gorman, B. K., & Summers, C. (2007). English literacy development for English language learners: Does Spanish instruction promote or hinder? *EBP Briefs, 2*(2), 1–15.

Thordardottir, E. (2010). Towards evidence-based practice in language intervention for bilingual children. *Journal of Communication Disorders, 43*, 523–537.

Thordardottir, E., Rothenberg, A., Rivard, M. E., & Naves, R. (2006). Bilingual assessment: Can overall proficiency be estimated from separate measurement of two languages? *Journal of Multilingual Communication Disorders, 4*, 1–21.

Thorndike, E. L. (1932). *The fundamentals of learning*. New York, NY: Teachers College, Columbia University. U.S. Department of Education. (2006, August 14). Rules and regulations. *Federal Register, 71*(156), 46540–46845.

Throneburg, R. N., Calvert, L. K., Strum, J. J., Paramboukas, A. A., & Paul, P. J. (2000). A comparison of service delivery models: Effects on curricular vocabulary skills in the school setting. *American Journal of Speech-Language Pathology, 9*(1), 10–20.

Thurlow, M., House, A., Boys, C., Scott, D., & Ysseldyke, J., (2000). *State participation and accommodation policies for students with disabilities: 1999 Update. Synthesis Report 33.* National Center on Educational Outcomes, Minneapolis, MN.; Council of Chief State School Officers, Washington, DC.: National Association of State Directors of Special Education, Alexandria, VA.

Thurlow, M. L., Lazarus, S., Thompson, S., & Robey, J. (2002). *2001 state policies on assessment participation and accommodations (Synthesis Report 46).* Minneapolis, MN: University of Minnesota, National Center on Educational Outcomes. Retrieved from https://nceo.info/ Resources/publications/OnlinePubs/Synthesis46.html

Trainor, A. A., Murray, A., & Kim, H. (2014). *Postsecondary transition and English language learners with disabilities: Data from the second National Longitudinal Transition Study* (WCER Working Paper No. 2014-4). Madison, WI: University of Wisconsin–Madison, Wisconsin Center for Education Research.

Tuckman, B., & Jensen, M. (1977). Stages of small group development revisited. *Group and Organizational Studies, 2,* 419–427.

Turkan, S., & Schramm-Possinger, M. (2014). Teaching content to English learners in the era of the common core standards. *R&D Connections, 23,* 1–10. Retrieved from https://www.ets.org/Media/Research/pdf/ RD_Connections_23.pdf

Ukrainetz, T. A., Ross, C. L., & Harm, H. M. (2009). An investigation of treatment scheduling for phonemic awareness with kindergarteners who are at risk for reading difficulties. *Language, Speech, and Hearing in Schools, 40*(1), 86–100.

Uro, G., & Barrio, A. (2013). *English language learners in America's great city schools: Demographics, achievement, and staffing.* Washington, DC: Council of the Great City Schools.

Urzua, C. (1987). You stopped too soon: Second language children composing and revising. *TESOL Quarterly, 21,* 279–304.

U.S. Census Bureau. (2015a). *2011–2015 American Community Survey 5-year estimates.* Retrieved from https://factfinder.census.gov/faces/ tableservices/jsf/pages/productview.xhtml?src=CF

U.S. Census Bureau. (2015b, November 3). *Census Bureau Reports at least 350 languages spoken in U.S. homes.* Retrieved from https: //www.census.gov/newsroom/press-releases/2015/cb15-185 .html

U.S. Department of Education. (1997). *1993–94 schools and staffing survey: A profile of policies and practices for limited English proficient students: Screening methods, program support, and teacher training* (NCES 97–472). Washington, DC: Author. Retrieved from http://nces.ed.gov/pubs97/97472.pdf

U.S. Department of Education. (1999). *Status of education reform in public elementary and secondary schools: Teachers' perspectives* (NCES, 1999-045). Washington, DC: Author. Retrieved from http://www.eric.ed.gov/ERICDocs/data/ericdocs2sql/content_storage_01/0000019b/80/29/c0/d8.pdf

U.S. Department of Education. (2001). *Teacher preparation and professional development: 2000* (NCES 2001-088). Washington, DC: Author.

U.S. Department of Education. (2002). *Executive summary: The No Child Left Behind Act of 2001.* Washington, DC: Author.

U.S. Department of Education. (2005). *To assure the free appropriate public education of all Americans: Twenty-seventh annual report to Congress on the implementation of the Individuals with Disabilities Education Act.* Retrieved from http://www.ed.gov/about/reports/anual/osep/2005/index.html

U.S. Department of Education. (2006, August 14). Rules and regulations. *Federal Register, 71*(156), 46540–46845.

U.S. Department of Education. (2009). *Office of Special Education and Rehabilitative Services, Office of Special Education Programs, 28th annual report to Congress on the implementation of the Individuals with Disabilities Education Act, 2006* (Vol. 2). Washington, DC: Author.

U.S. Department of Education. (2016a). *Non-regulatory guidance: English learners and Title III of the Elementary and Secondary Education Act (ESEA), as amended by Every Student Succeeds Act.* Retrieved from http://www2.ed.gov/policy/elsec/leg/essa/essatitleiiiguidenglishlearners92016.pdf

U.S. Department of Education. (2016b). *Tools and resources for identifying all English learners.* Retrieved from https://www2.ed.gov/about/offices/list/oela/english-learner-toolkit/chap1.pdf

U.S. Department of Education. (2018a, April). *The condition of education: Children and youth with disabilities.* Retrieved from https://nces.ed.gov/programs/coe/indicator_cgf.asp

U.S. Department of Education. (2018b, April). *The condition of education: English language learners in public schools.* Retrieved from https://nces.ed.gov/programs/coe/indicator_cgf.asp

U.S. Department of Education. (2018c). *The condition of education 2018.* Washington, DC: National Center for Education Statistics. Retrieved from https://nces.ed.gov/pubsearch/pubsinfo.asp?pubid=2018144

U.S. Department of Education, Office of English Language Acquisition. (2017). *English learner tool kit* (2nd rev. ed.). Washington, DC: Author.

U.S. Department of Education, Office of Planning, Evaluation and Policy Development, Policy and Program Studies Service, Language

Instruction Educational Programs (LIEPs). (2012). *A review of the foundational literature.* Retrieved from https://www2.ed.gov/rsch stat/eval/title-iii/language-instruction-ed-programs-report.pdf

U.S. Department of Education, Office of Special Education Programs. (2010). *Annual report to Congress on the Implementation of the Individuals with Disabilities Education Act, selected years, 1979 through 2006; and Individuals with Disabilities Education Act (IDEA) database.* Retrieved from http://www2.ed.gov/programs/osepidea/618-data/state-level-data-files/index.html#bcc

U.S. Department of Education, Office of Special Education and Rehabilitative Services, Office of Special Education Programs. (2018). *40th Annual Report to Congress on the implementation of the Individuals with Disabilities Education Act, 2018.* Retrieved from https://www2.ed.gov/about/reports/annual/osep/2018/parts-b-c/40th-arc-for-idea.pdf

U.S. Department of Education & U.S. Department of Justice. (2011, May 6). *Dear colleague letter: school enrollment procedures.* Retrieved from http://www.justice.gov/crt/about/edu/documents/plylerletter.pdf

Vacca, J., Vacca, R. T., Gove, M., Burkey, L., Henhard, L., & McKeon, C. (2018). *Reading and learning to read* (10th ed.). Boston, MA: Pearson.

Vacca, R. T., Vacca, J. L., & Mraz, M. (2016). *Content area reading: Literacy and learning across the curriculum* (12th ed.). Boston, MA: Pearson.

Valdés, G., & Figueroa, R. A. (1994). *Bilingualism and testing: A special case of bias.* Norwood, NJ: Ablex.

Valdés, G., Kibler, A., & Walqui, A. (2014, March). *Changes in the expertise of ESL professionals: Knowledge and action in an era of new standards.* Alexandria, VA: TESOL International Association. Retrieved from https://www.tesol.org/docs/default-source/papers-and-briefs/professional-paper-26-march-2014.pdf?sfvrsn=4

Valenzuela, A., & Rubio, B. (2018). Subtractive schooling. In J. I. Liontas, TESOL International Association, and M. DelliCarpini (Eds.), *The TESOL encyclopedia of English language.* New York, NY: Wiley.

VanDerHeyden, A. M., Witt, J. C., & Gilbertson, D. A. (2007). Multi-year evaluation of the effects of a response to intervention (RTI) model on identification of children for special education. *Journal of School Psychology, 45*, 225–256.

VanPatten, B., & Williams, J. (Eds.). (2015). *Theories in second language acquisition: An introduction* (2nd ed.). New York, NY: Routledge.

Vaughn, S., Linan-Thompson, S., Mathes, P. G., Cirino, P., Carlson, C. D., Pollard-Durodola, S. D., . . . Francis, D. J. (2006). Effectiveness of Spanish intervention for 1st grade English language learners at risk for reading difficulties. *Journal of Learning Disabilities, 39*, 56–73.

Verdon, S., Wong, S., & McLeod, W. (2016). Shared knowledge and mutual respect: Enhancing culturally competent practice through collaboration with families and communities. *Child Language Teaching and Therapy, 32*(2), 205–221.

Violand-Sanchez, E., Sutton, C. P., & Ware, H. W. (1991, Summer). *Fostering home-school cooperation: Involving language minority families as partners in education.* Washington, DC: National Clearinghouse on Bilingual Education.

Volterra, V., & Taeschner, T. (1978). The acquisition and development of language by bilingual children. *Journal of Child Language, 5,* 311–326.

Vygotsky, L. (1962). *Thought and language.* Cambridge, MA: MIT Press.

Vygotsky, L. (1986). *Thought and language* (Rev. ed.). Cambridge, MA: MIT Press.

Walker, J. D., & Barry, C. (2018). Assessing and supporting social-skill needs for students with high-incidence disabilities. *Teaching Exceptional Children, 51*(1), 18–30. doi:10.1177/0040059918790219

Waller, J. (2012). Preparing speech-language pathology students for school-based practice: The importance of graduate clinical experiences in universally designed classrooms. *ASHA Perspectives on School-Based Issues, 13*(4), 130–135.

Walmsley, S. A. (2008). *Closing the circle: A practical guide to implementing literacy reform, K–12.* San Francisco, CA: Jossey-Bass.

Walqui, A. (2000). Contextual factors in second language acquisition. *ERIC Clearinghouse on Language and Linguistics.* Retrieved from http://www.cal.org/resources/digest/0005contextual.html

Waters, G. S., & Doehring, D. G. (1990). Reading acquisition in congenitally deaf children who communicate orally: Insights from and analysis of component reading, language, and memory skills. In T. H. Carr & B. H. Levey (Eds.), *Reading and its development.* San Diego, CA: Academic Press.

Watson, G., & Bellon-Harn, M. (2013). Speech-language pathologist and general educator collaboration: A model for Tier 2 service delivery. *Intervention in School and Clinic, 49*(4), 237–243.

Waxman, H. C., Padrón, Y., Franco-Feunmayor, S., & Huang, S.Y. (2009). Observing classroom instruction for ELLs from student, teacher, and classroom perspectives. *Texas Association for Bilingual Education, 11*(1), 63–95.

Webster, M. J., & Shelton, R. L. (1964). Estimation of mean length of response in children of normal and below average intellectual capacity. *Journal of Speech and Hearing Research, 7,* 98–100.

Wei, L. (2006). *The bilingualism reader* (2nd ed.). New York, NY: Routledge.

Werner, E. O., & Kresheck, J. D. (1983). *Structured Photographic Expressive Language Test–2,* DeKalb, IL: Janelle.

Werner, E. O., & Kresheck, J. D. (1989). *Spanish Structured Photographic Expressive Language Test–Preschool.* Sandwich, IL: Janelle.

Whitmire, K. (2002). The evolution of school-based speech-language services: A half century of change and a new century of practice. *Communication Disorders Quarterly, 23*(2), 68–76.

Wiig, E., Semel, E., & Secord, W. (2013). *Clinical Evaluation of Language Fundamentals–Fifth Edition (CELF-5).* Bloomington, MN: NCS Pearson.

Wilkinson, B. R., & Payne, K. T. (2005). Effect of clinician's accent on verbal performance of preschool children. *ECHO: E-Journal for Black and Other Ethnic Group Research and Practices in Communication Sciences and Disorders, 1*(2), 11–28.

Winfield, F. E., & Barnes-Felfeli, P. (1982). The effects of familiar and unfamiliar cultural context on foreign language composition. *Modern Language Journal, 66,* 373–378.

Woodcock, R. W., Muñoz-Sandoval, A. F., Ruef, M., & Alvarado, C. G. (2005). *Woodcock-Muñoz Language Survey, Revised Normative Update.* Rolling Meadows, IL: Riverside.

Woodcock, R., Alvarado, C., Ruef, M., & Schrank, F. (2017). *The Woodcock-Muñoz Language Survey III.* Boston, MA: Houghton Mifflin Harcourt.

World-Class Instructional Design and Assessment (WIDA). (2012). *2012 amplification of the English language proficiency standards and resource guide, prekindergarten through Grade 12.* Madison, WI: Board of Regents of the University of Wisconsin System on behalf of the WIDA Consortium.

World Health Organization. (2010). *Framework for action on interprofessional education and collaborative practice.* Geneva, Switzerland: Author. Retrieved from http://www.who.int/hrh/resources/frame work_action/en/

Wright, W. (2015). *Foundations for teaching English language learners: Research, theory, policy, and practice* (2nd ed.). Philadelphia, PA: Caslon.

Xiao, Y. (2008). Building formal schemata with ESL student writers: Linking schema theory with contrastive rhetoric. *Asian EFL Journal, 32,* 13–40.

Yang, C., Crain, S., Berwick, R. C., Chomsky, N., & Bolhuis, J. J. (2017). The growth of language: Universal Grammar, experience, and principles of computation. *Neuroscience & Biobehavioral Reviews, 81,* 103–119. doi:10.1016/j.neubiorev.2016.12.023

Yule, G. (2016). *The study of language* (6th ed.). New York, NY: Cambridge University Press.

Zacrian, D., & Haynes, J. (2012). *The essential guide for educating beginning English learners.* Thousand Oaks, CA: Corwin Press.

Zehler, A., Fleischman, H., Hopstock, P., Stephenson, T., Pendzick, M., & Sapru, S. (2003). *Policy report: Summary of findings related to LEP and SPED-LEP students.* Arlington, VA: Development Associates.

Zimmerman, I. L., Steiner, V, G., & Pond, E. (2011). *Preschool Language Scales (5th ed.) (PLS-5).* San Antonio, TX: Pearson.

Zimmerman, I. L., Steiner, V, G., & Pond, E. (2012). *Preschool Language Scales (5th ed.) (PLS-5 Spanish).* San Antonio, TX: Pearson.

Zraick, R. I., Harten, A. C., & Hagstrom, F. (2014). Interprofessional education and practice: A primer for training future clinicians. *Perspectives on Issues in Higher Education, 17*(2), 39–46.

Zygouris-Coe, V. (2012). Disciplinary literacy and the Common Core State Standards. *Topics in Language Disorders, 32*(1), 35–50.

Zygouris-Coe, V., & Goodwiler, C. (2013). Language and literacy demands of content area courses in the era of the Common Core State Standards: Teachers' perspectives and the role of the SLP. *Perspectives on School-Based Issues, 14*(3), 61–67.

Index

Note: Page number in **bold** reference non-text material.

IPT (IDEA Language Proficiency Test), 203

J

Jazz chants, language learning activity, 272
Jose P. v. Ambach, 50–52, **51**

K

Kindergarten
  MODEL service, 200
  W-APT, 200
  WIDA-APT, 203, 215
Knowledge and Skills Needed by Speech Language Pathologists and Audiologists to Provide Culturally and Linguistically Appropriate Services, 63, 64
Korean rhetorical style, vs. English, 177–179
Krashen's Comprehension Hypothesis, 107–110

L

L1, first language acquisition, 81
  learning, to learn, 156–159
  reading, to learn, 156–159
  similarities and differences with L 2, 153–156
  writing, 173–175
L2, second language acquisition, 81
  language/reading problem, 160–164
  learning, to learn, 156–159
  reading, to learn, 156–159
  reading comprehension schema, 184–187
  reading model, 164–165
  similarities and differences with L1, 153–156
  writing, 173–175
  teaching contrastive rhetoric, 179–181
  writing proficiency schema, 187–189
LAD (Language Acquisition Device), 95–96
Language
  aptitude, 114
  assessment instruments
    considerations regarding, 241–244
    standardized testing/bias, 241–242
    test administration/interpretation, 242–243
    tests in primary language, 243–244
    translated tests, 243
  determination of disorder from difference, 53, 230–231
  difference, determination from language disorder, 53, 230–231
  disability, percentage of ELs with, **42**
  experience approach, reading skill and, 275
  impairment (LI), 21
    communication problems and, **139**
    defined, in Georgia, 140
  instruction, bilingual/dual-language, 88–91
  knowledge and skills learners must develop, K–3, **264**
  learning activity
    information gap, 271–272
    jazz chants, 272
    minimal pairs, 273

Workload, defined, 71
World-Class Instructional Design and Assessment (WIDA), 48
ACCESS Placement Test (W-APT), 289
Access Placement Test (W-APT), 289–290
Assessing Comprehension and Communication in English State-to-State for English Language Learners for ELLs (ACCESS for ELLs), 289
English language proficiency levels, **213**
levels of, 279
performance definitions, **120–123**
Screener, 200, 203, 211–215, 289
TESOL language proficiency standards, 289
Writing
clustering, 276
compensatory strategies, 287–288
defined, 171
dialogue journals, 275–276
L1 and L2, similarities and differences of, 173–175
Language Experience Approach (LEA), 275
letters, reading and, 259
leveled questioning, 278–279
mapping, 277
process of, 171–172
proficiency, schema, 187–189
purpose of, 172–173
sentences
combining/shortening, 277–278
frames, 279, 281–288
skills, developing, 274–288
structure of English, 175–179
structures of, **176**
systems, 153

Y

Y. S. v. School District of Philadelphia, 52

Z

Zero Reject, EAHCA and, 45
Zone of proximal development (ZPD), 111–114
ZPD (Zone of proximal development), 111–114